BASIC AND CLINICAL SCIENCE COURSE

Intraocular Inflammation and Uveitis

Section 9
2007–2008

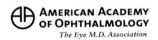

AMERICAN ACADEMY OF OPHTHALMOLOGY
The Eye M.D. Association

LEO

LIFELONG
EDUCATION for the
OPHTHALMOLOGIST®

The Basic and Clinical Science Course is one component of the Lifelong Education for the Ophthalmologist (LEO) framework, which assists members in planning their continuing medical education. LEO includes an array of clinical education products that members may select to form individualized, self-directed learning plans for updating their clinical knowledge. Active members or fellows who use LEO components may accumulate sufficient CME credits to earn the LEO Award. Contact the Academy's Clinical Education Division for further information on LEO.

The American Academy of Ophthalmology is accredited by the Accreditation Council for Continuing Medical Education to provide continuing medical education for physicians.

The American Academy of Ophthalmology designates this educational activity for a maximum of 30 *AMA PRA Category 1 Credits*™. Physicians should only claim credit commensurate with the extent of their participation in the activity.

The Academy provides this material for educational purposes only. It is not intended to represent the only or best method or procedure in every case, nor to replace a physician's own judgment or give specific advice for case management. Including all indications, contraindications, side effects, and alternative agents for each drug or treatment is beyond the scope of this material. All information and recommendations should be verified, prior to use, with current information included in the manufacturers' package inserts or other independent sources, and considered in light of the patient's condition and history. Reference to certain drugs, instruments, and other products in this course is made for illustrative purposes only and is not intended to constitute an endorsement of such. Some material may include information on applications that are not considered community standard, that reflect indications not included in approved FDA labeling, or that are approved for use only in restricted research settings. The FDA has stated that it is the responsibility of the physician to determine the FDA status of each drug or device he or she wishes to use, and to use them with appropriate patient consent in compliance with applicable law. The Academy specifically disclaims any and all liability for injury or other damages of any kind, from negligence or otherwise, for any and all claims that may arise from the use of any recommendations or other information contained herein.

Basic and Clinical Science Course

Thomas J. Liesegang, MD, Jacksonville, Florida, *Senior Secretary for Clinical Education*

Gregory L. Skuta, MD, Oklahoma City, Oklahoma, *Secretary for Ophthalmic Knowledge*

Louis B. Cantor, MD, Indianapolis, Indiana, *BCSC Course Chair*

Section 9

Faculty Responsible for This Edition

Ramana S. Moorthy, MD, *Chair,* Indianapolis, Indiana

Janet Davis, MD, Miami, Florida

C. Stephen Foster, MD, Cambridge, Massachusetts

Careen Yen Lowder, MD, PhD, Cleveland, Ohio

Albert T. Vitale, MD, Salt Lake City, Utah

Marta Lopatynsky, MD, Morristown, New Jersey
    Practicing Ophthalmologists Advisory Committee for Education

Bahram Bodaghi, MD, *Consultant,* Paris, France

Nalini S. Bora, PhD, *Consultant,* Little Rock, Arkansas

Dr Davis has received grant support from Bausch & Lomb, Inc, and is a consultant for Lux Biosciences.

Dr Foster has received speaking funds from and is a paid consultant for Alcon Laboratories; Allergan, Inc; and Bausch & Lomb, Inc; he is a paid consultant for Centocor, Inc; Genentech, Inc; and Inspire Pharmaceuticals, Inc.

Dr Vitale is a paid consultant for Bausch & Lomb, Inc.

The other authors state that they have no significant financial interest or other relationship with the manufacturer of any commercial product discussed in the chapters that they contributed to this publication or with the manufacturer of any competing commercial product.

Recent Past Faculty

Emmett T. Cunningham, Jr, MD

David Forster, MD

E. Mitchel Opremcak, MD

In addition, the Academy gratefully acknowledges the contributions of numerous past faculty and advisory committee members who have played an important role in the development of previous editions of the Basic and Clinical Science Course.

American Academy of Ophthalmology Staff

Richard A. Zorab, *Vice President, Ophthalmic Knowledge*
Hal Straus, *Director, Publications Department*
Carol L. Dondrea, *Publications Manager*
Christine Arturo, *Acquisitions Manager*
Nicole DuCharme, *Production Manager*
Stephanie Tanaka, *Medical Editor*
Steven Huebner, *Administrative Coordinator*

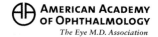

AMERICAN ACADEMY
OF OPHTHALMOLOGY
The Eye M.D. Association

655 Beach Street
Box 7424
San Francisco, CA 94120-7424

Contents

4   Mechanisms of Immune Effector Reactivity. **43**

5   Special Topics in Ocular Immunology. **87**

General Introduction

The Basic and Clinical Science Course (BCSC) is designed to meet the needs of residents and practitioners for a comprehensive yet concise curriculum of the field of ophthalmology. The BCSC has developed from its original brief outline format, which relied heavily on outside readings, to a more convenient and educationally useful self-contained text. The Academy updates and revises the course annually, with the goals of integrating the basic science and clinical practice of ophthalmology and of keeping ophthalmologists current with new developments in the various subspecialties.

The BCSC incorporates the effort and expertise of more than 80 ophthalmologists, organized into 13 Section faculties, working with Academy editorial staff. In addition, the course continues to benefit from many lasting contributions made by the faculties of previous editions. Members of the Academy's Practicing Ophthalmologists Advisory Committee for Education serve on each faculty and, as a group, review every volume before and after major revisions.

Organization of the Course

The Basic and Clinical Science Course comprises 13 volumes, incorporating fundamental ophthalmic knowledge, subspecialty areas, and special topics:

1 Update on General Medicine
2 Fundamentals and Principles of Ophthalmology
3 Clinical Optics
4 Ophthalmic Pathology and Intraocular Tumors
5 Neuro-Ophthalmology
6 Pediatric Ophthalmology and Strabismus
7 Orbit, Eyelids, and Lacrimal System
8 External Disease and Cornea
9 Intraocular Inflammation and Uveitis
10 Glaucoma
11 Lens and Cataract
12 Retina and Vitreous
13 Refractive Surgery

In addition, a comprehensive Master Index allows the reader to easily locate subjects throughout the entire series.

References

Readers who wish to explore specific topics in greater detail may consult the journal references cited within each chapter and the Basic Texts section at the back of the book. These references are intended to be selective rather than exhaustive, chosen by the BCSC faculty as being important, current, and readily available to residents and practitioners.

Related Academy educational materials are also listed in the appropriate sections. They include books, audiovisual materials, self-assessment programs, clinical modules, and interactive programs.

Study Questions and CME Credit

Each volume of the BCSC is designed as an independent study activity for ophthalmology residents and practitioners. The learning objectives for this volume are given on page 1. The text, illustrations, and references provide the information necessary to achieve the objectives; the study questions allow readers to test their understanding of the material and their mastery of the objectives. Physicians who wish to claim CME credit for this educational activity may do so by mail, by fax, or online. The necessary forms and instructions are given at the end of the book.

Conclusion

The Basic and Clinical Science Course has expanded greatly over the years, with the addition of much new text and numerous illustrations. Recent editions have sought to place a greater emphasis on clinical applicability while maintaining a solid foundation in basic science. As with any educational program, it reflects the experience of its authors. As its faculties change and as medicine progresses, new viewpoints are always emerging on controversial subjects and techniques. Not all alternate approaches can be included in this series; as with any educational endeavor, the learner should seek additional sources, including such carefully balanced opinions as the Academy's Preferred Practice Patterns.

The BCSC faculty and staff are continuously striving to improve the educational usefulness of the course; you, the reader, can contribute to this ongoing process. If you have any suggestions or questions about the series, please do not hesitate to contact the faculty or the editors.

The authors, editors, and reviewers hope that your study of the BCSC will be of lasting value and that each Section will serve as a practical resource for quality patient care.

Objectives

Upon completion of BCSC Section 9, *Intraocular Inflammation and Uveitis,* the reader should be able to

- outline the immunologic and infectious mechanisms involved in the occurrence and complications of uveitis and related inflammatory conditions, including acquired immunodeficiency syndrome (AIDS)

- identify general and specific pathophysiologic processes that affect the structure and function of the uvea, lens, intraocular cavities, retina, and other tissues in acute and chronic intraocular inflammation

- differentiate and identify infectious and noninfectious uveitic entities

- choose appropriate examination techniques and relevant ancillary studies based on whether an infectious or noninfectious cause is suspected

- develop appropriate differential diagnoses for ocular inflammatory disorders

- describe the principles of medical and surgical management of infectious and noninfectious uveitis and related intraocular inflammation, including indications for and complications of immunosuppressive agents

- describe criteria that can be applied to differentiate the masquerade syndromes from true uveitis

Introduction

This section of the BCSC is divided into 2 parts. Part II, Intraocular Inflammation and Uveitis, will come as no surprise to the reader opening a volume of the same name. Part II introduces the clinical approach to uveitis and devotes a chapter each to infectious and noninfectious forms of uveitis and to endophthalmitis. The chapter on noninfectious uveitis is organized anatomically. Because infectious uveitic conditions can involve any part of the uveal tract, the chapter on infectious uveitis is organized by causative agents. Part II then discusses the masquerade syndromes, both nonneoplastic and neoplastic. The following chapter discusses the complications of all forms of uveitis, and the final chapter of Part II covers ocular involvement in AIDS, offering the most complete summary of this topic in the BCSC series.

The reader may, however, not expect to find one third of the book, Part I, Immunology, going into such great depth. Why are so many pages given to this topic? What relevance does it have to Part II? Progress in basic immunology, as well as in the regional immunology of the eye, has translated into major advances in recent years. Our understanding of the mechanisms by which uveitis and other intraocular diseases develop has helped clinicians to identify and establish uveitis entities and to develop specific treatments directed at altered immune processes. These clinically relevant advances include the discovery of unique immune responses in the intraocular cavities and subretinal space; the delineation of the association between HLA and various uveitis entities; and the detection of infectious agents by immunologic methods such as Western blot, ELISA, and others. Lymphocytic studies for cell surface markers and in vitro studies based on antibodies have helped in clearly separating those uveitis entities that are mediated by immune mechanisms, in particular those resulting from organ-specific antibodies, from those caused by altered lymphocyte functions. The latter mechanism appears to be prevalent in posterior uveitis, and altered cell-mediated immunity can be directed to retinal proteins or other ocular antigens in these intraocular inflammations. Such findings have led to the introduction of potential therapeutic modalities such as oral tolerance, a promising though still experimental approach.

The section on immunology describes basic aspects of the human immune response, including responses specific to the ocular structures; the effector mechanisms of immunity, including antibody-mediated and lymphocyte-generated mechanisms; and the various pro- and anti-inflammatory cytokines and other effector molecules, including reactive oxygen species and nitric oxide products. Clinical examples are interspersed throughout the immunology text, discussing the clinical relevance of the issues covered in diagnosis and management of uveitis. A clear understanding of the immune mechanisms will enhance an appreciation of the clinical features and principles behind the management of uveitis triggered by either an infectious agent or another insult.

The authors would like to acknowledge Nalini Bora, PhD, for her assistance in reviewing Part I.

PART I

Immunology

Introduction to Immunology

Chapters 1 through 5 discuss the human immune system and its ocular effects in detail. Many specific terms are used, and some may be defined only briefly in an early chapter and then explained in depth in a later chapter. Similarly, abbreviations that may be unfamiliar to the reader often are used after the term has been spelled out at first mention. The following glossary and list of abbreviations are designed to provide the reader with a handy reference to terminology used in Part I, especially those terms discussed in later chapters and abbreviations that appear far from their original descriptions, and not as comprehensive listings.

Glossary

Antibody A glycoprotein that is able to bind biochemically to a specific antigenic substance.

Antigen Foreign substance that activates an adaptive immune response.

Antigen-presenting cells Specialized cells that carry antigen to a lymph node, process it into fragments, and present the fragments to T-cell antigen receptors.

Chemotaxis Attraction generated in macrophages, neutrophils, eosinophils, and lymphocytes by substances released at sites ot inflammatory reactions, such as lymphokines, complement, and various mediators.

Complement Effector molecules used to amplify inflammation for both innate and adaptive immunity.

Cytokine A generic term for any soluble polypeptide mediator synthesized and released by cells for the purposes of intercellular signaling and communication.

Epitope Each specific portion of an antigenic molecule to which the immune system responds.

Fc receptor The Fc domain of each immunoglobulin monomer contains the attachment site for effector cells and complement activation.

Hapten A small molecule, not antigenic by itself, that can react with antibodies when conjugated to a larger antigenic molecule.

Isotype Different subclasses of immunoglobulin.

Leukotriene A compound formed from arachidonic acid that functions as a regulator of allergic and inflammatory reactions, probably contributing significantly to inflammatory infiltration.

Lymphatics Common term for *afferent lymphatic channels,* which drain extracellular fluid to a regional lymph node, conveying immune cells and whole antigen, and *efferent lymphatic channels,* which drain to the circulatory system.

Mediator Substance released from cells as the result of the interaction of antigen with antibody or by the action of antigen with a sensitized lymphocyte.

Abbreviations

ACAID anterior chamber–associated immune deviation

ADCC antibody-dependent cellular cytotoxicity

ANCA antineutrophil cytoplasmic antibody

APC antigen-presenting cell(s)

CAM cell-adhesion molecule(s)

CTL cytotoxic T lymphocytes

DC dendritic cells

DH delayed hypersensitivity

HLA human leukocyte antigen

IFN interferon

IL interleukin

LC Langerhans cells

LPS lipopolysaccharide

MAC membrane attack complex

MALT mucosa-associated lymphoid tissue

MHC major histocompatibility complex

PAF platelet-activating factor(s)

PG prostaglandin

TGF transforming growth factor

Th helper T cell, as in *Th0, Th1,* etc.

TNF tumor necrosis factor

CHAPTER 1

Basic Concepts in Immunology

Definitions

In general, an immune response is a sequence of cellular and molecular events designed to rid the host of an offending stimulus, usually from a pathogenic organism, toxic substance, cellular debris, or neoplastic cell. Two broad categories of immune responses have been recognized: *adaptive* and *innate*. Simply put, adaptive (also called *specific* or *acquired immunity)* responses react to specific environmental stimuli (ie, unique antigens) with a stimulus-specific (ie, antigen-specific) immunologic response. In contrast, innate immune responses, also called *natural immunity,* require no prior contact with or "education" about the stimulus against which they mount an attack.

Adaptive Immune Response

Adaptive immunity is a host response set in motion by a specific environmental stimulus, or antigen. An antigen usually represents an alien substance completely foreign to the organism, and the immune system must generate, de novo, a specific receptor against it that must, in turn, recognize a unique molecular structure in the antigen for which no specific preexisting receptor was present. The organism attempts to defend itself by the following steps:

1. recognizing the unique foreign antigenic substance as distinguished from self
2. processing the unique antigen with receptors newly created by specialized tissues (the immune system)
3. generating unique antigen-specific immunologic effector cells (especially T and B lymphocytes) and unique antigen-specific soluble effector molecules, such as antibodies, that function to remove the specific stimulating antigenic substance from the organism while ignoring the presence of other, irrelevant antigenic stimuli

Thus, the adaptive immune system is not genetically predetermined but evolves as an ongoing way for an individual's T and B lymphocytes to continually generate new antigen receptors through recombination, rearrangement, and mutation of the germline genetic structure. This creates a vast repertoire of novel antigen receptor molecules that vary tremendously among individuals within a given species.

The immune response to a mutated virus is the classic example of this process. Viruses such as influenza virus are continuously mutating, thus developing new antigenic structures. The susceptible host could not possibly have evolved the receptors needed to recognize each of these new viral mutations. However, each new mutation serves as an antigen that stimulates a specific adaptive immune response by the host to the virus. The adaptive response recognizes the virus in question and not other organisms, such as polio virus. The adaptive immune response has been programmed to adapt to the new specific antigen following environmental exposure.

Innate Immune Response

Innate immunity is a pattern recognition response by the organism to

- identify various offensive stimuli (especially infectious agents, toxins, and cellular debris from injury) in an antigen-independent manner
- respond in a stereotyped, preprogrammed fashion determined by the preexistence of receptors for the stimulus
- generate biochemical mediators and cytokines that recruit nonspecific effector cells, especially macrophages and neutrophils, to remove the offending stimulus in a nonspecific manner through phagocytosis or enzymatic degradation

The stimuli of innate immunity interact with receptors that have been genetically predetermined by evolution to recognize and respond to molecular *motifs* on triggering stimuli. These motifs often include a specific amino acid sequence, certain lipoproteins, certain phospholipids, or other specific molecular patterns. The receptors of innate immunity are identical among all individuals within a species. In this way, the receptors on monocytes, neutrophils, and sometimes parenchymal tissues resemble the receptors for neurotransmitters or hormones.

The innate immune response to acute infection is the classic example of this process. For example, in endophthalmitis, bacteria-derived toxins or host cell debris stimulate the recruitment of neutrophils and monocytes, leading to the production of inflammatory mediators and phagocytosis of the bacteria. The triggering mechanisms and subsequent effector response to *Staphylococcus* are nearly identical to those mounted against other organisms. Nonspecific receptors that recognize families of related toxins or molecules in the environment determine this response.

Similarities Between Adaptive and Innate Immune Responses

Receptor activation

Both responses use receptors present on white blood cells to recognize offending stimuli, but the *recognition receptors* are fundamentally different.

Inflammatory or noninflammatory responses

Both responses can trigger inflammation, but they usually operate at a subclinical level so the individual is unaware of the response.

Nonspecific effector cells and molecules

Although only the adaptive immune response employs T and B lymphocytes as antigen-specific effector cells, both forms of immunity use neutrophils, eosinophils, and monocytes as nonspecific effector cells and the same chemical mediators as amplification systems.

Differences Between Adaptive and Innate Immune Responses

Triggering stimuli

Adaptive immunity is triggered by an antigen, usually in the form of a protein, although carbohydrates or lipids can sometimes be antigenic. Innate immunity is triggered by bacterial toxins and cell debris, often in the form of carbohydrate, phospholipid, or other nonprotein molecules.

Recognition receptors

The antigen receptors, or *paratopes,* of adaptive immunity, which are on antibody molecules and T lymphocytes, are specific for each antigen, recognizing unique molecular regions of an antigen called *epitopes.* The receptors used by innate immunity, such as scavenging receptors or toxin receptors, recognize conserved molecular patterns or motifs shared among various triggering stimuli.

Time of onset after triggering

Because adaptive immune responses are acquired, they require recognition, processing, and effector phases that need several days for activation. Therefore, onset is delayed. Innate immunity is preprogrammed, requiring only the direct activation of a cellular receptor to initiate an effector response, which induces release of mediators or recruitment of cells within hours.

Memory

Adaptive immune responses demonstrate memory, so that on second exposure to the same antigen, the release of effectors is more vigorous and more rapid than it was during the original response. Innate responses are genetically preprogrammed to react stereotypically to each encounter. Memory implies that the secondary, or repeat encounter, immune response is regulated by mechanisms different from the primary, or initial virgin encounter, immune response, specifically by memory T and B lymphocytes.

Specificity

Adaptive immune responses demonstrate specificity for each unique offending antigen. Innate responses do not. Specificity is maintained through the use of antibodies and antigen-specific T and B lymphocytes that recognize specific biochemical information, such as linear amino acid sequences for T lymphocytes and 3-dimensional geometry for B lymphocytes. Subtle biochemical changes (eg, amino acid substitutions) in the structure of the antigen remove specific recognition for memory responses but preserve overall antigenicity for a new primary response. In contrast, similar subtle changes in toxin structure or other stimuli for innate immunity do not necessarily alter the innate response if the changes do not involve the pattern recognition sites within the molecule.

Immunity Versus Inflammation

An immune response is the process for removing an offending stimulus. When this response becomes clinically apparent within a tissue, it can be termed an *inflammatory response*. More precisely, an inflammatory response is a sequence of molecular and cellular events triggered by innate or adaptive immunity resulting in 5 characteristic cardinal clinical manifestations:

1. pain
2. hyperemia
3. edema
4. heat
5. loss of function

These clinical signs reflect 2 main physiologic changes within a tissue: cellular recruitment and altered vascular permeability. Inflammatory response is associated with the following typical pathologic findings:

- infiltration of effector cells mediated by and resulting in the release of biochemical and molecular mediators/amplifiers of inflammation, such as cytokines (eg, interleukins and chemokines) and lipid mediators (eg, prostaglandins and platelet-activating factors)
- presence of oxygen metabolites (eg, superoxide and nitrogen radicals)
- presence of granule products as well as catalytic enzymes (eg, collagenases and elastases)
- activation of plasma-derived enzyme systems (ie, complement components such as anaphylatoxins)

See Chapter 3 for a more detailed discussion.

In practice, many clinicians use the term *immune response* to mean adaptive immunity and the term *inflammation* to imply innate immunity. However, it is important to remember that both adaptive and innate immune responses usually function physiologically at a subclinical level without overt manifestations. For example, in most persons, ocular surface allergen exposure, which occurs daily in all humans, or bacterial contamination during cataract surgery, which occurs in most eyes, is usually cleared by innate or adaptive mechanisms without overt inflammation. Similarly, both adaptive and innate immunity can trigger inflammation, and the physiologic changes induced by each form of immunity may be indistinguishable. For example, the hypopyon of bacterial endophthalmitis, which results from innate immunity against bacterial toxins, and the hypopyon of lens-associated uveitis, which presumably results from an inappropriate adaptive immune response against lens antigens, cannot be clearly distinguished clinically or histologically.

Delves PJ, Martin S, Burton D, Roitt IM. *Roitt's Essential Immunology.* 11th ed. Malden, MA: Blackwell Publishing; 2006.

Delves PJ, Roitt IM. The immune system. *N Engl J Med.* 2000;343:37–49 (part 1); 108–117 (part 2).

Goldsby RA, Kindt TJ, Osborne BA, Kuby J. *Immunology*. 5th ed. New York: W.H. Freeman; 2003.

Medzhitov R, Janeway C Jr. Innate immunity. *N Engl J Med*. 2000;343:338–344.

Components of the Immune System

Leukocytes

White blood cells, or *leukocytes,* are nucleated cells that can be distinguished from one another by the shape of their nuclei and the presence or absence of granules. They are further defined by uptake of various histologic stains.

Neutrophils

Neutrophils, 1 of the 3 types of polymorphonuclear leukocytes, are the most abundant granulocytes in the blood. They are efficient phagocytes that readily clear tissues and degrade ingested material. They act as important effector cells through the release of granule products and cytokines. Through specific receptors, such as complement receptors, neutrophils can be recruited and triggered by immune mechanisms. Nonimmune mechanisms also recruit neutrophils at sites of injury through poorly characterized receptor ligand interactions. Chapter 4 discusses neutrophil activation recruitment in greater detail.

Neutrophils dominate the infiltrate in experimental models and clinical examples of active bacterial infections of the conjunctiva, sclera (scleritis), cornea (keratitis), and vitreous (endophthalmitis). Neutrophils are also dominant in many models of active viral infections of the cornea (herpes simplex virus keratitis) and retina (herpes simplex virus retinitis) and in some human viral infections. Neutrophils also constitute the principal cell type in lipopolysaccharide-induced inflammation and after direct injection of most cytokines into various ocular tissues.

Eosinophils

Eosinophils, a second type of polymorphonuclear leukocyte, also contain abundant cytoplasmic granules and lysosomes. However, the biochemical nature of the granules in eosinophils consists of more basic and therefore more acid-binding protein (eg, acidic dye, such as eosin, will bind to these proteins), and eosinophils differ from neutrophils in the way they respond to certain triggering stimuli. Eosinophils have receptors for and become activated by many mediators; interleukin-5 (IL-5) is especially important. Eosinophil granule products, such as major basic protein or ribonucleases, are ideal for destroying parasites; not surprisingly, these cells accumulate at sites of parasitic infection. Eosinophils are numerous in skin infiltrates during the late-phase allergic response, in atopic lesions, and in lung infiltrates during asthma. T-lymphocyte production of IL-5 within the infiltrated site is probably an important regulator of eosinophil function locally, although many of the specific mechanisms for regulation of eosinophil recruitment, activation, and function remain unknown.

Eosinophils are abundant in the conjunctiva and tears in many forms of atopic conjunctivitis, especially vernal and allergic conjunctivitis. However, eosinophils are not considered major effectors for intraocular inflammation, except during helminthic infections of the eye, especially acute endophthalmitis caused by toxocariasis.

Basophils and mast cells

Basophils, a third type of polymorphonuclear leukocyte, are the bloodborne equivalent of the tissue-bound mast cell. Mast cells exist in 2 major subtypes—connective tissue and mucosal—both of which can release preformed granules and synthesize certain mediators de novo. *Connective tissue mast cells* contain abundant granules with histamine and heparin, and they synthesize prostaglandin D_2 upon stimulation. In contrast, *mucosal mast cells* require T-lymphocyte cytokine help for granule formation, and they therefore normally contain low levels of histamine. Mucosal mast cells synthesize mostly leukotrienes after stimulation. The tissue location can alter the granule type and functional activity, but the regulation of these important differences is not well understood.

Basophils and mast cells differ from other granulocytes in several important ways. The granule contents are different from those of neutrophils and eosinophils, and mast cells express high-affinity Fc receptors for the immunoglobulin IgE. *Fc,* from "*fragment, crystallizable,*" refers to the region of immunoglobulin that mediates cell surface receptors. Mast cells act as major effector cells in IgE-mediated, immune-triggered inflammatory reactions, especially allergy or immediate hypersensitivity. Mast cells may also participate in the induction of cell-mediated immunity, wound healing, and other functions not directly related to IgE-mediated degranulation (ie, release of cell contents). Thus, other stimuli, such as complement or certain cytokines, may also trigger degranulation.

The normal human conjunctiva contains significant numbers of mast cells localized in the substantia propria but not in the epithelium. In certain atopic and allergic disease states, such as vernal conjunctivitis, not only does the number of mast cells increase in the substantia propria, but the epithelium also becomes densely infiltrated. Careful anatomical studies have shown that the choroid and anterior uveal tract also contain significant densities of connective tissue–type mast cells; the cornea has none.

Monocytes and macrophages

Monocytes, the circulating cells, and macrophages, the tissue-infiltrating equivalents, are important effectors in all forms of immunity and inflammation. Monocytes are relatively large cells (12–20 μm in suspension but up to 40 μm in tissues) that travel through many normal sites. Most normal tissues have at least 2 identifiable macrophage populations: tissue-resident macrophages and blood-derived macrophages. Although many exceptions exist, in general, tissue-resident macrophages represent monocytes that migrated into a tissue during embryologic development, thereby acquiring tissue-specific properties and specific cellular markers. In many tissues, resident macrophages have been given tissue-specific names: Kupffer cells in the liver, alveolar macrophages in the lung, and microglia in the brain and retina. Blood-derived macrophages usually represent monocytes that have recently migrated from the blood into a fully developed tissue site.

Macrophages serve the following 3 primary functions:

1. as scavengers to clear cell debris and pathogens
2. as antigen-presenting cells (APCs) for T lymphocytes
3. as inflammatory effector cells

In vitro studies seem to indicate that resting monocytes can be primed through various signals into efficient APCs and, upon additional signals, activated into effector cells.

Effective activation stimuli include exposure to bacterial toxins such as lipopolysaccharide, phagocytosis of antibody-coated or complement-coated pathogens, or exposure to mediators released during inflammation, such as IL-1 or interferon-γ.

Only on full activation do macrophages become most efficient at the synthesis and release of inflammatory mediators and the killing and degradation of phagocytosed pathogens. At some sites of inflammation, macrophages undergo a morphologic change in size and histologic features into a cell called an *epithelioid cell*. Epithelioid cells can fuse into multinucleated *giant cells*. Macrophages are extremely important effector cells in both adaptive and innate immunity, with or without overt inflammation. They are often detectable in acute ocular infections, even if other cell types such as neutrophils are more numerous. Chapter 4 discusses these issues in more detail.

Dendritic cells and Langerhans cells

Dendritic cells (DCs) are terminally differentiated, bone marrow–derived, circulating mononuclear cells that are distinct from the macrophage–monocyte lineage. They make up approximately 0.1%–1.0% of blood mononuclear cells. However, in tissue sites, DCs become large (15–30 μm), with cytoplasmic veils that form extensions 2 to 3 times the diameter of the cell, and resemble the dendritic structure of neurons. In many nonlymphoid and lymphoid organs, DCs become a system of APCs. These sites recruit DCs by defined migration pathways, and DCs in each site share features of structure and function. Dendritic cells function as accessory cells important to the processing and presentation of antigens to T lymphocytes; the distinctive function of DCs is to initiate responses in quiescent lymphocytes. Thus, DCs may act as the most potent leukocytes for generating primary T-lymphocyte–dependent immune responses.

Epidermal Langerhans cells (LCs) are the best-characterized subset of DCs. LCs account for approximately 3%–8% of the cells in most human epithelia, including the skin, conjunctiva, nasopharyngeal mucosa, vaginal mucosa, and rectal mucosa. LCs are identified on the basis of their many dendrites, electron-dense cytoplasm, and Birbeck granules. They are not active APCs, although activity develops after in vitro culture with certain cytokines. As a result, LCs transform and lose their granules and thus fully resemble blood and lymphoid DCs. Evidence suggests that LCs can leave the skin and move along the afferent lymph to draining lymphoid organs. LCs are important components of the immune system and play a role in antigen presentation, control of lymphoid cell traffic, differentiation of T lymphocytes, and induction of delayed hypersensitivity. Elimination of LCs from skin before an antigen challenge inhibits the induction of the contact hypersensitivity response. In the conjunctiva and limbus, LCs are the only ones that constitutively express class II major histocompatibility molecules (MHC). Langerhans cells are present in the peripheral cornea, and any kind of irritation to the central cornea will result in central migration of the peripheral LCs.

Lymphocytes

Lymphocytes are small (10–20 μm) cells with large, dense nuclei also derived from stem cell precursors within the bone marrow. However, unlike other leukocytes, lymphocytes require subsequent maturation in peripheral lymphoid organs. Lymphocytes can be subdivided by the detection of specific cell-surface proteins (ie, *surface markers*). These markers are in turn related to the functional and molecular activity of individual subsets. Three broad categories of lymphocytes have been identified: T lymphocytes; B lymphocytes; and non-T, non-B lymphocytes. These subsets are discussed in greater detail in the following section.

Gallin JI, Snyderman R, eds. *Inflammation: Basic Principles and Clinical Correlates.* 3rd ed. Philadelphia: Lippincott Williams &Wilkins; 1999.

Lymphoid Tissues

Primary lymphoid tissues

The bone marrow is the site for replenishment and maturation of all leukocyte and lymphoid precursors. Thus, pluripotential stem cells differentiate into various myeloid or lymphoid precursor cells, which then differentiate into monocyte precursors, T- and B-lymphocyte precursors, and so on. B lymphocytes mature within the bone marrow, whereas immature T lymphocytes exit the bone marrow and mature within the thymus. Mature B and T lymphocytes then exit into the blood, where they enter secondary lymphoid tissues. Granulocytes and monocytes exit the bone marrow directly as functional effectors, although some monocyte subpopulations can further differentiate in peripheral tissues.

Secondary lymphoid tissues

The central lymphoid structures—lymph nodes and spleen—are very important to the adaptive immune response. Mature but naive lymphocytes, those that have not been exposed to antigens, enter lymph nodes through specialized postcapillary venules and take up residence in specialized areas (follicles for B lymphocytes and the paracortical region for T lymphocytes) until antigen exposure occurs. The lymphocytes can recirculate and travel between different nodes. Certain sites, termed *peripheral lymphoid structures,* especially mucosa and skin, are important for the initial interaction with antigen because of their location as a barrier to the outside world.

CHAPTER 2

Immunization and Adaptive Immunity: The Immune Response Arc

To understand the clinically relevant features of the adaptive immune response, the reader can consider the sequence of events that follows immunization with antigen using the skin, which is the classic experimental method of introducing antigen to the adaptive immune response. Several general immunologic concepts, especially the concept of the immune response arc, the primary adaptive immune response, and the secondary adaptive immune response, are involved in this process.

Overview of the Immune Response Arc

Interaction between antigen and the adaptive immune system at a peripheral site, such as the skin, can be subdivided, using the concept of the immune response arc, into 3 phases:

1. afferent
2. processing
3. effector

Each phase of the immune response arc is analogous to the 3 phases of the neural reflex arc (Fig 2-1). For example, in the neural response to the patellar deep tendon reflex, the *afferent response* begins with the recognition of a stimulus (the activation of the stretch receptor by percussion of the patellar tendon), followed by transformation of the stimulus into a neural signal that is conveyed along an afferent neuron into the central nervous system. In the central nervous system, complex neural *processing* occurs. Finally, along an efferent neuron, the neural signal is conveyed back to the site (quadriceps muscle), which is activated to contract (ie, an *effector response*).

Similarly, in the adaptive immune response, antigen is recognized during the *afferent* phase of the immune response, when the antigenic information is conveyed through the lymphatics and antigen-presenting cells (APCs) to the lymph node. There, *processing* of the antigenic signal occurs, resulting in the release of immune messengers (antibodies,

NEURAL REFLEX ARC

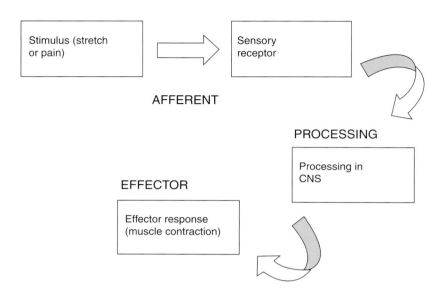

IMMUNE RESPONSE ARC

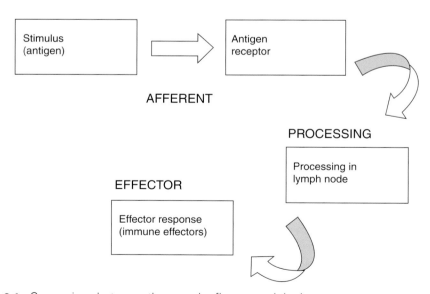

Figure 2-1 Comparison between the neural reflex arc and the immune response arc.

B lymphocytes, and T lymphocytes) into efferent lymphatics and venous circulation. The intent of the immune system is conveyed back to the original site, where an *effector response* occurs (ie, immune complex formation or delayed hypersensitivity reaction). The following discussion covers the important aspects of each phase in more detail.

Phases of the Immune Response Arc

Afferent Phase

The initial recognition, transport, and presentation of antigenic substances to the adaptive immune system constitute the afferent phase of the immune response arc. The term *antigen* refers to substances recognized by the immune system and resulting in antibody production and development of "sensitized" T lymphocytes. The term *epitope* refers to each specific portion of an antigen to which the immune system can respond. A complex 3-dimensional protein probably has multiple antigenic epitopes against which antibodies with different paratopes might bind, as well as many other sites that remain invisible to the immune system. The term *paratope* refers to the epitope-specific binding site on the Fab (*f*ragment, *a*ntigen-*b*inding) portion of the antibody. In addition, such a protein often can be enzymatically digested into many different peptide fragments, some of which contain molecular information to serve as antigenic epitopes for T-lymphocyte recognition and some of which are not recognized at all by the immune system.

Afferent lymphatic channels

Also simply called *lymphatics,* afferent lymphatic channels are veinlike structures that drain extracellular fluid (ie, lymph) from a site into a regional node. Lymphatics serve 2 major purposes: to convey immune cells and to carry whole antigen from the site of inoculation to a lymph node.

Antigen-presenting cells

Antigen-presenting cells are specialized cells that bind and phagocytize antigen at a site, carry it to a lymph node, then "process" the antigen, which is almost always in the form of a protein, into fragments (ie, uses intracellular enzymes to digest the antigen into peptides of 7–11 amino acids), transport the peptide antigen fragments into a specialized antigen-binding groove within human leukocyte antigen (HLA) molecules present on the APC cell surface, and "present" the peptide to T-lymphocyte antigen receptors, thereby beginning the activation process of adaptive immunity. Different HLA molecules vary in their capacity to bind various peptide fragments within the groove, and thus the HLA type determines the repertoire of peptide antigens capable of being presented to T lymphocytes. APCs from 1 individual cannot present to T lymphocytes derived from a second individual unless the 2 individuals share a common HLA haplotype that can bind the antigen in question. See Chapter 5 for a discussion of HLA molecules. Table 5-1, in Chapter 5, gives a short history of research on the HLA system.

Class II major histocompatibility complex (MHC) molecules (ie, HLA-DR, -DP, and -DQ) serve as the antigen-presenting platform for *CD4,* or *helper,* T lymphocytes (Fig 2-2). All APCs for CD4 T lymphocytes must express the class II MHC molecule, and the antigen receptor on the helper T lymphocyte can recognize peptide antigens only if they are presented with class II molecules simultaneously. However, only certain cell types express class II MHC on their plasma membrane. Macrophages and dendritic cells are the 2 most important class II APCs. B lymphocytes can also function as class II–dependent APCs, especially within a lymph node. Any cell that is induced to express class II MHC molecules also can potentially serve as an APC, although this topic is beyond the scope of this discussion. In general, class II–dependent APCs are the most efficient, "professional" APCs for processing extracellular protein antigens that have been endocytosed from the external environment (eg, bacterial or fungal antigens).

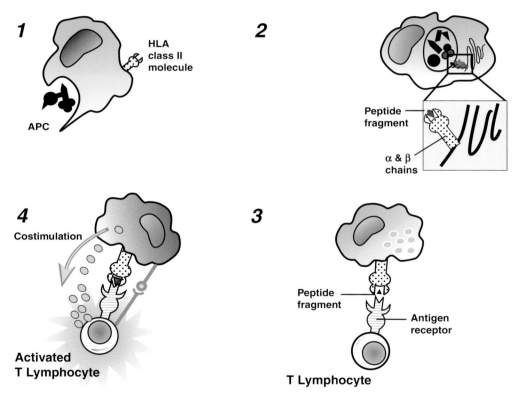

Figure 2-2 Class II–dependent antigen-processing cells (APCs). **1,** APCs endocytose exogenous antigens into the endosomal compartment. **2,** There, the antigen is digested into peptide fragments and placed into the groove formed by the α and β chains of the class II human leukocyte antigen (HLA) molecule. **3,** The CD4 T-lymphocyte receptor recognizes the fragment–class II complex. **4,** With the help of costimulatory molecules such as CD28/B7 interactions and cytokines, the CD4 T lymphocyte becomes primed, or partially activated. *(Illustration by Barb Cousins, modified by Joyce Zavarro.)*

Class I MHC molecules (ie, HLA-A, -B, and -C) serve as the antigen-presenting platform for *CD8,* or *regulatory,* T lymphocytes (Fig 2-3). Class I molecules are present on almost all nucleated cells, indicating that most cells have the potential to stimulate CD8 T lymphocytes. The CD8 T-lymphocyte antigen receptor must recognize its own class I type before it can respond to tumor or viral antigens on the appropriate target cell, and therefore CD8 T lymphocytes from 1 individual will not respond to a target cell

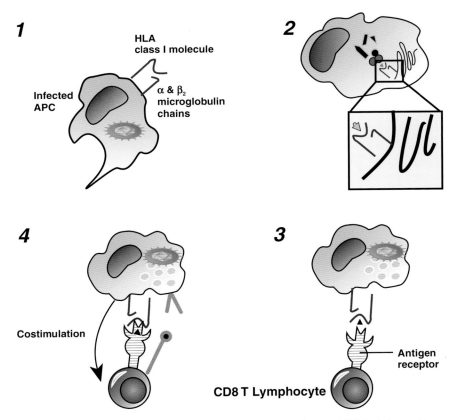

Figure 2-3 Class I–dependent antigen-presenting cells (APCs). **1,** APC is infected by a virus, which causes the cell to synthesize virus-associated peptides that are present in the cytosol. **2,** The viral antigen must be transported (through specialized transporter systems) into the endosomal compartment, where the antigen encounters class I human leukocyte antigen (HLA) molecules. The fragment is placed into the pocket formed by the α chain of the class I HLA molecule. Unlike class II molecules, the second chain, called β_2-microglobulin, is constant among all class I molecules. **3,** The CD8 T-lymphocyte receptor recognizes the fragment–class I complex. **4,** With the help of costimulatory molecules such as CD28/B7 interaction and cytokines, the CD8 T lymphocyte becomes primed, or partially activated. A similar mechanism is used to recognize tumor antigens that are produced by cells after malignant transformation. *(Illustration by Barb Cousins, modified by Joyce Zavarro.)*

from another individual if the class I MHC molecules do not correspond. In general, class I APCs are best for processing peptide antigens that have been synthesized by the host cell itself, including most tumor peptides or viral peptides after host cell invasion.

Several other important topics that greatly influence the afferent phase are beyond the scope of this book. The immunology texts listed as references can be consulted for more detail concerning the following:

- the nature of antigen
- the immunologic microenvironment of different tissues (eg, anatomical and functional differences among sites in APCs, growth factors, immunoregulatory molecules, blood–tissue barriers)
- the expression of HLA molecules on tissues other than leukocytes

Processing Phase

The conversion of the antigenic stimulus into an immunologic response through priming of naive B and T lymphocytes within the lymph nodes and spleen occurs during the processing phase of the immune response arc. This process is also called *activation,* or *sensitization,* of lymphocytes. Processing involves regulation of the interaction between antigen and naive lymphocytes, B lymphocytes or T lymphocytes that have not yet encountered their specific antigen, followed by their subsequent activation (Fig 2-4). The following discussion focuses on a few key concepts.

Preconditions necessary for processing

Helper T lymphocytes are the key functional cell type for immune processing. Most helper T lymphocytes express CD4 molecules on the cell membrane. T lymphocytes have an antigen receptor that detects antigen only when a trimolecular complex is formed consisting of an APC-HLA molecule, a processed antigen fragment, and a T-lymphocyte antigen receptor. The CD4 molecule stabilizes binding and enhances signaling between the HLA complex and the T-lymphocyte receptor. When helper T lymphocytes specific for an antigen become primed and partially activated, they acquire new functional properties, including cell division, cytokine synthesis, and cell membrane expression of *accessory molecules* such as cell-adhesion molecules and costimulatory molecules. The synthesis and release of immune cytokines, especially IL-2, by T lymphocytes is crucial for the progression of initial activation and the functional differentiation of T lymphocytes. The primed T lymphocyte produces IL-2, a potent mitogen, inducing mitosis, with resultant autocrine stimulation.

Helper T-lymphocyte differentiation

At the stage of initial priming, CD4 T lymphocytes are usually classified as *T helper 0,* or *Th0,* cells. However, CD4 T lymphocytes can differentiate into functional subsets as a consequence of differences in gene activation and the secretion of specific panels of cytokines. One subset, called *T helper 1,* or *Th1,* secretes interferon-γ (IFN-γ), tumor necrosis factor β, and IL-12 but *not* IL-4, IL-5, or IL-10. The other subset, *T helper 2,* or *Th2,* secretes IL-4, IL-5, and IL-10 but not Th1 cytokines.

Immune Processing

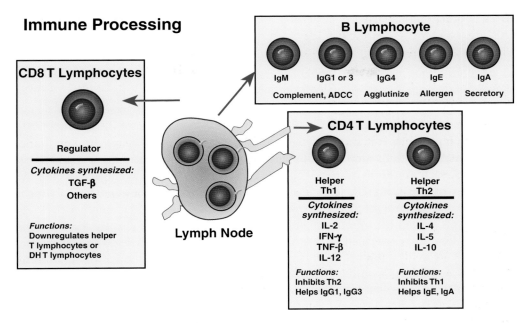

Figure 2-4 Schematic illustration of immune processing of antigen within the lymph node. On exposure to antigen and antigen-processing cells (APCs) within the lymph node, the 3 major lymphocyte subsets—B lymphocytes, CD4 T lymphocytes, and CD8 T lymphocytes—are activated to release specific cytokines and perform specific functional activities. B lymphocytes are stimulated to produce one of the various antibody isotypes, whose functions include complement activation, antibody-dependent cellular cytotoxicity, agglutinization, allergen recognition, and release into secretions. (See Chapter 4 for a detailed discussion.) CD4 T lymphocytes become activated into T helper 1 (Th1) or T helper 2 (Th2) subsets. Th1 lymphocytes function to help B lymphocytes secrete immunoglobulin G1 (IgG1) and IgG3; inhibit Th2; and release cytokines such as interleukin-2 (IL-2), interferon-γ (IFN-γ), tumor necrosis factor β (TNF-β), and interleukin-12 (IL-12). Th2 lymphocytes function to help B lymphocytes secrete IgE and IgA; inhibit Th1 lymphocytes; and synthesize cytokines such as IL-4, IL-5, and IL-10. CD8 T lymphocytes become activated into regulatory T lymphocytes that function by inhibiting other CD4 T lymphocytes, often by secreting cytokines such as TNF-β. *(Illustration by Barb Cousins, modified by Joyce Zavarro.)*

These subsets are important because the different cytokines produced by Th1 and Th2 profoundly influence subsequent "downstream" immune processing, B-lymphocyte antibody synthesis, and cell-mediated effector responses (see the following section). For example, IFN-γ, produced by Th1 lymphocytes, blocks the differentiation and activation of Th2 lymphocytes, and IL-4, produced by Th2 lymphocytes, blocks the differentiation of Th1 lymphocytes. The regulation determining whether a Th1 or a Th2 response develops consequent to exposure to a particular antigen is not entirely understood, but presumed variables include cytokines preexisting in the microenvironment, the nature of the antigen, the amount of antigen, and the type of APC. For example, IL-12, which is produced by macrophage APCs, might preferentially induce Th1 responses.

von Andrien UH, Mackay CR. T-cell function and migration—two sides of the same coin. *N Engl J Med.* 2000;343:1020–1034.

B-lymphocyte activation

One of the major regulatory functions for helper T lymphocytes is B-lymphocyte activation. B lymphocytes are responsible for producing antibodies, which are glycoproteins that bind to a specific antigen. B lymphocytes begin as naive lymphocytes with IgM and IgD on the cell surface; these serve as the B-lymphocyte antigen receptor. Through these surface antibodies, B lymphocytes can detect epitopes on intact antigens and thus do not require antigen processing by APCs. After appropriate stimulation of the B-lymphocyte antigen receptor, helper T lymphocyte–B lymphocyte interaction occurs, leading to further B-lymphocyte activation and differentiation. B lymphocytes acquire new functional properties, such as cell division, cell surface expression of accessory molecules, and the ability to synthesize and release large quantities of antibodies. Most important, activated B lymphocytes acquire the ability to change antibody class from IgM to another class (eg, to IgG1, IgA, or another immunoglobulin). This shift requires a molecular change of the immunoglobulin heavy chain class at the genetic level, and this is regulated by specific cytokines released by the helper T lymphocyte. For example, treatment of an antigen-primed B lymphocyte with IFN-γ induces a switch from IgM to IgG1 production. Treatment with IL-4 induces a switch from IgM to IgE production. Chapter 4 discusses the importance of the different antibody classes in immune reactivity.

Role of regulatory (suppressor) T lymphocytes

The regulation of the B-lymphocyte and helper T-lymphocyte response has recently been clarified, and the roles of antigen receptors and tolerance are discussed in Chapter 5; immunologic microenvironments are discussed later in this chapter and in Chapter 3. The immunoregulatory role of regulatory, or suppressor, T lymphocytes has become partially clarified, especially through the induction of immunomodulatory cytokine synthesis by regulatory T lymphocytes. Originally, regulatory T lymphocytes were observed to express the CD8 marker and to become activated during the initial phases of processing. More recently, certain CD4 T lymphocytes have also been observed to have regulatory, or suppressive, functions. In many cases, both CD8 and CD4 regulatory T lymphocytes appear to operate by the release of immunomodulatory cytokines such as transforming growth factor β, which can inhibit or alter the helper or effector function of other T lymphocytes. Other classic mechanisms of regulatory T-lymphocyte function, such as complicated antigen-specific T-lymphocyte circuits and release of antigen-specific suppressor molecules, have received less attention. Administration of antigen orally or via the anterior chamber preferentially induces regulatory T lymphocytes (see the following section). The relationship between CD8 regulatory T lymphocytes and CD8 cytotoxic effector cells is not entirely clear.

Effector Phase

During the effector phase, the adaptive immune response (eg, eliminate offending foreign antigen) is physically carried out. Antigen-specific effectors exist in 2 major subsets:

1. T lymphocytes
2. B lymphocytes plus their antibodies

A third population of *non-T, non-B effector lymphocytes,* formerly called *null cells,* is sometimes also grouped with immune effectors, although these cells are not antigen-specific and might be considered part of the innate immune system.

In general, effector lymphocytes require 2 exposures to antigen:

1. the initial exposure, often called *priming* or *activation,* occurring in the lymph node
2. a second exposure, often called *restimulation,* happening in the peripheral tissue in which the initial antigen contact occurred

This second exposure is usually necessary to fully exploit the effector mechanism within a local tissue. All of these effector mechanisms are described in more detail in Chapter 4.

Subsets of effector T lymphocytes can be distinguished into 2 main types by functional differences in experimental assays or by differences in cell surface molecules (Fig 2-5). *Delayed hypersensitivity (DH) T lymphocytes* usually express CD4 and release IFN-γ and tumor necrosis factor β. They function by homing to a tissue, recognizing antigen and APCs, becoming fully activated, and releasing cytokines and mediators that then recruit other

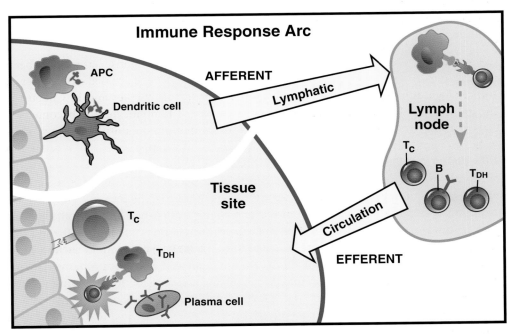

Figure 2-5 Schematic representation of effector mechanisms during adaptive immunity. Not only is the immune response initiated within the tissue site, but ultimately the immune response arc is completed when effectors encounter antigen within the tissue after release into the circulation from the lymph node. The 3 most important effector mechanisms of adaptive immunity include cytotoxic T lymphocytes (T$_C$), delayed hypersensitivity T lymphocytes (T$_{DH}$), and antibody-producing B lymphocytes, especially plasma cells. APC = antigen-processing cells. *(Illustration by Barb Cousins, modified by Joyce Zavarro.)*

nonspecific, antigen-independent effector cells such as neutrophils, basophils, or monocytes. As with helper T lymphocytes, Th1 and Th2 types of DH effector cells have been identified.

Cytotoxic T lymphocytes are the other major type of effector T lymphocyte. Cytotoxic T lymphocytes express CD8 and serve as effector cells for killing tumors or virally infected host cells through release of cytotoxic cytokines or specialized pore-forming molecules. The subset of effector lymphocytes now grouped as non-T, non-B lymphocytes includes natural killer cells, lymphokine-activated cells, and killer cells.

Antibodies, or *immunoglobulins,* are soluble antigen-specific effector molecules of adaptive immunity. After appropriate antigenic stimulation with T-lymphocyte help, B lymphocytes secrete IgM antibodies, and later other isotypes, into the efferent lymph fluid draining into the venous circulation. Antibodies then mediate a variety of immune effector activities by combining with antigen in the blood or in tissues.

Immune Response Arc and Primary or Secondary Immune Response

Concept of Immunologic Memory

Immunologic memory is probably the most distinctive feature of adaptive immune responses; protective immunization is the prototypical example of this powerful phenomenon. Classically, immunologic memory was the concept used to explain why serum antibody production for a specific antigen began much more quickly and rose to much higher levels after reexposure to that antigen but not after exposure to a different antigen. Later it was learned that the concept of memory applied not only to antibody production by B lymphocytes but also to that by T lymphocytes.

Differences in primary and secondary responses

The concept of an anamnestic response posits that the second encounter with an antigen is regulated differently from the first encounter. Differences in the primary and secondary immune response arc, especially in the processing and effector phases, offer partial explanation. During the processing phase of the primary response, antigen must find the relatively rare specific B lymphocyte (perhaps 1 in 100,000) and T lymphocyte (perhaps 1 in 10,000) and then stimulate these cells from a completely resting and naive state, a sequence that requires days. The secondary processing response for T and B lymphocytes is shorter for at least 3 reasons:

1. Upon removal of antigen, T and B lymphocytes activated during the primary response may gradually return to a resting state, but they retain the capacity to become reactivated within 12–24 hours of antigen exposure. That is, they are now memory cells rather than naive cells.
2. Because stimulated lymphocytes divide, the population of potential antigen-responsive T or B lymphocytes will have increased manyfold, and these cells will have migrated to other sites of potential encounters with antigen.

3. In some cases, such as in mycobacterial infection, low doses of antigen may remain in the node or site, producing a chronic, low-level, continuous antigenic stimulation of T and B lymphocytes.

For antibody responses, another memory function dependent on antibody requires even less time and operates primarily at the level of the effector phase. IgM produced during the effector phase of the primary response and released into the blood is often too large to passively leak into a peripheral site. However, during the secondary response, antibody class switching has occurred so that IgG or other isotypes that have passively leaked into a site or have been actively produced there can immediately combine with an antigen, causing the secondary response triggered by antibody to be very rapid (*immediate hypersensitivity*).

Homing

Memory also requires that lymphocytes demonstrate a complex migratory pattern called *homing*. Thus, lymphocytes pass from the circulation into various tissues, from which they subsequently depart, and then pass by way of lymphatics to reenter the circulation. Homing involves the variable interaction between lymphocytes and endothelial cells using multiple *cell-adhesion molecules,* which are discussed in Chapter 4. Usually, the major types of lymphocytes that migrate into tissue sites are memory lymphocytes that express higher levels of certain cell-adhesion molecules, such as the integrins, than do naive cells. Naive lymphocytes tend to migrate to lymphoid tissues, where they have the chance of meeting their cognate antigen. Inflammation, however, changes the rules and serves to break down homing patterns. At inflammatory sites, the volume of lymphocyte migration is far greater and selection much less precise, although migration of memory cells or activated lymphocytes still exceeds that of naive cells.

Regional Immunity and Immunologic Microenvironments

Regional Immunity

The idea that each organ and tissue site has its own particular immune response arc, which may vary significantly from the classic cutaneous response, is called *regional immunity*. Regional immunity of the tissue site can characterize all 3 phases—afferent, processing, and efferent—of the responses involved. For instance, the immune response arc for oral immunization (eg, polio vaccine) differs from that for intramuscular immunization (eg, mumps/measles/rubella vaccine), which differs from that for cutaneous vaccination (eg, bacille Calmette-Guérin vaccine). Regional immunity also affects the transplantation of donor tissue, such as a kidney or cornea. Such transplantations require the recipient to produce afferent, processing, and effector responses to the transplant, all modified by the unique location. Chapter 3 describes regional immune concepts relevant to the eye. See also BCSC Section 8, *External Disease and Cornea,* for a discussion of the regional immunity of the cornea in Part XI, Corneal Transplantation.

Immunologic Microenvironments

Regional immunologic differences occur because different tissue sites are composed of different *immunologic microenvironments*. The concept of immunologic microenvironment incorporates a broad range of anatomical and physiologic differences among tissues or organs that regulate the immune response:

- the presence of well-formed lymphatics
- specialized immunologic structures (Peyer patches or conjunctival follicles)
- blood–tissue barriers to macromolecules or cell migration
- type of resident APC
- constitutive synthesis of immunoregulatory cytokines or molecules by the parenchymal cell types
- many other factors

The analysis of immunologic microenvironments has become important for understanding the immunology of transplantation, infection, and autoimmunity for gene therapy or many organ systems.

Clinical Examples of the Concept of the Immune Response Arc

The concept of the immune response arc is a powerful tool for understanding clinically relevant immunologic phenomena. The 2 examples of cutaneous immunity (see Clinical Examples 2-1) illustrate this feature. Throughout the discussion in Chapters 3, 4, and 5, such clinical examples are interspersed with the text to provide similar illustrations.

Delves PJ, Martin S, Burton D, Roitt IM. *Roitt's Essential Immunology.* 11th ed. Malden, MA: Blackwell; 2006.

Male DK, Cooke A, Owen M, Trowsdale J, Champion B. *Advanced Immunology.* 3rd ed. St Louis: Mosby; 1996.

CLINICAL EXAMPLES 2-1

Primary response to poison ivy toxin The first contact between the poison ivy resin urushiol and the epidermal surface of an exposed extremity, such as the forearm, triggers the immunologic mechanisms of poison ivy dermatitis. The *afferent phase* of this primary response begins when the toxin permeates into the epidermis, where much of it binds to extracellular proteins, forming a protein–toxin conjugate technically called a *hapten*. Some of the toxin is taken up by antigen-presenting cells (APCs), especially Langerhans cells (LCs), and over the next 4–18 hours the toxin-stimulated LCs leave their normal location in the basal epidermis and migrate along afferent lymphatics into the draining lymph nodes. During this time, the toxin is internalized into endocytic compartments and processed by the LCs so that it can be recognized by helper T lymphocytes within the node. Some of the free toxin or hapten is also carried by lymph into the node.

In the lymph node, the *processing phase* begins. The urushiol-stimulated LCs interact with T lymphocytes, seeking over the next 3–5 days the rare T lymphocyte that has the correct specific antigen receptor. Once located, the naive T lymphocyte becomes primed. It is induced to undergo cell division, to acquire new functions such as cytokine secretion, and to upregulate certain surface molecules and receptors of the plasma membrane. These primed cells ultimately either function as helper cells or become effector cells, which leave the node through efferent lymphatics, accumulate in the thoracic duct, and then enter venous blood, where they recirculate.

Free toxin or hapten not taken up by APCs experiences a different fate during the processing phase. It enters a zone of the lymph node populated by B lymphocytes. These naive B lymphocytes express membrane-bound antibody (IgM and IgD) that serves as an antigen receptor. If a chance encounter occurs between the correct antibody and the toxin, the B lymphocyte becomes partially activated. However, completion of B-lymphocyte activation requires further interaction with helper T lymphocytes, which release cytokines, inducing B lymphocytes to undergo cell division and to increase production of antibodies, thus releasing antitoxin antibodies into the lymph fluid and ultimately the venous circulation.

The *effector phase* begins when the primed T lymphocytes, primed B lymphocytes, or antibodies leave the lymphatics and enter the peripheral site of the original antigen encounter. By 5–7 days after exposure, much of the urushiol toxin might have already been removed through nonspecific clearance mechanisms such as desquamation of exposed epidermis, washing of involved skin, and subclinical effects of innate immunity. When toxin-stimulated APCs do remain at the site, primed T lymphocytes become further activated into effector cells, releasing inflammatory mediators to recruit other leukocyte populations. This represents the contact hypersensitivity type of delayed hypersensitivity. Rarely, if adequate free toxin is present, IgG antitoxin immune complexes can form and mediate inflammation (see the following example). However, if most of the antigen is already cleared, then the primed T lymphocyte may enter the skin but become inactive, retaining memory. Or the T lymphocyte may exit the skin through afferent lymphatics to reenter the lymph node. Similarly, antibodies or antibody-producing B lymphocytes may remain in the skin or reach the lymph nodes.

Secondary response to poison ivy toxin The immunologic mechanisms work much faster after the second encounter with poison ivy toxin. The *afferent phase* of this secondary response begins when the toxin permeates the epidermis. Again, some of the toxin is taken up by the LCs, internalized over the next 4–18 hours into endocytic compartments, and processed in a way that can be recognized by T lymphocytes. If a memory T lymphocyte is present at the cutaneous site, then the *processing* and *effector phases* occur within 24 hours at the site, as the memory T lymphocyte becomes activated upon interacting with the LC. In addition, some LCs leave the skin, enter the draining node, and encounter memory T lymphocytes there.

Processing during the secondary response is much quicker, and within 24 hours restimulated memory cells enter the circulation and migrate to the toxin-exposed cutaneous site. Because abundant toxin remains, additional T lymphocyte–LC stimulation occurs, inducing vigorous T-lymphocyte cytokine production. The inflammatory mediators, in turn, recruit neutrophils and monocytes, leading to a severe inflammatory reaction within 12–36 hours after exposure, causing the typical epidermal blisters of poison ivy. Because the response is delayed by 24 hours, it is considered delayed hypersensitivity and, in this case, a specific form of delayed hypersensitivity called *contact hypersensitivity*.

Primary and secondary response to tuberculosis The primary and secondary immune response arcs can occur at different sites, as with the immunologic mechanisms of the first and second encounter with *Mycobacterium tuberculosis* antigens. The *afferent phase* of the primary response occurs after the inhalation of the live organisms, which proliferate slowly within the lung. Alveolar macrophages ingest the bacteria and transport the organisms to the hilar lymph nodes, where the *processsing phase* begins. Over the next few days, as T and B lymphocytes are primed, the hilar nodes become enlarged because of the increased number of dividing T and B lymphocytes as well as by the generalized increased trafficking of other lymphocytes through the nodes. The *effector phase* begins when the primed T lymphocytes recirculate and enter the infected lung. The T lymphocytes interact with the macrophage-ingested bacteria, and cytokines are released that activate neighboring macrophages to fuse into giant cells, forming caseating granulomas. Meanwhile, some of the effector T lymphocytes home to other lymph nodes throughout the body, where they become inactive memory T lymphocytes, trafficking and recirculating throughout the secondary lymphoid tissue.

A secondary response using the immune response arc of the skin is the basis of the tuberculin skin test to diagnose TB. The *afferent phase* of the secondary response begins when purified protein derivative (PPD) reagent, antigens purified from mycobacteria, is injected into the dermis, where the PPD is taken up by dermal macrophages. The secondary *processing phase* begins when these PPD-stimulated macrophages migrate into the draining lymph node, where they encounter memory T lymphocytes from the previous lung infection, leading to memory T-lymphocyte reactivation. The secondary *effector phase* commences when these reactivated memory T lymphocytes recirculate and home back into the dermis and encounter additional antigen/macrophages at the site, causing the T lymphocytes to become fully activated and release cytokines. Within 24–72 hours, these cytokines induce infiltration of additional lymphocytes and monocytes as well as fibrin clotting. This process produces the typical indurated dermal lesion of the tuberculosis skin test, called the *tuberculin form* of delayed hypersensitivity.

CHAPTER 3

Ocular Immune Responses

Just as regional differences in immune responses occur because of differences in the immunologic microenvironments of various tissue sites, regional differences can be identified for specific locations within and around the eye. Immune responses in health and disease are affected by differences in the immunologic microenvironment (Table 3-1) in such areas as the

- conjunctiva
- anterior chamber, anterior uvea (iris and ciliary body), and vitreous
- cornea and sclera
- retina/retinal pigment epithelium (RPE)/choriocapillaris
- choroid

Immune Responses of the Conjunctiva

Features of the Immunologic Microenvironment

The conjunctiva shares many of the features typical of mucosal sites. It is composed of 2 layers: an epithelial layer and a connective tissue layer called the *substantia propria*. The conjunctiva is well vascularized and has good lymphatic drainage to preauricular and submandibular nodes. The tissue is richly invested with Langerhans cells, other dendritic cells, and macrophages that serve as potential *antigen-presenting cells (APCs)*. Conjunctival follicles that enlarge after certain types of ocular surface infection or inflammation represent collections of T lymphocytes, B lymphocytes, and APCs. Observation of the function of similar sites, such as Peyer patches of the intestine, suggests that follicles might represent a site for localized immune processing of antigens that permeate through the thin overlying epithelium to be processed by T lymphocytes and B lymphocytes locally within the follicle.

The conjunctiva, especially the substantia propria, is richly infiltrated with potential effector cells, predominately mast cells. All antibody isotypes are represented, and presumably local production as well as passive leakage occurs. IgA is the most abundant antibody in the tear film. Soluble molecules of the innate immune system are also represented, especially complement. The conjunctiva appears to support most adaptive and innate immune effector responses, especially antibody-mediated and lymphocyte-mediated responses, although IgE-mediated mast-cell degranulation is one of the most common

Table 3-1 Comparison of Immune Microenvironments in Various Normal Ocular Sites

	Conjunctiva	Cornea/Sclera	Anterior Chamber, Anterior Uvea, Vitreous	Subretina/RPE/Choroid
Anatomical features	Lymphatics, follicles	Lymphatics at limbus, none centrally Macromolecules diffuse through stroma	No lymphatics, antigen clearance through trabecular meshwork Partial blood–uveal barrier	No lymphatics Blood–retina barrier Uveal circulation permeable
Resident APC	Dendritic and Langerhans cells, macrophages	Langerhans cells at limbus No APC in central cornea No APC in sclera Epithelium/endothelium can be induced to express class II MHC	Many dendritic cells and macrophages in iris and ciliary body Hyalocytes are macrophage-derived	Microglia in the retina Dendritic cells and macrophages in choriocapillaris RPE can be induced to express class II MHC
Specialized immune compartments for localized immune processing	?? Follicles	None	None	None
Resident effector cells	Mast cells, T lymphocytes, B lymphocytes, plasma cells, rare neutrophil	Centrally—none Sclera—none	Rare to no T lymphocytes or B lymphocytes, rare mast cells	Retina—normally no lymphocytes Choroid—mast cells, some lymphocytes
Resident effector molecules	All antibody iso-types, especially IgE, IgG sub-classes, IgA in tears Complement and kininogen precursors present	Peripherally Igs but minimal IgM Centrally minimal antibody, some complement present Sclera: low antibody concentration, minimal IgM	Kallikrein but not kininogen precursors Some complement present, but less than in blood Minimal Igs in iris, some IgG in ciliary body and aqueous humor	Retina—minimal to no Igs Choroid—IgGs and IgA
Immunoregulatory systems	Mucosa-associated lymphoid tissue	Immune privilege—Fas ligand, avascularity, lack of central APC	Immune privilege—anterior chamber–associated immune deviation, immunosuppressive factors in aqueous, Fas ligand	Immune privilege— ?? mechanisms

APC = antigen-presenting cells

and important. Chapter 4 discusses these mechanisms in greater detail. See also Part IV of BCSC Section 8, *External Disease and Cornea*.

Immunoregulatory Systems

The most important immunoregulatory system for the conjunctiva is called *mucosa-associated lymphoid tissue (MALT)*. The MALT concept refers to the interconnected network of mucosal sites (the epithelial lining of the respiratory tract, gut, and genitourinary tract and the ocular surface and its adnexae) that share certain specific immunologic features:

- rich investment of APCs
- specialized structures for localized antigen processing (eg, Peyer patches and tonsils)
- unique effector cells (eg, intraepithelial T lymphocytes and abundant mast cells)

However, the most distinctive aspect of MALT is the distribution and homing of effector T and B lymphocytes induced by immunization at 1 mucosal site to all MALT sites because of the shared expression of specific cell-adhesion molecules on postcapillary venules of the mucosal vasculature. MALT immune response arcs tend to favor T helper 2 (Th2)–dominated responses that result in the production of predominantly IgA and IgE antibodies. Immunization of soluble antigens through MALT, especially in the gut sites, often produces oral tolerance, presumably by activating Th2-like regulatory T lymphocytes that suppress Th1–delayed hypersensitivity (DH) effector cells.

Clinical Example 3-1 gives an example of a conjunctival immune response.

CLINICAL EXAMPLE 3-1

Immune response to viral conjunctivitis Conjunctivitis caused by adenovirus infection is a common ocular infection (see BCSC Section 8, *External Disease and Cornea*). Although details of the immune response after conjunctival adenovirus infection remain unknown, they can be inferred from knowledge of viral infection at other mucosal sites and from animal studies. After infection with adenovirus, the epithelial cells begin to die within 36 hours. Innate immune mechanisms that can assist in limiting infection become activated soon after infection. For example, infected cells produce cytokines such as interferons that limit spread of infectious virus and recruit nonspecific effector cells such as macrophages and neutrophils.

However, the adaptive immune response to adenovirus infection is considered more important in viral clearance. The primary adaptive response begins when macrophages and dendritic cells presumably become infected or take up cell debris and viral antigens. Both APCs and extracellular antigenic material are conveyed to the preauricular and submandibular nodes along lymphatics, where vigorous helper T-lymphocyte and antibody responses are activated, producing lymphadenopathy. Local immune processing may also occur within the follicle if virus invades the epithelial capsule. During the early effector phase of the primary B-lymphocyte response, IgM antibodies are released into the blood that will *not* be very effective in controlling surface infection, although they will prevent widespread viremia. However, IgM-bearing B lymphocytes eventually infiltrate the conjunctival stroma and may release antibodies locally in the conjunctiva. Later, during the primary effector response, class switching to IgG or IgA may occur to mediate local effector responses, such as neutralization or complement-mediated lysis of infected cells.

The most active effector response later in acute viral infection comes from natural killer cells and CD8 cytotoxic T lymphocytes (CTLs), which kill infected epithelium. However, adenovirus can block the expression of class I MHC on infected cells and thereby escape being killed by CTLs. Adaptive immunity can also activate macrophages by antiviral delayed hypersensitivity (DH) mechanisms later during infection. DH response to viral antigens is thought to contribute to the development of the corneal subepithelial infiltrates that occur in some patients late in adenovirus infection.

The secondary response of the conjunctiva, assuming a prior primary exposure to the same virus at some other mucosal site, differs in that antibody-mediated effector mechanisms dominate. Because of MALT, antivirus IgA is present not only in blood but also in tears as a result of differentiated IgA-secreting B lymphocytes in the lacrimal gland, the substantia propria, and follicles. Thus, recurrent infection is often prevented by preexisting neutralizing antibodies that had disseminated into tears or follicles following the primary infection. However, if the inoculum of recurrent virus overwhelms this antibody barrier, or if the virus has mutated its surface glycoproteins recognized by antibodies, then epithelial infection does occur. Additional immune processing can occur in the follicle and draining nodes. Specific memory effector CTLs are effective in clearing infection within a few days.

Nathanson N, ed. *Viral Pathogenesis and Immunity.* Philadelphia: Lippincott; 2002.

Pepose JS, Holland GN, Wilhelmus KR, eds. *Ocular Infection and Immunity.* St Louis: Mosby; 1996.

Immune Responses of the Anterior Chamber, Anterior Uvea, and Vitreous

Features of the Immunologic Microenvironment

Numerous specialized anatomical features of the anterior region of the eye affect ocular immune responses. The anterior chamber is a fluid-filled cavity; circulating aqueous humor provides a unique medium for intercellular communication among cytokines, immune cells, and resident tissue cells of the iris, ciliary body, and corneal endothelium. Although aqueous humor is relatively protein-depleted compared to serum (about 0.1%–1.0% of total serum protein concentration), even normal aqueous humor contains a complex mixture of biological factors, such as immunomodulatory cytokines, neuropeptides, and complement inhibitors, that can influence immunologic events within the eye.

A partial blood–ocular barrier is present. Fenestrated capillaries in the ciliary body allow a size-dependent concentration gradient of plasma macromolecules to permeate the interstitial tissue; smaller plasma-derived molecules are present in higher concentration than are larger molecules. The tight junctions between the pigmented and the nonpigmented ciliary epithelium provide a more exclusive barrier, preventing interstitial macromolecules from permeating directly through the ciliary body into the aqueous humor. Nevertheless, low numbers of plasma macromolecules bypass the nonpigmented epithelium barrier and may permeate by diffusion anteriorly through the uvea to enter the anterior chamber through the anterior iris surface.

The inner eye does not contain well-developed lymphatics. Rather, clearance of soluble substances depends on the aqueous humor outflow channels; clearance of particulates depends on endocytosis by trabecular meshwork endothelial cells or macrophages. Nevertheless, antigen inoculation into the anterior chamber results in efficient communication with the systemic immune response. Intact soluble antigens gain entrance to the venous circulation, where they communicate with the spleen.

The iris and ciliary body contain a rich investment of macrophages and dendritic cells that serve as APCs and possible effector cells. Immune processing is unlikely to occur locally, but APCs leave the eye by the trabecular meshwork and home to the spleen, where processing occurs that favors a Th2 response and preferential activation of CD8 regulatory T lymphocytes. Few resident T lymphocytes and some mast cells are present in the normal anterior uvea; B lymphocytes, eosinophils, and neutrophils are not present. Very low concentrations of IgG, complement components, and kallikrein occur in normal eyes.

The vitreous has not been described as carefully as the anterior chamber, but the vitreous probably manifests most of the same properties, with several notable exceptions. The vitreous gel can electrostatically bind charged protein substances and may thus serve as an antigen depot as well as a substrate for leukocyte cell adhesion. Because the vitreous contains type II collagen, it may serve as a depot of potential autoantigen in some forms of uveitis related to arthritis in which type II collagen in the joint is an autoantigen. See also BCSC Section 12, *Retina and Vitreous*.

Immunoregulatory Systems

The anterior uvea has an immunoregulatory system that has been described as *immune privilege*. The modern concept of immune privilege refers to the observation that tumor implants or allografts survive better within an immunologically privileged region, whereas a similar implant or graft is rapidly rejected by immune mechanisms within the skin or other nonprivileged sites. Other immune-privileged sites are the subretinal space, the brain, and the testes. Although the nature of the antigen involved is probably important, immune privilege of the anterior uvea has been observed with a wide variety of antigens, including alloantigens (eg, transplantation antigens), tumor antigens, haptens, soluble proteins, autoantigens, bacteria, and viruses.

Immune privilege is mediated by influences on both the afferent and the effector phases of the immune response arc. Immunization using the anterior segment as the afferent phase of a primary immune response arc results in a unique generation of immunologic effectors. Immunization as with lens protein or other autoantigens through the anterior chamber does not result in the same pattern of systemic immunity as does immunization by skin. Immunization by an anterior chamber injection in experimental animals results in an altered form of systemic immunity to that antigen called *anterior chamber–associated immune deviation (ACAID)*. The "deviant" immune response is characterized by robust systemic antibody response to the encounter with antigen but the absence of any elicitable DH response to that antigen.

Following injection of antigen into the anterior chamber, the afferent phase begins when specialized macrophages residing in the iris recognize and take up the antigen. The APC function of these uveal macrophages has been altered by exposure to immunoregulatory cytokines normally present within aqueous humor and uveal tissue, especially transforming growth factor β2 (TGF-β2). The process by which aqueous humor factors convert macrophages into ACAID-inducing APCs is unknown. The TGF-β2–exposed antigen-stimulated ocular macrophages leave by the trabecular meshwork and the Schlemm canal to enter the venous circulation, where they preferentially migrate to the spleen. Here, the antigen signal is processed, with activation of not only helper T lymphocytes and B lymphocytes but also regulatory T lymphocytes. The CD8 regulatory cells serve to alter CD4 helper T-lymphocyte responses in the spleen and to downregulate CD4 T-lymphocyte DH responses to the specific *immunizing* antigen at all body sites. Thus, the resulting effector response is characterized by a selective suppression of antigen-specific DH and a selectively diminished production of complement-fixing isotypes of antibodies. The other antibody isotypes and cytotoxic T-lymphocyte precursors are the same as those occurring after conventional cutaneous immunization.

Several other mechanisms for ACAID have been proposed. A small percentage of intact antigen can leave the eye to enter the blood, where it tends to be processed within the spleen. Low doses of intravenous antigens produce a form of immunomodulation that has been called *low-zone tolerance*. Various mechanisms for immunoregulatory T-lymphocyte activation within the eye have been suggested as well.

Especially important to the clinician is the capacity of a tissue site to sustain the secondary effector phase of the immune response arc, because the primary immune response arc in autoimmune diseases might have occurred outside of the eye. In this regard, the secondary effector phase of the anterior segment is also immunomodulatory and has been termed the *effector blockade*. Because various immunoregulatory systems are normally present within the eye, intact immunologic effectors that are functional elsewhere—in the skin, for example—are *partially* blocked from activation and function within the anterior segment. Thus, Th1 DH T lymphocytes, cytotoxic T lymphocytes, natural killer cells, and complement activation appear to function less effectively in the anterior uvea than elsewhere. For instance, the anterior uvea is *relatively* resistant to induction of a secondary purified protein derivative DH response after primary immunization with mycobacteria in the skin. Mechanisms for effector blockade are multifactorial but include production of the following:

- immunomodulatory cytokines, produced by ocular tissues
- immunomodulatory neuropeptides, produced by ocular nerves
- functionally unique APCs
- complement inhibitors in aqueous humor
- other factors

Fas ligand (FasL), or CD95 ligand, is constitutively expressed on iris and corneal endothelium. FasL is normally expressed in the thymus and a few other immune-privileged sites, such as the testes. FasL is a potent trigger of programmed cell death, or *apoptosis,* of lymphocytes. Thus, FasL can induce apoptotic killing of infiltrating T lymphocytes, thereby preventing T-lymphocyte effector function. The loss of these protective mechanisms may occur prior to the development of uveitis.

The vitreous cavity has not been as well characterized immunologically, but preliminary experimental evidence suggests that an ACAID-like primary immune response arc probably applies to the vitreous as well, especially in an eye that has undergone vitrectomy. The existence of effector blockade in the vitreous is controversial, but it seems clear that soluble (as opposed to particulate) antigen injected into the vitreous can elicit a phenomenon similar to ACAID; this form of immunomodulation may also be facilitated by vitrectomy, even for particulate antigens. Other rationales for performing vitrectomy in eyes with uveitis are

- to remove any depot of antigen, including type II collagen, trapped in the gel
- to remove the gel substrate for cell-adhesion molecules to recruit and adhere leukocytes
- to allow circulation of immunomodulatory factors in aqueous humor

See Clinical Example 3-2.

Foster CS, Streilein JW. Basic immunology. In: Foster CS, Vitale AT, eds. *Diagnosis and Treatment of Uveitis.* Philadelphia: Saunders; 2002:34–78.

Sugita S, Ng TF, Lucas PJ, Gress RE, Streilein JW. B7⁺ iris pigment epithelium induce CD8⁺ T regulatory cells; both suppress CTLA-4⁺ T cells. *J Immunol.* 2006;176:118–127.

Zamiri P, Masli S, Kitaichi N, Taylor AW, Streilein JW. Thrombospondin plays a vital role in the immune privilege of the eye. *Invest Ophthalmol Vis Sci.* 2005;46:908–919.

CLINICAL EXAMPLE 3-2

Therapeutic potential of immune privilege It is unknown whether ACAID has practical consequences for clinical diseases, although it is thought to play a role in immunologic tolerance to lens crystallins after cataract surgery and in immunologic acceptance of corneal transplantation. ACAID can influence the immune response to ocular autoantigens. Animals immunized through the anterior chamber with the retinal autoantigens S-antigen or interphotoreceptor retinol-binding protein develop ACAID, and they are then protected from experimental autoimmune uveitis in the contralateral eye after subsequent conventional cutaneous immunization. Recently, ACAID has been reproduced by infusion of monocytes that were first treated extracorporeally with TGF-β and antigen, suggesting a potential clinically relevant method for immunotherapy.

Ferguson TA, Griffith TS. A vision of cell death: insights into immune privilege. *Immunol Rev.* 1997;156:167–184.

Immune Responses of the Cornea

Features of the Immunologic Microenvironment

The cornea is unique in that the periphery and the central portions of the tissue represent distinctly different immunologic microenvironments (Fig 3-1). Obviously, only the limbus is vascularized. Whereas the limbus is richly invested with Langerhans cells, the paracentral and central cornea are normally devoid of APCs. However, various stimuli, such as mild trauma, certain cytokines (eg, IL-1), or infection, can recruit APCs to the central cornea. Plasma-derived enzymes (eg, complement), IgM, and IgG are present in moderate concentrations in the periphery, but only low levels of the IgM are present centrally.

Corneal cells also appear to synthesize various antimicrobial and immunoregulatory proteins. Effector cells are absent or scarce in the normal cornea, but neutrophils, monocytes, and lymphocytes can readily migrate through the stroma if appropriate chemotactic stimuli are activated. Lymphocytes, monocytes, and neutrophils can also adhere to the endothelial surface during inflammation, giving rise to keratic precipitates or the classic Khodadoust line of endothelial rejection (Fig 3-2). Localized immune processing probably does not occur in the cornea. See also BCSC Section 8, *External Disease and Cornea*.

Immunoregulatory Systems

The cornea also demonstrates a form of immune privilege different from that observed in the anterior uvea. Immune privilege of the cornea is multifactorial. Normal limbal physiology is a major component, especially the maintenance of avascularity and lack of APCs in the mid- and central cornea. The absence of APCs and lymphatics partially inhibits afferent recognition in the central cornea, and the absence of postcapillary venules centrally can limit the efficiency of effector recruitment, although both effector cells and molecules can ultimately infiltrate even

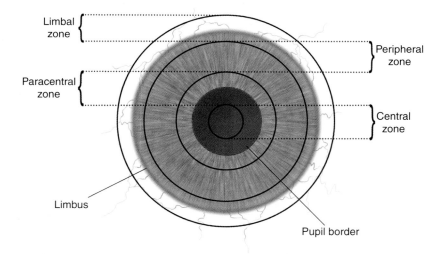

Figure 3-1 Topographic zones of the cornea. *(Illustration by Christine Gralapp.)*

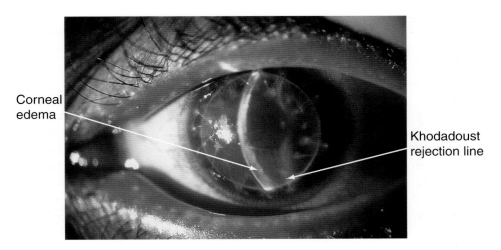

Corneal edema

Khodadoust rejection line

Figure 3-2 Endothelial graft rejection with stromal and epithelial edema on the trailing aspect of the migrating Khodadoust line.

avascular cornea. Another factor is the presence of intact immunoregulatory systems of the anterior chamber (ie, ACAID), to which the corneal endothelium is exposed.

See Clinical Example 3-3.

CLINICAL EXAMPLE 3-3

Corneal allograft rejection Penetrating keratoplasty, the transplantation of foreign corneal allografts, enjoys an extremely high success rate (>90%) even in the absence of systemic immunomodulation. This rate compares favorably to the transplantation rates of other donor tissues. The mechanisms of corneal graft survival have been attributed to immune privilege. In experimental models, factors contributing to rejection include the following:

- presence of central corneal vascularization
- induction of MHC molecule expression by the stroma, which is normally quite low
- contamination of the donor graft with donor-derived APCs prior to transplantation
- MHC disparity between the host and the donor
- preimmunization of the recipient to donor transplantation antigens

In addition, loss of immunoregulatory systems of the anterior chamber can apparently influence corneal allograft immunity, and the expression of FasL on corneal endothelium has been observed to greatly influence allograft protection. Rapid replacement of donor epithelium by host epithelium removes this layer as an antigenic stimulus. Once activated, however, antibody-dependent DH and CTL-related mechanisms can target transplantation antigens in all corneal layers.

Streilein JW. Regulation of ocular immune responses. *Eye.* 1997;11:171–175.

Immune Responses of the Retina, RPE, Choriocapillaris, and Choroid

Features of the Immunologic Microenvironment

The immunologic microenvironments of the retina, RPE, choriocapillaris, and choroid have not been well described. The retinal circulation demonstrates a blood–ocular barrier at the level of tight junctions between adjacent endothelial cells. The vessels of the choriocapillaris are highly permeable to macromolecules and allow transudation of most plasma macromolecules into the extravascular spaces of the choroid and choriocapillaris. The tight junctions between the RPE cells probably provide the true physiologic barrier between the choroid and the retina. Well-developed lymphatics are absent, although both the retina and the choroid have abundant potential APCs. In the retina, resident microglia (bone marrow–derived cells related to monocytes) are interspersed within all layers and can undergo physical changes and migration in response to various stimuli. The choriocapillaris and choroid are richly invested with certain potential APCs, especially macrophages and dendritic cells.

RPE can be induced to express class II major histocompatibility complex (MHC) molecules, suggesting that RPE may also interact with T lymphocytes. The presence of T lymphocytes or B lymphocytes within the normal posterior segment has not been carefully addressed, but effector cells appear to be absent from the normal retina. The density of mast cells is moderate in the choroid, especially around the arterioles, but lymphocytes are present only in very low density. Eosinophils and neutrophils appear to be absent. Under various clinical or experimental conditions, however, high densities of T lymphocytes, B lymphocytes, macrophages, and neutrophils can infiltrate the choroid, choriocapillaris, and retina. The RPE and various cell types within the retina and the choroid (eg, pericytes) can synthesize many different cytokines (eg, TGF-β) that may alter the subsequent immune response. Local immune processing does not appear to occur. See also BCSC Section 12, *Retina and Vitreous*.

Streilein JW, Ma N, Wenkel H, Ng TF, Zamiri P. Immunobiology and privilege of neuronal retina and pigment epithelium transplants. *Vision Res.* 2002;42:487–495.

Wenkel H, Streilein JW. Evidence that retinal pigment epithelium functions as an immune-privileged tissue. *Invest Ophthalmol Vis Sci.* 2000;41:3467–3473.

Immunoregulatory Systems

Recently, it has been demonstrated that a form of immune privilege is present after subretinal injection of antigen. The mechanism is unclear but is probably similar to ACAID. This observation may be important because of growing interest in retinal transplantation and gene therapy. (See Clinical Examples 3-4.) The capacity of the choriocapillaris and choroid to function as unique environments for the afferent or effector phases has not yet been evaluated.

Stein-Streilein J, Streilein JW. Anterior chamber-associated immune deviation (ACAID): regulation, biological relevance, and implications for therapy. *Int Rev Immunol.* 2002;21:123–152.

CLINICAL EXAMPLES 3-4

Retinal transplantation Transplantation of retina or RPE is being investigated as a method for regenerating retinal function in various disorders. In experimental animals, subretinal transplantation of fetal retinal tissue or various kinds of RPE allografts often show longer survival than the same grafts implanted elsewhere, even without systemic immunomodulation. The afferent phase recognition of alloantigens is likely performed by retinal microglia or recruited blood-derived macrophages from the choriocapillaris.

The subretinal cytokine environment remains unknown because transplantation is performed in the setting of retinal diseases, such as retinitis pigmentosa or macular degeneration, in which the blood–retina barrier is altered and retinal cell/RPE injury is present. However, injured RPE can still synthesize either immunomodulatory or inflammatory cytokines. The site of immune processing is unknown, but the spleen or some other secondary compartment outside of the eye is probably involved. When rejection does occur, the effector mechanisms are also unclear. In mice with fetal retinal grafts, immune rejection occurs by an unusual, slowly progressive cytotoxic mechanism not involving typical antibody-mediated cytolysis or DH T lymphocytes. In humans and nonhuman primates, rejection of RPE allografts has occurred in both subacute and chronic forms.

Retinal gene therapy Retinal gene therapy is the therapeutic use of intentional transfection of photoreceptors or RPE with a replication-defective virus that has been genetically altered to carry a replacement gene of choice. This gene becomes expressed in any cell infected by the virus. Immune clearance of the virus has been shown to cause loss of expression of the transferred gene in other body sites. If immune privilege protects the viral vector or the protein synthesized by the transferred gene from immune clearance, then subretinal gene therapy might enjoy greater success in the eye than elsewhere. This topic is currently under intense investigation.

CHAPTER 4

Mechanisms of Immune Effector Reactivity

Immunologists have long been fascinated with all 3 phases of the adaptive immune response, as well as related issues such as developmental biology and the ontogeny of lymphoid precursors. From the clinician's perspective, however, the effector phase is the most important aspect of both innate and adaptive immune responses, because patients who present with inflammation presumably have already experienced the afferent and processing phases of adaptive immunity or they are in the midst of the triggering mechanisms of innate immunity. In the following discussion, immune effector responses are subdivided into 3 categories:

1. *innate immune effector responses:* bacterial triggers, nonspecific effector molecules, neutrophil activation, macrophage activation
2. *adaptive immune effector responses:* antibody-dependent responses, lymphocyte-dependent responses, combination antibody/cellular responses
3. *amplification mechanisms relevant to both immune responses:* inflammatory mediators, cytokines, related topics

Effector Reactivities of Innate Immunity

Whereas adaptive immune responses use a complex afferent and processing system to activate effector responses, innate immune responses generally use more direct triggering mechanisms. Four of the most important triggering or response mechanisms to initiate an effector response of innate immunity are reviewed here (Table 4-1).

Bacteria-Derived Molecules That Trigger Innate Immunity

Bacterial lipopolysaccharide

Bacterial lipopolysaccharide (LPS), also known as *endotoxin,* is an intrinsic component of most gram-negative bacterial cell walls. One of the most important triggering molecules of innate immunity, LPS consists of 3 components:

1. lipid A
2. lipopolysaccharide
3. a protein core

Table 4-1 Effector Reactivities of the Innate Immune Response in the Eye

Bacteria-derived molecules that trigger innate immunity
    Lipopolysaccharide (LPS)
    Other cell wall components
    Exotoxins and secreted toxins

Nonspecific soluble molecules that trigger or modulate innate immunity
    Plasma-derived enzymes
    Acute phase reactants
    Local production of cytokines by parenchymal cells within a tissue site

Innate mechanisms for recruitment and activation of neutrophils
    Cell adhesion and transmigration
    Activation mechanisms
        Phagocytosis of bacteria

Innate mechanisms for recruitment and activation of macrophages
    Cell adhesion and transmigration
    Activation mechanisms
        Scavenging
        Priming
        Activation

Lipid A is responsible for most of the inflammatory effects of LPS.

LPS is an important cause of morbidity and mortality during infections with gram-negative bacteria and is the major cause of shock, fever, and other pathophysiologic responses to bacterial sepsis. The pleiotropic effects of LPS include activation of monocytes and neutrophils, leading to upregulation of genes for various cytokines (IL-1, IL-6, tumor necrosis factor [TNF]); degranulation; activation of complement through the alternative pathway; and direct impact on vascular endothelium. The cellular effects of LPS are the result of interactions with specific cell receptors, such as CD18/CR3, an LPS scavenger receptor on macrophages and lymphocytes. In addition, a circulating LPS-binding protein has been identified. Binding by the LPS-binding protein complex with the CD14 molecule on the macrophage surface leads to activation. See Clinical Examples 4-1 and 4-2.

Other bacterial cell wall components

The bacterial cell wall and membrane are complex, with numerous polysaccharide, lipid, and protein structures that can initiate the innate immune response whether or not they act as antigens for adaptive immunity. Such toxins may include

- muramyl dipeptide
- lipoteichoic acids, in gram-positive bacteria
- lipoarabinomannan, in mycobacteria
- other poorly characterized soluble factors, such as heat shock proteins, common to all bacteria

Killed lysates of many types of gram-positive bacteria or mycobacteria have been demonstrated to directly activate macrophages, making them useful as adjuvants. Some of these components have been implicated in various models for arthritis and uveitis. In many cases, the molecular mechanisms are probably similar to LPS.

CLINICAL EXAMPLE 4-1

Lipopolysaccharide-induced uveitis Humans are intermittently exposed to low doses of LPS that are released from the gut, especially during episodes of diarrhea and dysentery, and exposure to LPS may play a role in dysentery-related uveitis, arthritis, and Reiter syndrome. Systemic administration of a low dose of LPS in rabbits, rats, and mice produces a mild acute uveitis; this effect occurs at doses of LPS lower than those that cause apparent systemic shock. In rabbits, a breakdown of the blood–ocular barrier occurs because of leakage of plasma proteins through uveal vessels and loosening of the tight junctions between the nonpigmented ciliary epithelial cells. Rats and mice develop an acute neutrophil and monocytic infiltrate in the iris and ciliary body within 24 hours.

The precise mechanism of LPS-induced ocular effects after systemic administration is unknown. One possibility is that LPS circulates and binds to the vascular endothelium or other sites within the anterior uvea. Alternatively, LPS might cause activation of uveal macrophages or circulating leukocytes, leading them to preferentially adhere to the anterior uveal vascular endothelium. It is clear that TLR2, a toll-like receptor, recognizes LPS, and binding of LPS by TLR2 on macrophages results in macrophage activation and secretion of a wide array of inflammatory cytokines. Degranulation of platelets is among the first of histologic changes in LPS uveitis, probably mediated by eicosanoids, platelet-activating factors, and vasoactive amines. The subsequent intraocular generation of several mediators, especially leukotriene B_4, thromboxane B_2, prostaglandin E_2, and IL-6, correlates with the development of the cellular infiltrate and vascular leakage.

Not surprisingly, direct injection of LPS into various ocular sites can initiate a severe localized inflammatory response. For example, intravitreal injection of LPS triggers a dose-dependent infiltration of the uveal tract, retina, and vitreous with neutrophils and monocytes. Injection of LPS into the central cornea causes development of a ring infiltrate as a result of the infiltration of neutrophils circumferentially from the limbus.

Exotoxins and other secretory products of bacteria

Various bacteria are known to secrete products such as *exotoxins* into the microenvironment in which the bacterium is growing. Many of these products are enzymes that, although not directly inflammatory, can cause tissue damage that subsequently results in inflammation. Examples include

- collagenases
- hemolysins such as streptolysin O, which can kill neutrophils by causing cytoplasmic and extracellular release of their granules
- phospholipases such as the *Clostridium perfringens* α-toxins, which kill cells and cause necrosis by disrupting cell membranes

Intravitreal injection of a cytolytic toxin derived from *Bacillus cereus* can cause direct necrosis of retinal cells. In addition, the metabolic by-products of bacterial physiology can

---

CLINICAL EXAMPLE 4-2

Role of bacterial toxin production and severity of endophthalmitis The effect of toxin production by various bacterial strains on the severity of endophthalmitis has recently been evaluated in experimental studies. It has been known for nearly a century that intraocular injection of LPS is highly inflammatory and accounts for much of the enhanced pathogenicity of gram-negative infections of the eye. Using clinical isolates or bacteria genetically altered to diminish production of the various types of bacterial toxins, investigators have recently demonstrated that toxin elaboration by the living organism in gram-positive or -negative endophthalmitis greatly influences inflammatory cell infiltration and retinal cytotoxicity. This research suggests that sterilization with antibiotic therapy alone, in the absence of antitoxin therapy, may not prevent activation of innate immunity, ocular inflammation, and vision loss in eyes infected by toxin-producing strains.

> Booth MC, Atkuri RV, Gilmore MS. Toxin production contributes to severity of *Staphylococcus aureus* endophthalmitis. In: Nussenblatt RB, Whitcup SM, Caspi RR, et al, eds. *Advances in Ocular Immunology: Proceedings of the 6th International Symposium on the Immunology and Immunopathology of the Eye.* New York: Elsevier; 1994:269–272.
> Jett BD, Parke DW 2nd, Booth MC, Gilmore MS. Host/parasite interactions in bacterial endophthalmitis. *Zentralbl Bakteriol.* 1997;285:341–367.

---

result in nonspecific tissue alterations that predispose to inflammation, such as altered tissue pH.

Some bacteria secrete small formyl peptide molecules related to the tripeptide *N*-formylmethionylleucylphenylalanine (FMLP). These formyl peptides are potent triggering stimuli for innate immunity. FMLP interacts with specific receptors on leukocytes, resulting in their recruitment into the site. In vitro FMLP activates neutrophils, causes degranulation, and stimulates chemotaxis. Injection of FMLP into the cornea, conjunctiva, or vitreous produces infiltration with neutrophils and monocytes, which can be prevented by pretreatment with corticosteroids, cyclooxygenase (COX) inhibitors, and competitive inhibitors of FMLP.

> Gallin JI, Snyderman R, eds. *Inflammation: Basic Principles and Clinical Correlates.* 3rd ed. Philadelphia: Lippincott Williams & Wilkins; 1999.
> Medzhitov R, Janeway C. Innate immunity. *N Engl J Med.* 2000;343:338–344.

Other Triggers or Modulators of Innate Immunity

As discussed in earlier chapters, the adaptive immune response employs 1 main family of soluble effector molecules: antibodies specific for antigen. Although no similar mechanism exists for innate immunity, various *nonspecific* soluble protein molecules are used by the innate immune response.

Plasma-derived enzyme systems, especially *complement,* are discussed later in the chapter under amplification systems because they are effector molecules used to amplify inflammation for both innate and adaptive immunity. However, it is important to emphasize that complement, especially when activated through the alternative pathway, is a major effector molecule for innate immunity. Thus, stimuli that activate the alternative pathway, such as microbial cell walls, plastic surfaces of IOLs, or traumatized tissues, are potential triggering mechanisms of innate immunity. See Clinical Example 4-3.

Another important family of molecules for innate immunity is the group of *acute-phase reactants,* such as C-reactive protein and α_2-macroglobulin. Although generally synthesized by the liver and released into blood, many of these molecules are also made by macrophages or produced locally in tissues. α_2-Macroglobulin is especially interesting. It is a natural scavenging molecule, capable of binding various types of proteins and substances, presumably for clearance from the host. α_2-Macroglobulin is present in aqueous humor during uveitis and is synthesized by various ocular parenchymal cells of the eye as well. Enzyme systems in tears, such as lysozyme and lactoferrin, also play a role in ocular surface defenses.

Finally, various traumatic or toxic stimuli within ocular sites can trigger innate immunity. For example, trauma or toxins interacting directly with nonimmune ocular parenchymal cells, especially iris or ciliary body epithelium, retinal pigment epithelium, retinal Müller cells, or corneal or conjunctival epithelium, can result in a wide range of mediator, cytokine, and eicosanoid synthesis (see Table 4-7 later in the chapter), and this mechanism probably should be considered a form of innate immunity. Thus, phagocytosis of

CLINICAL EXAMPLE 4-3

Uveitis-glaucoma-hyphema syndrome One cause of postoperative inflammation following cataract surgery, uveitis-glaucoma-hyphema (UGH) syndrome is related to the physical presence of certain intraocular lens (IOL) styles. Although UGH syndrome was more common when rigid anterior chamber lenses were used during the early 1980s, it has also been reported with posterior chamber lenses. The pathogenesis of UGH syndrome appears to be related to various mechanisms for activation of innate immunity. One of the most likely mechanisms is cytokine and eicosanoid synthesis triggered by mechanical chafing or trauma to the iris or ciliary body. Plasma-derived enzymes, especially complement or fibrin, can enter the eye through vascular permeability altered by surgery or trauma and can then be activated by the surface of IOLs, especially those composed of polymethylmethacrylate (PMMA). Adherence of bacteria and leukocytes to the surface has also been implicated. Toxicity caused by contaminants on the lens surface during manufacturing has become rare. Recent research suggests that surface modification of IOLs, such as coating with heparin, might diminish the capacity of IOL materials to activate innate immune effector mechanisms. Nevertheless, even many noninflamed eyes with IOLs can demonstrate histologic evidence of low-grade foreign-body reactions around the haptics.

Pepose JS, Holland GN, Wilhelmus KR, eds. *Ocular Infection and Immunity.* St Louis: Mosby; 1996.

staphylococcus by corneal epithelium, microtrauma to ocular surface epithelium by contact lenses, chafing of iris or ciliary epithelium by an IOL, or laser treatment of the retina can stimulate ocular cells to produce mediators that assist in the recruitment of innate effector cells such as neutrophils or macrophages.

Innate Mechanisms for the Recruitment and Activation of Neutrophils

Neutrophils are among the most efficient effectors of innate immunity following trauma or acute infection. Neutrophils are categorized as either *resting* or *activated,* based on secretory and cell membrane activity. Cellular recruitment of resting, circulating neutrophils by the innate immune response occurs rapidly in a tightly controlled process requiring 2 main mechanisms:

1. neutrophil adhesion to the vascular endothelium through cell-adhesion molecules (CAMs) on leukocytes as well as on endothelial cells in postcapillary venules
2. transmigration of the neutrophils through the endothelium and its extracellular matrix, mediated by various chemotactic factors

For resting neutrophils to escape from blood vessels, an essential adhesion with activated vascular endothelial cells must occur; this is triggered by various innate stimuli, such as LPS, physical injury, thrombin, histamine, or leukotriene release, as well as other agonists.

The initial phase involves *neutrophil rolling,* a process by which neutrophils bind loosely but reversibly to nonactivated endothelial cells (Fig 4-1). Involved are molecules on both cell types belonging to at least 3 sets of CAM families:

1. the *selectins,* especially L-, P-, and E-selectin
2. the *integrins,* especially leukocyte function–associated antigen 1 (LFA-1) and Mac-1
3. molecules in the immunoglobulin (Ig) superfamily, especially intercellular adhesion molecule 1 (ICAM-1) and ICAM-2

The primary events are mediated largely by members of the selectin family and occur within minutes of stimulation. The ligands for selectin molecules are as yet poorly characterized oligosaccharides found in the cell membranes. Nonactivated neutrophils express L-selectin, which mediates a weak bond to endothelial cells. Upon exposure to the activating factors just mentioned, endothelial cells become activated, expressing in turn at least 2 other selectins (E and P) by which they can bind to the neutrophils and help stabilize the interaction by a process called *adhesion.* Subsequently, other factors, such as platelet-activating factor (PAF), various cytokines, and bacterial products, can induce the upregulation of the β-integrin family. As integrins are expressed, the selectins are shed, and neutrophils then bind firmly to endothelial cells through the immunoglobulin superfamily molecules.

Subsequent to adhesion, various chemotactic factors are required to induce *transmigration* of neutrophils across the endothelial barrier and extracellular matrix into the tissue site. Chemotactic factors are short-range signaling molecules that diffuse in a

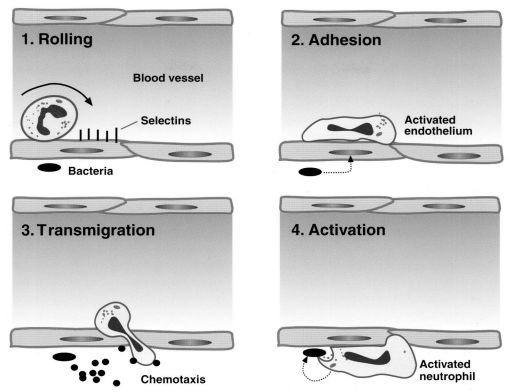

Figure 4-1 Four steps of neutrophil migration and activation. **1,** In response to innate stimuli, such as bacterial invasion of tissue, *rolling* neutrophils within the blood vessel bind loosely but reversibly to nonactivated endothelial cells by selectins. **2,** Exposure to innate activating factors and bacterial products *(dotted arrow)* activates endothelial cells, which in turn express E- and P-selectins, β-integrins, and immunoglobulin superfamily molecules to enhance and stabilize the interaction by a process called *adhesion.* **3,** Chemotactic factors triggered by the infection induce *transmigration* of neutrophils across the endothelial barrier into the extracellular matrix of the tissue. **4,** Finally, neutrophils are fully *activated* into functional effector cells upon stimulation by bacterial toxins and phagocytosis. *(Illustration by Barb Cousins, modified by Joyce Zavarro.)*

declining concentration gradient from the source of production within a tissue to the vessel itself. Neutrophils have receptors for these molecules, and they are induced to undergo membrane changes so they can migrate in the direction of highest concentration. A large number of such factors have been identified:

- complement products (C5a)
- fibrin split products
- certain neuropeptides, such as substance P
- bacteria-derived formyl tripeptides, such as FMLP

- leukotrienes
- α-chemokines, such as IL-8
- many others

Another function of certain chemotactic factors is that they may also enhance endothelial cell activation to upregulate CAM and to synthesize additional chemotactic factors.

Activation of neutrophils into functional effector cells begins during adhesion and transmigration but is fully exploited upon interaction with specific signals within the injured or infected site. Perhaps the most effective triggers of activation are bacteria and their toxins, especially LPS. Other innate or adaptive mechanisms (especially complement) and chemical mediators (such as leukotrienes and PAF) can also contribute to neutrophil activation. Unlike monocytes or lymphocytes, neutrophils do not leave a tissue to recirculate but remain and die.

Phagocytosis

Phagocytosis of bacteria and other pathogens is a selective receptor-mediated process, and the 2 most important receptors are the *antibody Fc receptors* and the *complement receptors.* Thus, those pathogens in complexes with antibody or with activated complement components are specifically bound to the cell-surface membrane–expressed Fc or complement (C) receptors and are effectively ingested. Other, less well characterized receptors may also mediate attachment to phagocytes. Particle ingestion is an energy-requiring process that is modulated by several biochemical events within the cells. Concomitant processes that occur in the cells during ingestion include

- membrane synthesis
- lysosomal enzyme synthesis
- generation of metabolic products of oxygen and nitrogen
- migration of the various types of granules toward the phagosome

Ultimately, several granules fuse with the phagosomes, a process that may occur prior to complete invagination, spilling certain granule contents outside of the phagocyte. Phagocytes are endowed with multiple means of destroying microorganisms, especially antimicrobial polypeptides that reside within cytoplasmic granules, reactive oxygen radicals generated from oxygen during the respiratory burst, and reactive nitrogen radicals, which are discussed later in this chapter. Although these mechanisms are primarily designed to destroy pathogens, released contents such as lysosomal enzymes may contribute to the amplification of inflammation and tissue damage.

Innate Mechanisms for the Recruitment and Activation of Macrophages

Monocyte-derived macrophages are the second important type of effector cell for the innate immune response following trauma or acute infection. The various molecules involved in monocyte adhesion and transmigration from blood into tissues are probably similar to those discussed with neutrophils, although they have not been studied as thoroughly. However, the functional activation of macrophages is more complex. Macrophages exist in different levels or stages of metabolic and functional activity, each representing different "programs" of gene activation and synthesis of macrophage-derived cytokines and mediators:

- resting (immature or quiescent)
- primed
- activated

A fourth category of macrophages, often called *stimulated, reparative,* or *inflammatory,* is used by some authorities to refer to those macrophages that are not quite fully activated. This multilevel model is clearly oversimplified, but it does provide a framework for conceptualizing different levels of macrophage activation in terms of acute inflammation (Fig 4-2).

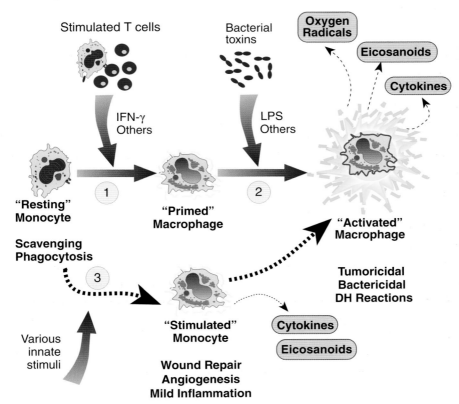

Figure 4-2 Schematic representation of macrophage activation pathway. Classically, *resting monocytes* are thought to be the principal noninflammatory scavenging phagocyte. **1,** Upon exposure to low levels of interferon-γ from T lymphocytes, monocytes become primed, upregulating class II major histocompatibility complex molecules and performing other functions. *Primed monocytes* function in antigen presentation. **2,** *Fully activated macrophages,* after exposure to bacterial lipopolysaccharide and interferon, are tumoricidal and bactericidal and mediate severe inflammation. **3,** *Stimulated monocytes* are incompletely activated, producing low levels of cytokines and eicosanoids but not reactive oxygen intermediates. These cells participate in wound healing, angiogenesis, and low-level inflammatory reactions. *(Illustration by Barb Cousins, modified by Joyce Zavarro.)*

Resting and scavenging macrophages

Host cell debris is cleared from a tissue site by phagocytosis in a process called *scavenging*. Resting macrophages are the classic scavenging cell, capable of phagocytosis and uptake of the following:

- dead cell membranes, by recognition of phosphatidyl serine
- chemically modified extracellular protein, through acetylated or oxidized lipo-proteins
- sugar ligands, through mannose receptors
- naked nucleic acids as well as bacterial pathogens

Resting monocytes express scavenging receptors of at least 3 types but synthesize very low levels of proinflammatory cytokines. In general, scavenging can occur in the absence of inflammation. See Clinical Example 4-4.

Primed macrophages

Resting macrophages become primed by exposure to certain cytokines. Upon priming, these cells become positive for major histocompatibility complex (MHC) class II antigen and capable of functioning as antigen-presenting cells (APCs) to T lymphocytes. Priming implies activation of specialized lysosomal enzymes such as cathepsins D and E for degrading proteins into peptide fragments, upregulation of certain specific genes, such as class II MHC, and costimulatory molecules, such as B7.1, and increased cycling of proteins between endosomes and the surface membrane. Prototypically, primed macrophages resemble dendritic cells. They can exit tissue sites by the afferent lymphatics to reenter the lymph node. Classically, T-lymphocyte–derived IFN-γ was thought to be the most important priming signal. It is now known, however, that many cytokines not necessarily of T-lymphocyte origin can also prime macrophages, and the cellular response to the priming stimulus has tissue-specific variations.

CLINICAL EXAMPLE 4-4

Phacolytic glaucoma Mild infiltration of scavenging macrophages centered around retained lens cortex or nucleus fragments occurs in nearly all eyes with lens injury, including those subjected to routine cataract surgery. This infiltrate is notable for the *absence* of both prominent neutrophil infiltration and significant nongranulomatous inflammation. An occasional giant cell may be present, but granulomatous changes are not extensive.

Phacolytic glaucoma is a variant of scavenging macrophage infiltration in which glaucoma occurs in the setting of a hypermature cataract that leaks lens protein through an *intact* capsule. Lens protein–engorged scavenging macrophages are present in the anterior chamber, and glaucoma develops as these cells block the trabecular meshwork outflow channels. Other signs of typical lens-associated uveitis are conspicuously absent. Experimental studies suggest that lens proteins may be chemotactic stimuli for monocytes.

Activated and stimulated macrophages

Activated macrophages are classically defined as macrophages producing the full spectrum of inflammatory and cytotoxic cytokines; thus, they are the cells that mediate and amplify acute inflammation (delayed hypersensitivity [DH]), tumor killing, and major antibacterial activity. *Epithelioid cells* and *giant cells* represent the terminal differentiation of the activated macrophage. Activated macrophages synthesize numerous mediators to amplify inflammation:

- inflammatory or cytotoxic cytokines, such as IL-1, IL-6, TNF-α
- reactive oxygen or nitrogen intermediates
- lipid mediators
- other products

See Clinical Example 4-5.

Traditionally, full activation was observed to require stimulation by 2 signals: IFN-γ from DH T lymphocytes and LPS from gram-negative bacteria. However, the level of macrophage activation can vary tremendously and can be regulated much more precisely than is implied by the monolithic term *activated*.

It is now thought that macrophages can be partially activated by many different innate stimuli, such as

- cytokines not derived from T lymphocytes, such as the chemokines
- bacterial cell walls or toxins from gram-positive or acid-fast organisms
- complement activated through the alternative pathway
- foreign bodies composed of potentially toxic substances, such as talc or beryllium
- exposure to certain surfaces, such as some plastics

CLINICAL EXAMPLE 4-5

Propionibacterium acnes endophthalmitis Infection of the capsular bag and residual lens material with the anaerobic organism *P acnes* has been found to cause some cases of chronic postoperative uveitis after cataract surgery and IOL implantation. This bacterium, presumably introduced at the time of surgery, replicates very slowly and fails to produce a significant purulent infection. Thus, the initial infection is noninflammatory and clinically inapparent. However, some clinical event, such as additional surgery with the Nd:YAG laser or other unknown trigger, results in inflammation apparently related to enhanced replication or release of the bacterium. Granulomatous inflammation ultimately develops that spreads to involve the residual lens and vitreous.

No clear explanation for the pattern of inflammation in the *P acnes* syndrome is presently known. Some investigators speculate that the infective plaque of organisms is growing, initially, within an anaerobic environment formed by a sequestered pocket of capsular flap and IOL, and the bacteria are thus isolated from the immune response. After release of the toxins, especially cell wall components, macrophages are directly activated through innate immunity to initiate a subacute inflammatory reaction. Activated macrophages then produce mediators and cytokines that amplify the inflammation.

Thus, macrophages that are partially activated to produce some inflammatory cytokines—but perhaps not fully activated to antimicrobial or tumoricidal function—are sometimes termed *stimulated* or *reparative* macrophages. Such partially activated macrophages also contribute to fibrosis and wound healing through the synthesis of mitogens such as platelet-derived growth factors, metalloproteinases, and other matrix degradation factors and to angiogenesis through synthesis of angiogenic factors such as vascular endothelial growth factor.

Effector Reactivities of Adaptive Immunity

Although most adaptive (or innate) immune responses are protective and occur subclinically, when adaptive immune responses do cause inflammation, these responses have classically been called *immune hypersensitivity reactions*. The traditional classification for describing the 4 mechanisms of adaptive immune-triggered inflammatory responses— namely, anaphylactoid, cytotoxic antibodies, immune complex reactions, and cell-mediated—was elaborated by Coombs and Gell in 1962, and a fifth category, *stimulatory hypersensitivity*, was added later (Table 4-2). Although this system is still useful, it was developed before T lymphocytes had been discovered, in a time when understanding was limited to antibody-triggered mechanisms. In addition, it is unlikely that any effector mechanism in a disease process is purely 1 type. For example, all antibody-dependent mechanisms require a processing phase using helper T lymphocytes, which may also contribute to effector responses. Finally, the term *hypersensitivity* may obscure the concept that many of these same mechanisms are often protective and noninflammatory. Thus, in some ways, this traditional classification is inadequate. This discussion introduces an expanded classification system that incorporates modern concepts for immune effector reactivities and, when appropriate, points out where the classic Coombs and Gell system applies (Table 4-3).

Delves PJ, Martin S, Burton D, Roitt IM. *Roitt's Essential Immunology.* 11th ed. Malden, MA: Blackwell; 2006.

Goldsby RA, Kindt TJ, Osborne BA, Kuby J. *Immunology.* 5th ed. New York: W.H. Freeman; 2003.

Male DK, Cooke A, Owen M, et al. *Advanced Immunology.* 3rd ed. St Louis: Mosby; 1996.

Table 4-2 Types of Hypersensitivity (Coombs and Gell)

Type I	Anaphylactoid
Type II	Cytotoxic antibodies
Type III	Immune complex reactions
Type IV	Cell-mediated
Type V	Stimulatory

Table 4-3 Effector Reactivities of the Adaptive Immune Response in the Eye

Predominantly antibody-mediated soluble effectors

Intravascular circulating antibodies that form circulating immune complexes with bloodborne antigen (Type III)

Passive leakage of antibody into a tissue followed by complex formation with tissue-bound antigen causing

    Complement-mediated cell lysis (Type II)

    Complement activation with inflammation (a variant of Type III)

    Novel cytotoxic mechanisms

    Stimulation of cell activities (Type V)

Local infiltration of circulating B cells into a tissue with local secretion of antibody and other cell activities (a variant of Type III)

Predominantly lymphocyte-mediated (cellular) effectors

Delayed hypersensitivity T cells (Type IV)

    Th1 type of delayed hypersensitivity

    Th2 type of delayed hypersensitivity

Cytotoxic lymphocytes

    Cytotoxic T lymphocytes

    Natural killer cells

    Lymphokine-activated killer cells

Combined antibody and cellular effector mechanisms

Antibody-dependent cellular cytotoxicity (ADCC) with killer cells or macrophages

Acute IgE-mediated mast-cell degranulation (Type I)

Chronic mast-cell degranulation and Th2-delayed hypersensitivity

Antibody-Mediated Immune Effector Responses

Structural and functional properties of antibody molecules

Structural features of immunoglobulins Five major classes (M, G, A, E, and D) of immunoglobulin exist in 9 different subclasses, or *isotypes* (IgG1, IgG2, IgG3, IgG4, IgM, IgA1, IgA2, IgE, and IgD). The basic immunoglobulin structure is composed of 4 covalently bonded glycoprotein chains that form a monomer of approximately 150,000–180,000 daltons (Fig 4-3). This monomer is about 2½ to 3 times the size of albumin. Each antibody monomer contains 2 identical *light chains,* either kappa (κ) or lambda (λ), and 2 identical *heavy chains* from 1 of the 9 structurally distinct subclasses of immunoglobulins. Thus, the heavy chain type defines the specific isotype (Table 4-4). IgM can form pentamers or hexamers in vivo, and IgA can form dimers in secretions, so the molecular size of these 2 classes in vivo is much larger than those of the others.

Each monomer has analogous regions called *domains.* Certain domains carry out specific functions of the antibody molecule. In particular, the *Fab region* on each molecule contains the antigen recognition/combining domain, called the *hypervariable region.* The opposite end of the molecule, on the heavy chain portion, contains the attachment site for effector cells *(Fc portion);* it also contains the site of other effector functions, such as complement activation (eg, as for IgG3) or binding to the secretory component so it can be transported through epithelia and secreted into tears (eg, as for

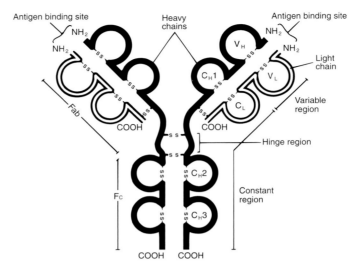

Figure 4-3 Schematic representation of an immunoglobulin molecule. The *solid lines* indicate the identical 2 heavy chains; the *open lines* indicate the identical light chains; *-s-s-* indicates intra- and interchain covalent disulfide bonds. *(Reprinted with permission from* Dorland's Illustrated Medical Dictionary. *28th ed. Philadelphia: Saunders; 1994:824.)*

IgA). Table 4-4 summarizes the important structural differences among immunoglobulin isotypes.

Functional properties of immunoglobulins The immunoglobulin isotypes do not all mediate the effector functions of antibody activity equally. For example, human IgM and IgG3 are good complement activators, but IgG4 is not. Only IgA1 and IgA2 can bind secretory component and thus be actively passed into mucosal secretions after transport through the epithelial cell from the subepithelial location, where they are synthesized by B lymphocytes. Other isotypes must remain in the subepithelial tissue. A partial list of isotype-specific functions is included in Table 4-4. The importance of these differences is that 2 antibodies with the identical capacity to bind to an antigen, but of different isotype, will have different effector and inflammatory outcomes.

Terminology

Various regions of an antibody can themselves be antigenic. These antigenic sites are called *idiotopes,* as distinguished from *epitopes,* the antigenic sites on foreign molecules. Antibodies to idiotopes are called *idiotypes.* Anti-idiotypic antibodies might be important feedback mechanisms for immune regulation.

The concept of *monoclonal antibodies* has become very important in research and diagnostic medicine. After immunization with a particular antigen, a high frequency of B lymphocytes producing antibodies specific for that antigen will be present in the spleen or lymph nodes. Although 1 B lymphocyte synthesizes antibody of 1 antigenic specificity, different B lymphocytes responding to different epitopes of the same antigen produce

Table 4-4   Structural and Functional Properties of Immunoglobulin Isotypes

Immunoglobulin Isotype (Heavy Chain)	Structural Properties			Functional Properties		
	% of Total Serum Igs	Relative Size	Other Structural Features	Activates Complement	Fc Receptor Binding Preferences	Other Functions
IgD δ	<1%	Monomer	Mostly on surface of B lymphocytes	No		B-lymphocyte antigen receptor
IgM μ	5%	Pentamer or hexamer	Mostly on B lymphocytes or intravascular	Strong (classic pathway)		B-lymphocyte antigen receptor, agglutinization, neutralization, intravascular cytolysis
IgG1 γ	50%	Monomer	Intravascular, in tissues, crosses placenta	Moderate (classic pathway)	Monocytes	Cytolysis
IgG2 γ	18%	Monomer	Same as IgG1	Weak (classic pathway)	Neutrophil monocytes, killer lymphocytes	ADCC
IgG3 γ	6%	Monomer	Same as IgG1	Strong (classic pathway)	Neutrophil monocytes, killer lymphocytes	ADCC, agglutinization, cytolysis
IgG4 γ	3%	Monomer	Same as IgG1	No		
IgE ε	<<1%	Monomer	Mostly in skin or mucosa, bound to mast cells	No	Mast cells	Neutralization Mast-cell degranulation
IgA1 α	15%	Mostly monomer in serum, dimer in secretions	In mucosal secretions, binds secretory component in subepithelial tissues for transepithelial transport and protection from proteolysis	Moderate (alternative pathway)		Mucosal immunity, neutralization
IgA2 α	3%	Same as IgA1	Same as IgA1	Same as IgA1		

ADCC = antibody-dependent cellular cytotoxicity

specific antibodies to each different epitope. The population of all antigen-specific antibodies to the various epitopes is termed *polyclonal,* as these antibodies derive from different B lymphocyte clones or progeny from 1 initial parental B lymphocyte, each producing antibodies of different specificities.

Myeloma cells are immortal tumor cells that have the cellular machinery for producing an unlimited amount of 1 antibody without additional helper stimulation by T lymphocytes, antigen, or cytokines. If activated B lymphocytes from an immunized host and myeloma cells are fused by various laboratory manipulations, then a population of *hybridomas* is formed. Each hybridoma makes an unlimited amount of the original lymphocyte's single antibody, yet it is immortal and therefore easy to grow and care for in the laboratory. Thus, the antibody is *monoclonal,* because it represents the product of 1 specific parental B lymphocyte fused to the myeloma tumor. The population of hybridomas produced by this fusion can be screened for selection of the ones that may be synthesizing the monoclonal antibody of interest.

Intravascular circulating antibodies that form circulating immune complexes with bloodborne antigen

Systemic release of antibody into the circulation or into external secretions occurs frequently after immunization, and antibody interactions with antigen solubilized in plasma or secretions are important effector mechanisms in this setting (Fig 4-4).

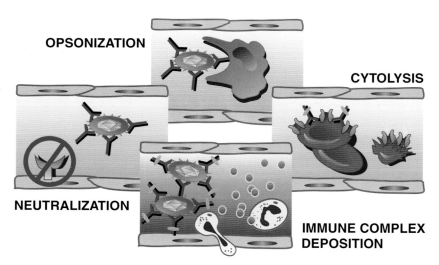

Figure 4-4 Schematic representation of the 4 most important antibody effector mechanisms in the blood. *Neutralization:* When an antibody combines with a live pathogen, it neutralizes the ability of the pathogen to bind to most cell receptors. *Opsonization:* When an antibody coats a soluble antigen or pathogen in blood, the antibody enhances clearance by macrophages or similar cells in the liver or spleen. *Cytolysis:* Antibodies can coat cells and activate complement, which can result in cytolysis via formation of porelike membrane attack complexes (MACs). *Immune complex deposition* occurs when soluble antibody–antigen complexes deposit on tissues, resulting in complement activation and inflammation. *(Illustration by Barb Cousins, modified by Joyce Zavarro.)*

Neutralization, opsonization, and agglutinization When antibody combines with a live pathogen such as a virus or bacteria, it can block, or *neutralize,* the ability of the pathogen to bind to host cell receptors, thereby preventing infection of host cells. This process can occur in the blood or in external secretions such as tears. The role of this process in preventing reinfection with adenovirus is discussed in Clinical Example 3-1, Immune response to viral conjunctivitis, in Chapter 3. When an antibody coats a soluble pathogen or antigen in blood, the antibody can enhance phagocytosis or reticuloendothelial clearance by macrophage-like cells in the spleen or liver in a process called *opsonization.* Opsonization is usually facilitated by Fc receptor recognition by the phagocyte. In some cases, such as in certain bacterial cell wall antigens, an antigen contains multiple identical antigenic sites on 1 molecule so more than 1 antibody can bind each molecule. In these cases, the antibody/antigen complex may *agglutinize,* causing the complex to precipitate out of solution.

Deposition of circulating soluble immune complexes Usually, when antigen is soluble within blood, as during viremia or bacteremia, soluble immune complexes formed between antigen and antibody bind to erythrocytes and are efficiently removed from the circulation, then cleared by the reticuloendothelial system. However, in some cases, soluble immune complexes can passively deposit within the blood vessels, kidneys, and other vascular structures, usually facilitated by predisposing stimuli that cause altered vascular permeability (eg, mast-cell degranulation). This mechanism must be differentiated from the in situ formation of immune complexes within a tissue, which is discussed next. Tissue deposition of circulating immune complexes can trigger an inflammatory response by activating complement, one variant of Coombs and Gell Type III.

The classic clinical setting in which circulating immune complexes caused a systemic disease was *serum sickness,* a disease occurring in the preantibiotic and presteroid era that was caused by a late primary or secondary immune response following intravenous treatment with animal serum in a patient suffering from infection or inflammation. Massive intravascular immune complex formation caused severe systemic vasculitis and chronic inflammation in many organs. Now, serum sickness occurs rarely, after certain infections such as Lyme disease, or in rare individuals treated with certain drugs, such as antibiotics. In these cases, the drug binds to self-proteins to form a drug/protein *neoantigen,* or *hapten,* that inadvertently initiates an immune response. Deposition of circulating immune complexes may occur in some forms of systemic vasculitis. See Clinical Examples 4-6 and 4-7.

Passive leakage of antibody into peripheral tissues followed by complex formation with tissue-bound antigen

Antibody in serum, especially of the IgG subclasses, can passively leak into peripheral tissues, particularly those with fenestrated capillaries, leading to formation of a local complex of antibody with tissue-associated antigens. Figure 4-5 illustrates the antibody effector mechanisms discussed next.

Complement-mediated cell lysis, or immune cytolysis If an antigen is associated with the external surface of the plasma membrane, antibody binding might activate the complement cascade to induce cell lysis through formation of specialized porelike structures called the *membrane attack complex (MAC)* (ie, Coombs and Gell Type II). Hemolytic

CLINICAL EXAMPLE 4-6

Anterior uveitis is probably not caused by circulating immune complexes Following observations that uveitis developed in some animal models of serum sickness, investigators in the 1970s and 1980s sought to confirm a role for circulating immune complexes as a cause of anterior uveitis. Although elevated levels of immune complexes were detected in many patients, a convincing correlation with disease activity was never established. Now, most immunologists and clinicians think that the ocular deposition of circulating immune complexes is *not* an important pathogenic mechanism for uveitis in humans.

CLINICAL EXAMPLES 4-7

Retinal vasculitis in systemic lupus erythematosus Although rare, retinal vasculitis can develop in patients with systemic lupus erythematosus (SLE) (see Chapter 7). Observation of the probable mechanism for vasculitis elsewhere in SLE suggests that local immune complex formation plays a role in this development. DNA and histones released from injured cells can become trapped in the basement membrane of the blood vessel wall, perhaps as a result of electrostatic binding by matrix proteins. Circulating cationic anti-DNA IgG autoantibodies permeate into the vessel wall, bind the autoantigen, and activate complement. These cationic IgG antibodies are thought to have a stronger affinity for anionic extracellular matrix and therefore permeate tissues efficiently.

Complement fragments, or *anaphylatoxins,* initiate an Arthus reaction. The observed vascular sheathing in the retinal vessels is presumed to be caused by infiltration of neutrophils and macrophages in response to complement activation. However, helper T-lymphocyte responses and innate mechanisms may also contribute. In addition to DNA, other potential autoantigens in SLE include collagen and phospholipids.

Alternatively, molecular mimicry between basement membrane components and DNA may occur. The mechanism for the initiation of afferent events causing the induction of aberrant autoimmunity to DNA and other antigens is unknown. A similar effector mechanism has been postulated for scleritis in rheumatoid arthritis.

Cancer-associated retinopathy Cancer-associated retinopathy is a paraneoplastic syndrome in which some patients with carcinoma, especially small cell carcinoma of the lung or occasionally cutaneous melanoma, develop antibodies against a tumor-associated antigen that happens to cross-react with an ocular autoantigen. For example, some small cell carcinomas aberrantly synthesize recoverin, a normal protein in photoreceptors. The immune system inappropriately recognizes and processes recoverin and produces an antibody effector response, releasing antirecoverin antibodies into the circulation. These antibodies passively permeate the retina, are taken up by photoreceptors, and cause slowly progressive photoreceptor degeneration by a novel, poorly understood cytotoxic mechanism. Current research speculates that induction of programmed cell death may be caused by intracellular antibody/antigen complex formation after photoreceptor uptake of antirecoverin antibodies.

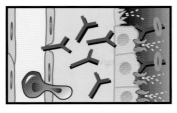

CYTOLYSIS

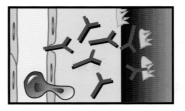

CELL DEGENERATION

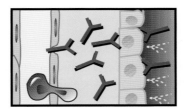

STIMULATORY

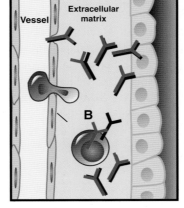

ANTIBODY DEPOSITION

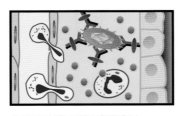

ARTHUS REACTION

Figure 4-5 Schematic representation of the most important antibody effector mechanisms caused by passive leakage of antibody into tissues. *(Illustration by Barb Cousins, modified by Joyce Zavarro.)*

anemia of a newborn as a result of Rh incompatibility is the classic example of this process. Others include Hashimoto thyroiditis, glomerulonephritis of Goodpasture syndrome, and autoimmune thrombocytopenia. This mechanism does not appear to be very important in uveitis or ocular inflammation, although it may play a role in killing virus-infected cells during viral conjunctivitis.

Tissue-bound immune complexes and the acute Arthus reaction When free antibody passively leaks from the serum into a tissue, it can combine with tissue-bound antigens trapped in the extracellular matrix or with cell-associated antigens such as a viral protein expressed on the surface of an infected cell. These in situ, or locally formed, complexes sometimes activate the complement pathway to produce complement fragments called *anaphylatoxins* (a second variant of Coombs and Gell Type III). This mechanism should be differentiated from the deposition of circulating immune complexes, which are preformed in the blood. Typically, the histology is dominated by neutrophils and monocytes. The resultant lesion, called the *acute Arthus reaction,* can be produced experimentally by injection of antigen into a tissue site of an animal previously immunized in a way to optimize antibody rather than T-lymphocyte production. In general, many types of glomerulonephritis and vasculitis are thought to represent this mechanism. See Clinical Examples 4-7.

Novel cytotoxic mechanisms Circulating antibodies can cause tissue injury by mechanisms different from cytolysis or complement activation, using pathogenic mechanisms not yet understood. For example, some autoantibodies in systemic lupus erythematosus appear to be taken up by renal cells, leading to loss of function, and these may cause some cases of nephritis in the absence of immune complex activation. In paraneoplastic syndromes, autoantibodies to various tissues can develop and mediate *cellular degeneration* or other manifestations. See Clinical Examples 4-7.

Stimulatory antibodies Tissue- or cell-bound immune complexes that stimulate receptors on target cells are known as *stimulatory antibodies.* In some cases, antibody leaking into tissues or binding to cells in the blood can cross-react with and bind to a receptor or molecule expressed on the surface of normal parenchymal cells, thereby activating the receptor as if the antibody were the natural ligand for that receptor (Coombs and Gell Type V). For example, in Graves disease, antibodies to the thyroid-stimulating hormone receptor activate the thyroid gland as if the patient had taken an overdose of thyroid-stimulating hormone. Immunologists have used this information to develop many antibodies to activate cell receptors in the absence of the natural ligand and to develop antibodies with enzymatic or other metabolic functions. In other cases, the autoantibody can block the function of the receptor, as in myasthenia gravis, wherein antiacetylcholine antibodies cause internalization of the normal receptor without activation, thereby depleting functional receptors from the nerve ending. Many other examples of stimulatory, or metabolically active, antibodies have been identified. See Clinical Example 4-8.

Infiltration of B lymphocytes into tissues and local production of antibody

B-lymphocyte infiltration B lymphocytes can infiltrate the site of an immunologic reaction in response to persistent antigenic stimulus, leading to a clinical picture of moderate to severe inflammation. If the process becomes chronic, plasma cell formation occurs, representing fully differentiated B lymphocytes that have become dedicated to antibody synthesis. In both of these cases, local production of antibody specific for the inciting antigen(s) occurs within the site. If the antigen is known, as for certain presumed infections, local antibody formation can be used as a diagnostic test.

Differentiation between local production of antibody and passive leakage from the blood involves calculation of the *Goldmann-Witmer (GW) coefficient,* which is generated by comparison of the ratio of intraocular fluid/serum antibody concentration for the specific antibody in question to the intraocular fluid/serum ratio of total immunoglobulin levels. Theoretically, a coefficient above 1.0 would indicate local production of antibodies within the eye. In practice, however, positive quotients above 3.0 are used most often to improve specificity and positive predictive value. See Clinical Example 4-9.

Local antibody production within a tissue and chronic inflammation Persistence of antigen within a site, coupled with infiltration of specific B lymphocytes and local antibody formation, can produce a chronic inflammatory reaction with a complicated histologic pattern,

CLINICAL EXAMPLE 4-8

Scleritis or retinal vasculitis in Wegener granulomatosis Necrotizing scleritis is a common feature in Wegener granulomatosis, and retinal vasculitis can, rarely, develop in some of these patients as well (see Chapter 7). Although the mechanism for scleritis and retinal vasculitis in Wegener granulomatosis is unknown, the primary pathogenesis can be inferred from experimental studies of systemic disease to be a vasculitis mediated in part by stimulatory autoantibodies. The autoantigen is thought to be the neutrophil-derived serine protease *proteinase-3*. The initial effector process is thought to require the translocation of proteinase-3 from cytoplasmic granules to the cell surface after neutrophil exposure to various innate activational stimuli, such as a predisposing infection or systemic cytokine release. Then, antineutrophil cytoplasmic antibodies can bind surface proteinase-3, further activating and stimulating the neutrophils. This process, in turn, causes the neutrophils to bind to endothelium and to release granules and other mediators that injure the vessel wall. The endothelial cells then synthesize cytokines to recruit additional inflammatory cells, especially T lymphocytes, which amplify the process. The mechanism for the initiation of afferent events causing the induction of aberrant autoimmunity to proteinase-3 is unknown. However, the processing phase must also include proteinase-specific helper T lymphocytes, which are responsible for providing cytokine help to B lymphocytes; DH effector cells presumably contribute to granuloma formation in tissue sites.

Kallenberg CG, Brouwer E, Mulder AH, Stegeman CA, Weening JJ, Tervaert JW. ANCA—pathophysiology revisited. *Clin Exp Immunol.* 1995;100:1–3.

CLINICAL EXAMPLE 4-9

Diagnosis of atypical necrotizing retinitis The sensitivity, specificity, and accuracy of aqueous humor antibody levels (intraocular antibody synthesis) were compared in the diagnoses of atypical retinitis ultimately caused by *Toxoplasma gondii,* varicella-zoster virus, herpes simplex virus, cytomegalovirus, and noninfectious causes. In general, the authors found that results were best (78% diagnostic accuracy) when the highest quotient greater than 1.0 was used for diagnosis even in the face of multiple positive quotients. False-positive quotients for cytomegalovirus were the most frequent confounding finding, causing 4 of 6 false diagnoses.

Davis JL, Feuer W, Culbertson WW, Pflugfelder SC. Interpretation of intraocular and serum antibody levels in necrotizing retinitis. *Retina.* 1995;15:233–240.

often demonstrating lymphocytic infiltration, plasma cell infiltration, and granulomatous features (a third variant of Coombs and Gell Type III). This process is sometimes called the *chronic Arthus reaction.* This mechanism may contribute to the pathophysiology of certain chronic autoimmune disorders, such as rheumatoid arthritis, which feature formation of pathogenic antibody. See Clinical Example 4-10.

CLINICAL EXAMPLE 4-10

Phacoantigenic endophthalmitis Phacoantigenic endophthalmitis is a form of lens-associated uveitis with 3 distinct zones of inflammation centered around the lens:

1. an inner zone of neutrophils invading the lens substance
2. a secondary zone of macrophages, epithelioid cells, or giant cells (or a combination thereof) surrounding the capsule injury site
3. an outer zone of fibrotic reparative or granulation tissue infiltrated with nongranulomatous inflammation and plasma cells, presumably secreting specific antibodies into ocular fluids

Antibody-mediated autoimmunity has been well demonstrated in rats immunized against whole-lens proteins. The mechanism for the initiation of afferent events causing the induction of aberrant autoimmunity to lens crystallins is unknown. The adaptive immune system of unaffected patients has already been exposed to crystallins in a "tolerizing" manner (see Chapter 5).

Because lens-associated uveitis almost always occurs in a severely traumatized or congenitally abnormal eye, it has been suggested that the disease is initiated in eyes with an atypical immunologic microenvironment that allows a secondary afferent response to override tolerance. The effector phase appears to be dominated by complement-fixing antibodies specific for lens crystallins, which are either produced locally by B lymphocytes or plasma cells within the eye or leaked passively from the blood. Presumably, generation of the anaphylatoxin C5a by complement-activating immune complexes *within the lens substance* explains the neutrophil infiltration into the lens. Diffusion of anaphylatoxins into the anterior chamber probably results in a chemotactic gradient, yielding a zonal pattern. Activated macrophages must also contribute, because epithelioid and giant cells that are subsets of activated, differentiated macrophages are classic features. The mechanism for giant cell formation has not been totally resolved, but phagocytosis of immune complexes coated with complement can contribute to macrophage activation and induce giant cell formation. Injury to retina or other tissues is probably exacerbated by toxic oxygen radicals. It has been suggested that T-lymphocyte and innate effector mechanisms may also be involved.

Foster CS, Streilein JW. Immune-mediated tissue injury. In: Albert DM, Jakobiec FA. *Principles and Practice of Ophthalmology.* 2nd ed. Philadelphia: Saunders; 2000:74–82.

Samson CM, Foster CS. Hypersensitivity: antibody-mediated cytotoxic (type II). *Encyclopedia of Life Sciences.* London: John Wiley & Sons; 2001.

Lymphocyte-Mediated Effector Responses

Delayed hypersensitivity T lymphocytes

Delayed hypersensitivity (Coombs and Gell Type IV) represents the prototypical adaptive immune mechanism for lymphocyte-triggered inflammation. It is especially powerful in secondary immune responses. Previously primed DH CD4 T lymphocytes leave the lymph node, home into local tissues where antigen persists, and become activated by further restimulation with the specific priming antigen and class II MHC–expressing APCs. Fully activated DH T lymphocytes secrete mediators and cytokines, leading to the recruitment and activation of macrophages or other nonspecific leukocytes (Fig 4-6). The term *delayed* for this type of hypersensitivity refers to the fact that the reaction becomes maximal 12–48 hours after antigen exposure.

Analysis of experimental animal models and the histopathologic changes of human inflammation suggest that different subtypes of DH might exist. One of the most important determinants of the pattern of DH reaction is the subtype of DH CD4 T effector cells that mediate the reaction. Just as helper T lymphocytes can be differentiated into 2 groups—Th1 and Th2 subsets—according to the spectrum of cytokines secreted, DH T lymphocytes can also be grouped by the same criteria. Experimentally, the Th1 subset of cytokines, especially IFN-γ, also known as *macrophage-activating factor,* and TNF-β, activates macrophages to secrete inflammatory mediators and kill pathogens, thus amplifying inflammation. Th1-mediated DH mechanisms, therefore, are thought to produce the following:

- the classic delayed hypersensitivity reaction (eg, the purified protein derivative [PPD] skin reaction)
- immunity to intracellular infections (eg, to mycobacteria or pneumocystis)

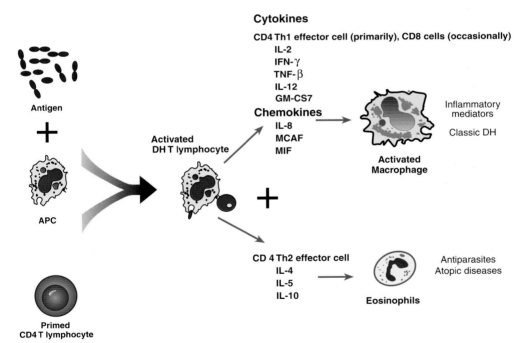

Figure 4-6 Schematic representation of the 2 major forms of delayed hypersensitivity (DH). CD4 T lymphocytes, having undergone initial priming in the lymph node, enter the tissue site, where they again encounter antigen-presenting cells (APC) and antigen. Upon restimulation, they become activated into either Th1 or Th2 effector cells. Th1 lymphocytes are the classic DH effector cells, which are associated with most severe forms of inflammation. Th2 lymphocytes are thought to be less intensively inflammatory, but they have been associated with parasite-induced granulomas and atopic diseases. *(Illustration by Barb Cousins, modified by Joyce Zavarro.)*

- immunity to fungi
- most forms of severe T-lymphocyte–mediated autoimmune diseases
- chronic transplant rejection

The Th2 subset of DH cells secretes IL-4 and IL-5 and other cytokines. IL-4 can induce B lymphocytes to synthesize IgE, and IL-5 can recruit and activate eosinophils within a site. IL-4 can also induce macrophage granulomas in response to parasite-derived antigens. Thus, Th2-mediated DH mechanisms are thought to play a major role in the following:

- response to parasite infections
- late-phase responses of allergic reactions
- asthma
- atopic dermatitis or other manifestations of atopic diseases

The inciting antigen and the immunologic microenvironment of the tissue site are other important variables in determining the pattern of DH, affecting the afferent and efferent phases, respectively. Some of these variables probably influence the development of a Th1 versus Th2 pattern of cytokine production as well. Some soluble antigens, especially in mucosal sites, can induce a type of DH with features of immediate hypersensitivity and basophil infiltration called *cutaneous basophil hypersensitivity*. Most epidermal toxins, especially heavy metals, plant toxins, and chemical toxins, cause monocyte infiltration and epidermal desquamation of the skin, the *contact hypersensitivity* type of Th1 DH. Deposition of certain insoluble antigens (bacterial or fungal debris) or immunization with soluble proteins using adjuvants causes the classic *tuberculin* type of Th1 DH that is characterized by fibrin deposition and monocyte and lymphocyte infiltration.

The persistence of certain infectious agents, especially bacteria within intracellular compartments of APCs or certain extracellular parasites, can cause destructive induration with granuloma formation and giant cells, the *granulomatous* form of DH. However, immune complex deposition (see "Lens-associated uveitis" in Chapter 7) and innate immune mechanisms in response to heavy metal or foreign-body reactions can also cause granulomatous inflammation, in which the inflammatory cascade (resulting in DH) is triggered in the absence of specific T lymphocytes. Unfortunately, for most clinical entities in which T-lymphocyte responses are suspected, especially autoimmune disorders such as multiple sclerosis or arthritis, the precise immunologic mechanism remains highly speculative. See Clinical Examples 4-11.

Cytotoxic lymphocytes

Cytotoxic T lymphocytes Cytotoxic T lymphocytes (CTLs) are a subset of antigen-specific T lymphocytes, usually bearing the CD8 marker, that are especially good at killing tumor cells and virus-infected cells. CTLs can also mediate graft rejection and some cases of autoimmunity. In most cases, the ideal antigen for CTLs is an intracellular protein that either occurs naturally or is produced as a result of viral infection. CTLs appear to require help from CD4 helper T-lymphocyte signals to fully differentiate. Primed *precursor* CTLs leave the lymph node and migrate to the target tissue, where they are restimulated by the interaction of the CTL antigen receptor and foreign antigens within the antigen pocket

CLINICAL EXAMPLES 4-11

Toxocara granuloma (Th2 DH) *Toxocara canis* is a nematode parasite that infects up to 2% of all children worldwide and may occasionally produce vitreoretinal inflammatory manifestations. Although the ocular immunology of this disorder is not clearly delineated, animal models and a study of the immunopathogenesis of human nematode infections at other sites suggest the following scenario. The primary immune response begins in the gut after ingestion of viable eggs, which mature into larvae within the intestine. The primary processing phase produces a strong Th2 response, leading to a primary effector response that includes production of IgM, IgG, and IgE antibodies, as well as Th2-mediated DH T lymphocytes. Hematogenous dissemination of a few larvae may result from accidental avoidance of immune effector mechanisms, leading to choroidal or retinal dissemination followed by invasion into the retina and vitreous. There, a Th2-mediated T-lymphocyte effector response recognizes larva antigens and releases Th2-derived cytokines to induce eosinophil and macrophage infiltration, causing the characteristic eosinophilic granuloma seen in the eye. In addition, antilarval B lymphocytes can infiltrate the eye and are induced to secrete various immunoglobulins, especially IgE. Finally, eosinophils, in part by attachment through Fc receptors, can recognize IgE or IgG bound to parasites and release cytotoxic granules containing the antiparasitic cationic protein directly in the vicinity of the larvae, using a mechanism similar to antibody-dependent cellular cytotoxicity.

> Grencis RK. Th2-mediated host protective immunity to intestinal nematode infections. *Philos Trans R Soc Lond Biol Sci.* 1997;352:1377–1384.

Sympathetic ophthalmia (Th1 DH) Sympathetic ophthalmia is a bilateral panuveitis that follows penetrating trauma to 1 eye (see Chapter 7 for a more detailed discussion). This disorder represents one of the few human diseases in which autoimmunity can be directly linked to an initiating event. In most cases, penetrating injury activates the afferent phase. It is unclear whether the injury causes a de novo primary immunization to self-antigens, perhaps because of externalization of sequestered uveal antigens through the wound and exposure to the afferent immune response arc of the conjunctiva/extraocular sites, or if it instead somehow changes the immunologic microenvironment of the retina, RPE, and uvea so that a secondary afferent response is initiated that serves to alter preexisting tolerance to retinal and uveal self-antigens.

It is generally thought that the inflammatory effector response is dominated by a Th1-mediated DH mechanism generated in response to uveal or retinal antigens. CD4 T lymphocytes predominate early in the disease course, although CD8, or suppressor, T lymphocytes can be numerous in chronic cases. Activated macrophages are also numerous in granulomas, and Th1 cytokines have been identified in the vitreous or produced by T lymphocytes recovered from the eyes of affected patients. Although the target antigen for sympathetic ophthalmia is unknown, cutaneous immunization in experimental animals with certain retinal antigens (arrestin, rhodopsin, interphotoreceptor retinol–binding protein), RPE-associated antigens, and melanocyte-associated tyrosinase can induce autoimmune uveitis with physiology or features suggestive of sympathetic ophthalmia. Th1-mediated DH is thought to mediate many forms of ocular inflammation. Table 4-5 lists other examples.

Rao NA. Mechanisms of inflammatory response in sympathetic ophthalmia and VKH syndrome. *Eye.* 1997;11:213–216.

of class I molecules (HLA-A, -B, or -C) on the target cell. Additional CD4 T lymphocytes help at the site, and expression of other accessory costimulatory molecules on the target is often required to obtain maximal killing.

CTLs kill cells in 1 of 2 ways: assassination or suicide induction (Fig 4-7). *Assassination* refers to CTL-mediated *lysis* of targets; a specialized pore-forming protein called *perforin,* which puts pores, or holes, into cell membranes, causes osmotic lysis of the cell. *Suicide induction* refers to the capability of CTLs to stimulate *programmed cell death* of target cells, called *apoptosis,* using the CD95 ligand, the *FasL,* to activate its receptor on targets. Alternatively, CTLs can release cytotoxic cytokines like TNF to induce apoptosis. Activation of the apoptosis pathway induces the release of target cell enzymes and nucleases that cause fragmentation of chromosomal DNA and blebbing of the cell membrane, ultimately killing the cell. CTLs produce low-grade lymphocytic infiltrate within tumors or infected tissues and usually kill without causing significant inflammation.

Natural killer cells Natural killer (NK) cells—a subset of non-T, non-B lymphocytes— were originally called *null cells,* or *large granular lymphocytes.* They too kill tumor cells and virally infected cells, but, unlike CTLs, NK cells do not have a specific antigen receptor. Instead, they are triggered by a less well characterized NK cell receptor. Once triggered, however, NK cells kill target cells using the same molecular mechanisms as CTLs. Because NK cells are not antigen-specific, they theoretically have the advantage of not requiring the

Table 4-5 Ocular Inflammatory Diseases Thought to Require a Major Contribution of Th1-Mediated DH Effector Mechanisms

Site	Disease	Presumed Antigen
Conjunctiva	Contact hypersensitivity to contact lens solutions	Thimerosal or other chemicals
	Giant papillary conjunctivitis	Unknown
	Phlyctenulosis	Bacterial antigens
Cornea and sclera	Chronic allograft rejection	Histocompatibility antigens
	Marginal infiltrates of blepharitis	Bacterial antigens
	Disciform keratitis after viral infection	Viral antigens
Anterior uvea	Acute anterior uveitis	Uveal autoantigens, bacterial antigens
	Sarcoid-associated uveitis	Unknown
	Intermediate uveitis	Unknown
Retina and choroid	Sympathetic ophthalmia	Retinal or uveal autoantigens
	Vogt-Koyanagi-Harada syndrome	Retinal or uveal autoantigens
	Birdshot choroiditis	Unknown
Orbit	Acute thyroid orbitopathy	Unknown
	Giant cell arteritis	Unknown

CTL FUNCTION

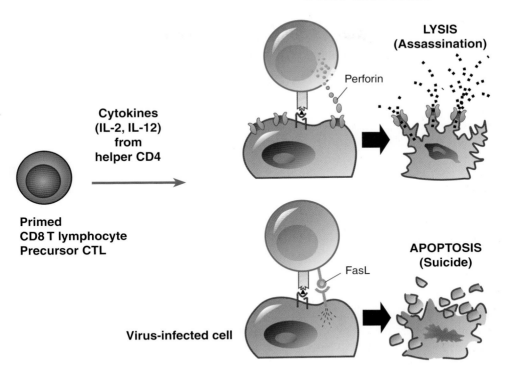

Figure 4-7 Schematic representation of the 2 major mechanisms of CD8 T-lymphocyte cyto-toxicity. CD8 T lymphocytes, having undergone initial priming in the lymph node, enter the tissue site, where they again encounter antigen in the form of infected target cells. Upon restimulation, usually requiring CD4 helper T-lymphocyte factors, they become activated into fully cytolytic T lymphocytes. CD8 T lymphocytes can kill by lysing the infected cell, using a pore-forming protein called *perforin*, or cytotoxic lymphocytes (CTLs) can kill by inducing *programmed cell death*, or *apoptosis*, using either FasL or cytokine-mediated mechanisms. *(Illustration by Barb Cousins, modified by Joyce Zavarro.)*

time delay caused by induction of the adaptive, antigen-specific CTL immune response. However, NK cells do seem to require some of the same effector activational signals at the tissue site, especially cytokine stimulation. Thus, NK cells are probably most effective in combination with adaptive effector responses.

In some ways, NK cells and CTLs are complementary in that they are inversely regulated—that is, cell processes, such as diminished class I molecule expression, that inhibit CTL function often enhance activation of NK cells, and vice versa. NK cells thereby provide another layer of protection against pathogens that interfere with class I expression, as do many viruses, especially cytomegalovirus. Experimental evidence suggests that NK cells may contribute to antiviral protection in cytomegalovirus and herpes simplex virus infections of the eye. See Clinical Example 4-12.

Lymphokine-activated killer cells Lymphokine-activated killer (LAK) cells are T lymphocytes that have become nonspecifically activated by iatrogenic administration of immune cytokines such as IL-2 and others. LAK cells kill by various mechanisms, including those

CLINICAL EXAMPLE 4-12

Antiviral immunity in cytomegalovirus retinitis Cytomegalovirus (CMV) retinitis is the most frequent opportunistic ocular infection in patients with AIDS. The majority of most populations have serologic evidence of prior CMV infection, which is typically thought to occur during chldhood or after contact with infected children. The pathophysiology of CMV infection is not entirely understood, but it can be inferred from analysis of animal experiments and human epidemiologic studies. The primary afferent phase is usually initiated after upper respiratory tract infection, not uncommonly associated with viremia. The site of processing is unknown. Innate effectors, such as macrophages, natural killer cells, and neutrophils, provide some antiviral activity. However, most investigators think that virus-specific CD8 T lymphocytes are the best antiviral effector for controlling active infection. Some evidence also suggests a role for DH T lymphocytes. Antibodies are also generated, but they do not seem to play a major role in controlling virus infection, spread, or clearance. Antibodies may limit reinfection, however.

During the primary infection, virus is not completely cleared from the infected host but remains in a chronic state. It was originally thought that virus disseminated to various target tissues, such as eye, gut, or kidney, and became latent. More recent research suggests that the virus chronically infects the bone marrow and lung, probably persisting in certain macrophage precursor cells. Alternatively, CMV might infect the salivary gland, where it remains in epithelial cells. CMV appears to persist in these sites in a chronic but nonproductive state, and the existence of true latency is debated. However, as long as the host immune response is intact, the virus does not replicate effectively to infect the eye or other target organs.

Immunomodulation allows the virus to reactivate into a productive infection. Virus infects neutrophils, macrophages, and other leukocytes and spreads through the blood to susceptible target sites such as the retina. Alternatively, viremia during a primary CMV infection that occurs in previously uninfected immunomodulated persons, especially after organ transplantation, can spread virus by a similar mechanism. It is thought that virus-specific CD8 T lymphocytes are the most important effector cells in preventing spread, but natural killer cells might also be effective. CD4 T lymphocytes play a role primarily by providing helper cytokines to fully activate CD8 T lymphocytes. Thus, in AIDS, CMV retinitis presumably occurs late in the disease because CD8 effectors become diminished later in the course of infection than do CD4 T lymphocytes. Transfusion of virus-specific CD8 T lymphocytes in organ transplant patients and replacement of helper cytokines to activate CD8 T lymphocytes in a mouse model of AIDS have both been shown to prevent CMV. Highly active antiretroviral therapy to suppress the HIV viral load has dramatically decreased the incidence of new cases of CMV retinitis in AIDS. The role of intravenous immune globulins, polyclonal antibodies enriched from human sera, in prophylaxis or treatment is controversial, but they may help prevent CMV disease after organ transplantation.

Riddell SR. Pathogenesis of cytomegalovirus pneumonia in immunocompromised hosts. *Semin Respir Infect.* 1995;10:199–208.

described earlier. Once it was learned that T lymphocytes are produced and become activated upon exposure to immune cytokines, or *lymphokines,* clinicians began to evaluate the clinical efficacy of treatment with cytokine immunotherapy. Originally, it was discovered that patients with certain tumors, especially metastatic malignant melanoma, who were treated with large doses of intravenous IL-2, sometimes responded with immune-mediated rejection of the tumor. Efficacy was subsequently improved when CTLs were removed from the blood or even from within metastatic tumor foci (ie, tumor-infiltrating lymphocytes) and treated with cytokines extracorporeally, then reinfused. Currently, numerous biotechnological approaches are being developed to enhance immunotherapy of LAK function for the treatment of tumors and viral infections. See Clinical Example 4-13.

> Streilein JW. T lymphocyte responses. In: Albert DM, Jakobiec FA. *Principles and Practice of Ophthalmology.* 2nd ed. Philadelphia: Saunders; 2000:61–65.

Combined Antibody and Cellular Effector Mechanisms

Antibody-dependent cellular cytotoxicity

Antibody can combine with a cell-associated antigen such as a tumor or viral antigen, but if the antibody is not a subclass that activates complement, it may not induce any apparent cytotoxicity. However, because the Fc tail of the antibody is externally exposed, various

---

CLINICAL EXAMPLE 4-13

Immune responses to malignant melanoma Several investigators have evaluated the immune response to human uveal melanomas. Although controversial, data suggest that most primary or metastatic uveal melanomas demonstrate *melanoma antigen genes (MAGE)* and that these growing tumors express at least 1 family of tumor-associated antigens that should be recognized by CD8 cytolytic adaptive immune responses. Tumor-infiltrating lymphocytes were isolated from eyes undergoing enucleation because of large, growing melanomas. Numerous CD8 T lymphocytes could be isolated from all tumors, including tumor-specific T lymphocytes (indicating that afferent and processing phases had been initiated).

In cell culture, the cytolytic T lymphocytes failed to effectively kill melanoma cells. After treatment with the cytokine (or lymphokine) IL-2, however, the CD8 T lymphocytes became fully cytolytic and did effectively kill the melanoma cells. The investigators concluded that uveal melanomas might create an immunologic microenvironment that prevents activation of the antitumor effector responses even though sensitized CTLs may be present in the tumor. Lymphokine activation may be a method to overcome this suppressive microenvironment and to upregulate the host's antitumor response to melanoma in order to prevent or control metastases.

> Chen PW, Murray TG, Uno T, Salgaller ML, Reddy R, Ksander BR. Expression of MAGE genes in ocular melanoma during progression from primary to metastatic disease. *Clin Exp Metastasis.* 1997;15:509–518.
> Niederkorn JY. Immunoregulation of intraocular tumours. *Eye.* 1997;11:249–254.

leukocytes can recognize the Fc domain of the antibody molecule and be directed to the cell through the antibody. When this happens, binding to the antibody activates various leukocyte cytotoxic mechanisms, including degranulation and cytokine production.

Because human leukocytes can express various types of Fc receptors—IgG subclasses have 3 different Fcg receptors, IgE has 2 different Fce receptors, and so on—leukocyte subsets differ in their capacity to recognize and bind different antibody isotypes. Classically, *antibody-dependent cellular cytotoxicity (ADCC)* was observed to be mediated by a special subset of large granular (non-T, non-B) lymphocytes, called *killer cells,* that induce cell death in a manner similar to that of CTLs. The killer cell itself is nonspecific but gains antigen specificity through interaction with specific antibody. Macrophages, NK cells, certain T lymphocytes, and neutrophils can also participate in ADCC using other Fc receptor types. An IgE-dependent form of ADCC might also exist for eosinophils.

ADCC is presumed to be important in tumor surveillance, antimicrobial host protection, graft rejection, and certain autoimmune diseases such as cutaneous systemic lupus erythematosus. However, this effector mechanism probably does not play an important role in uveitis, although it might contribute to corneal graft rejection and antiparasitic immunity.

Acute IgE-mediated mast-cell degranulation

Mast cells can bind IgE antibodies to their surface through a high-affinity Fc receptor specific for IgE molecules, positioning the antigen-combining site of the bound IgE externally (Fig 4-8). The combining of 2 adjacent IgE antibody molecules with a specific allergen (see Clinical Examples 4-14) causes degranulation of the mast cell and release of mediators within min-

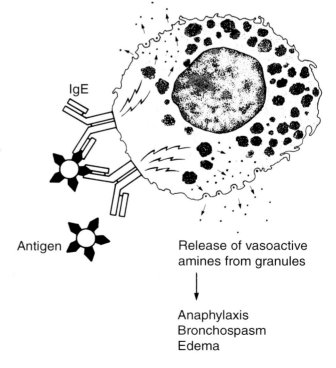

MAST CELL

IgE

Antigen

Release of vasoactive amines from granules

Anaphylaxis
Bronchospasm
Edema

Figure 4-8 Schematic representation of IgE-mediated mast cell degranulation.

CLINICAL EXAMPLES 4-14

Allergic conjunctivitis Allergic conjunctivitis is an atopic (out of place or inappropriate) immune response to a family of antigens called *allergens,* ordinarily harmless and tolerated by most humans, that induce predominantly an acute IgE–mast-cell effector response in individuals genetically destined to be "allergic" to such substances. The primary response presumably has occurred during a prior exposure to the allergen, often within the nasopharynx, in which afferent and processing phases were initiated. During this primary response, allergen-specific B lymphocytes were distributed to specialized areas in various MALT sites. At these sites, the B lymphocytes, with T-lymphocyte help, switch from IgM-antiallergen production to IgE-antiallergen production. IgE released at the site then combines with Fc receptors of mast cells, thereby "arming" the mast cells with a specific allergen receptor (ie, the antigen-recognizing Fab portion of the IgE). Thus, 1 mast cell may have bound IgE specific for numerous different allergens.

When reexposure to allergen occurs, allergen must permeate beyond the superficial conjunctival epithelium to the subepithelial region, where the antigen binds allergen-specific IgE on the surface of mast cells. Degranulation occurs within 60 minutes, leading to the release of mediators, most particularly histamine, causing chemosis and itching. A late response, within 4–24 hours, is characterized by the recruitment of lymphocytes, eosinophils, and neutrophils. The role of Th2 DH or helper T lymphocytes in the effector response has not been confirmed for allergic conjunctivitis, but presumably both play a role, especially in B-lymphocyte differentiation, because the IgE is thought to be produced locally within the conjunctiva.

Atopic keratoconjunctivitis Atopic keratoconjunctivitis (AKC) is a complex, vision-threatening ocular allergy with chronic inflammation of the palpebral and bulbar conjunctiva with both immediate and delayed cell-mediated inflammation (see BCSC Section 8, *External Disease and Cornea*). Analysis of biopsy specimens reveals the inflammatory infiltration to consist of mast cells and eosinophils, as well as activated CD4 T lymphocytes and B lymphocytes. Although immunopathogenesis is not clearly defined, a mechanism similar to that of atopic dermatitis can be inferred, combining poorly understood genetic mechanisms, chronic mast-cell degranulation, and features of Th2-type DH. Immunopathogenesis of vernal conjunctivitis and giant papillary conjunctivitis is probably also similar. The eosinophil, with its highly toxic cytokines, eosinophil major basic protein and eosinophil cationic protein, is the effector cell most responsible for corneal damage and vision loss in patients with AKC.

utes, producing an acute inflammatory reaction called *immediate hypersensitivity* (Coombs and Gell Type I), which is characterized by local plasma leakage and itching. When severe, this response can produce a systemic reaction called *anaphylaxis,* which ranges in severity from generalized skin lesions such as erythema, urticaria, or angioedema to severe altered vascular permeability with plasma leakage into tissues that causes airway obstruction or hypotensive shock. Mast cells and vasoactive amines are discussed in greater detail later in the chapter.

Chronic mast-cell degranulation plus Th2 DH

Recent research has suggested that mast cells, B lymphocytes, and T lymphocytes can cooperate in atopic diseases to mediate chronic inflammatory reactions with a pattern that represents a mixture of acute allergy and DH. As discussed earlier, a Th2 subset of CD4$^+$ DH cells not only releases inflammatory mediators but also secretes certain cytokines (IL-4) that induce B lymphocytes to synthesize IgE and to recruit and activate eosinophils within a site (IL-5). Because mast cells can degranulate in response to stimuli other than IgE, the precise contributions of IgE-mediated mast-cell degranulation in these chronic reactions have not been clarified. This pathogenic mechanism is thought to be especially important in the skin and at mucosal sites.

Mediator Systems That Amplify Innate and Adaptive Immune Responses

Although innate or adaptive effector responses may directly induce inflammation, in most cases these effectors instead initiate a process that must be amplified to produce overt clinical manifestations. Molecules generated within the host that induce and amplify inflammation are termed *inflammatory mediators,* and mediator systems include several categories of these molecules (Table 4-6). Most act on target cells through receptor-mediated processes, although some act in enzymatic cascades that interact in a complex fashion.

Plasma-Derived Enzyme Systems

Complement factors

Complement is an important inflammatory mediator in the eye. Components and fragments of the complement cascade, which account for approximately 5% of plasma protein and more than 30 different proteins, represent important endogenous amplifiers of innate and adaptive immunity, as well as mediators of inflammatory responses. Both adaptive and innate immune responses can initiate complement activation pathways, which generate products that contribute to the inflammatory process (Fig 4-9). Adaptive immunity

---

Table 4-6 Mediator Systems That Amplify Innate and Adaptive Immune Responses

Plasma-derived enzyme systems: complement, kinins, and fibrin
Vasoactive amines: serotonin and histamine
Lipid mediators: eicosanoids and platelet-activating factors
Cytokines
Reactive oxygen intermediates
Reactive nitrogen products
Neutrophil-derived granules and products

Three of the most important oxygen intermediates are superoxide anion, hydrogen peroxide, and the hydroxyl radical:

$O_2 + e^- \rightarrow O_2^-$ superoxide anion

$O_2^- + O_2^- + 2H^+ \rightarrow O_2 + H_2O_2$ superoxide dismutase catalyzes anions to form hydrogen peroxide

$H_2O_2 + e^- \rightarrow OH^- + OH\bullet$ hydroxyl anion and hydroxyl radical

Oxygen metabolites that are generated by leukocytes, especially neutrophils and macrophages, and triggered by immune responses are the most important source of free radicals during inflammation. A wide variety of stimuli can trigger leukocyte oxygen metabolism, including

- innate triggers such as LPS or formyl methionine-leucine-proline
- adaptive effectors such as complement-fixing antibodies or certain cytokines produced by DH T lymphocytes
- other chemical mediator systems, such as C5a, PAF, and leukotrienes

Reactive oxygen intermediates can also be generated as part of noninflammatory cellular biochemical processes, especially by electron transport in the mitochondria, detoxification of certain chemicals, or interactions with environmental light or radiation.

The principal mechanism by which oxygen metabolites are activated during inflammation is the induction of various oxidases in neutrophils or macrophage cell membranes, especially NADPH (the reduced form of nicotinamide-adenine dinucleotide phosphate) oxidase, but also NADH (the reduced form of nicotinamide-adenine dinucleotide) oxidase, xanthine oxidase, and aldehyde oxidase. NADPH oxidase catalyzes the transfer of electrons from NADPH or from NADH to oxygen or hydrogen peroxide (H_2O_2) to form intermediates such as the reactive oxygen radical superoxide anion. As shown in the formulas, the transfer of a single electron to oxygen forms a superoxide anion, an unstable radical that may dismutate spontaneously; that is, one of the molecules gains an electron and the other loses one. Otherwise, the reaction can be catalyzed by the enzyme superoxide dismutase to form H_2O_2 and oxygen.

Alternatively, 2 electrons can be transferred to molecular oxygen, a process that normally occurs in the peroxisomes. This process also results in formation of H_2O_2, a molecule that by itself has feeble inflammatory and microbicidal activity. Moreover, H_2O_2 can be readily neutralized into water and oxygen by enzymes such as catalase in peroxisomes and glutathione peroxidase in the cytosol, as shown in Figure 4-11.

H_2O_2, however, can be converted into molecules with potential inflammatory and antimicrobial activity by at least 3 chemical processes:

1. The Fenton and the Haber-Weiss reactions can add 1 electron to form the hydroxyl anion (OH^-) as well as the highly reactive hydroxyl radical ($OH\bullet$).
2. H_2O_2 may be catalyzed by myeloperoxidase, a protein found in neutrophils, to react with halide or pseudohalide (thiocyanate) substrates to form extremely toxic products that are highly damaging to bacteria and tissues. These include hypohalous acids, halogens, chloramines, and hydroxyl radicals. Hydroxyl radicals interact with several potential cellular targets to cause enzyme and protein damage as a

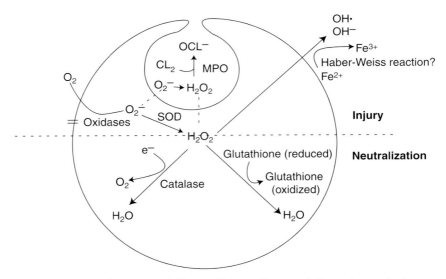

Figure 4-11 Overview of the essential intracellular and extracellular pathways in the generation of reactive oxygen intermediates. Activation of oxidases catalyzes the production of superoxide anion (O_2^-), which can be converted into H_2O_2 by superoxide dismutase (SOD). Catalase (in the peroxisome) and glutathione can neutralize H_2O_2. However, H_2O_2 can be converted into hydroxyl ion (OH^+) or hydroxyl radical ($OH^•$) by the Haber-Weiss reaction. Alternatively, H_2O_2 can be catalyzed by myeloperoxidase (MPO) into hypochlorous anion and other reactive intermediates. *(Reprinted with permission from Pepose JS, Holland GN, Wilhelmus KR, eds.* Ocular Infection and Immunity. *St Louis: Mosby; 1996.)*

result of cross-linking of sulfhydryl groups; cell membrane injury by lipid peroxidation of the lipid bilayers; loss of energization and cellular stores of adenosine triphosphate as a result of loss of integrity of the inner membrane of the mitochondria; and breaks or cross-links in DNA from chemical alterations of nucleotides.

3. Peroxynitrite is formed after chemical interaction between superoxide and nitric oxide (see the following section).

See Clinical Example 4-15.

Reactive Nitrogen Products

Another important pathway of host defenses and inflammation involves the toxic products of nitrogen, especially *nitric oxide (NO)*. NO is a highly reactive chemical species that, like reactive oxygen intermediates, can react with various important biochemical functions in microorganisms and host cells. This pathway was first observed in patients with a deficiency of the respiratory burst enzymes. Because of this deficiency, their neutrophils and macrophages were unable to generate reactive oxygen intermediates, but they were still able to mount effective antimicrobial function through a toxic nitrogen product, NO.

The formation of NO depends on the enzyme nitric oxide synthetase (NOS), which is located in the cytosol and is NADPH-dependent. NO is formed from the terminal guanidino-nitrogen atoms of L-arginine. Several forms of NO synthetase are known, including several constitutive forms of NOS (cNOS) and an inducible NOS (iNOS). Many

The precise role of clonal deletion in immunologic tolerance to ocular autoantigens remains uncertain. Intriguingly, a crystallin protein and S-antigen have been detected within the thymus, suggesting the possibility of crystallin-specific and S-antigen–specific deletion of T lymphocytes. However, actual clonal deletion of autoreactive T lymphocytes has not yet been demonstrated for ocular autoantigens. If clonal deletion were complete, lens- or retinal-responsive T lymphocytes would be absent during uveitis. Because such T lymphocytes can indeed be demonstrated under certain experimental conditions, clonal deletion, if present, must be incomplete.

Anergy

Anergy and *clonal inactivation* are terms that have been used to describe the situation in which antigen-specific T lymphocytes or B lymphocytes are rendered incapable of mounting a normal inflammation-triggering response to that antigen. For example, when B lymphocytes of mice are exposed to antigen early in the developmental process, they are rendered unresponsive to that antigen after maturation. Similarly, several different mechanisms that "tolerize" T lymphocytes have been demonstrated. When T lymphocytes are presented antigen by "nonprofessional" antigen-presenting cells such as corneal endothelium or Müller cells, they become inactivated from further differentiation into inflammatory effector cells. Although these T lymphocytes survive, they are incapable of initiating inflammatory immune responses. Anergy therefore provides an additional mechanism for immunologic unresponsiveness.

Regulation

Regulation, the third classic mechanism for tolerance, postulates that a population of *regulatory T lymphocytes* exists to balance the population of helper and inflammation-enhancing T lymphocytes. These regulatory T lymphocytes modulate and diminish the level of activation by the effector or helper T lymphocytes. Whereas clonal deletion or anergy supports immunologic unresponsiveness, regulation indicates an active but tolerizing immune response to a specific antigen. The best-described mechanism involves the release of immunomodulatory cytokines such as transforming growth factor (TGF)–β2 by CD8 regulatory T lymphocytes, but several other mechanisms have also been supported by experimental data. Although the physiologic importance and mechanism(s) by which regulation is induced have been challenged, regulation is clearly an important mechanism for the immune system in general and for ocular immune responses in particular. See Chapter 3 for a discussion of regulation induced during anterior chamber–associated immune deviation (ACAID).

Potential role of antibody isotype

An interesting paradox can be demonstrated in many healthy people: antiself-antibodies to many major autoantigens can be demonstrated in sera, but these autoantibodies do not seem to cause inflammation. One explanation may be related to the different effector functions of various antibody isotypes (see Table 4-4 in Chapter 4). The major inflammation-inducing mechanism of antibody is brought about by complement activation, which in turn is a function of the isotype of the antibody molecule itself. As discussed in Chapter 4, isotypes vary in their capacity to activate complement. Preferential activation of B lymphocytes that produce complement-fixing antibodies results in inflammation-inducing immunity, because complement activation is initiated following immune complex formation.

Conversely, preferential activation of non–complement-fixing antibodies results in high antibody titers but not severe inflammation. Immune complexes opsonize or agglutinate the antigen, but complement is not activated. Therefore, one key to B-lymphocyte effector function is determined by the regulation of the class switch from an IgM-synthesizing B lymphocyte to one producing an antibody of the other isotypes. This switch is controlled by different T-lymphocyte–derived cytokines. By inference, the regulation of this form of B-lymphocyte tolerance is passive and under the control of helper T-lymphocyte signals.

Delves PJ, Martin S, Burton D, Roitt IM. *Roitt's Essential Immunology.* 11th ed. Malden, MA: Blackwell; 2006.

Male DK, Cooke A, Owen M, Trowsdale J, Champion B. *Advanced Immunology.* 3rd ed. St Louis: Mosby; 1996.

Molecular Mimicry

Autoimmunity may play an important role in the pathogenesis of inflammatory ocular diseases. One mechanism through which autoimmunity to self-antigens in the eye may be triggered is *molecular mimicry,* the immunologic cross-reaction between epitopes of an unrelated foreign antigen and self-epitopes with similar structures. Theoretically, these epitopes would be similar enough to stimulate an immune response, yet different enough to cause a breakdown of immunologic tolerance.

For example, a foreign antigen such as those present within yeast, viruses, or bacteria can induce an appropriate afferent, processing, and effector immune response. A self-antigen with similar epitopes may induce antimicrobial antibodies or effector lymphocytes to inappropriately cross-react. A dynamic process would then be initiated, causing tissue injury by an autoimmune response that would induce additional lymphocyte responses directed at other self-antigens. Thus, the process would not require the ongoing replication of a pathogen or the continuous presence of the inciting antigen.

See Clinical Example 5-2.

CLINICAL EXAMPLE 5-2

Molecular mimicry and autoimmune uveitis Molecular mimicry was suggested as a mechanism for uveitis after it was found that the primary amino acid sequence of a variety of foreign antigens (including those of baker's yeast histone, *Escherichia coli,* hepatitis B virus, and certain murine and primate retroviruses) showed sequence homology to a pathogenic epitope of the ocular autoantigen S-antigen. Immunization of rats with crude extracts prepared from these organisms or synthetic peptides corresponding to the homologous epitopes induced retinal inflammation. In addition, T lymphocytes isolated from rats immunized with foreign substances cross-reacted with retinal autoantigens, providing evidence of molecular mimicry between self and nonself proteins. Currently, no definitive clinical evidence suggests that molecular mimicry contributes to autoimmune diseases of the human eye.

HLA Associations and Disease

Normal Function of HLA Molecules

All animals with white blood cells express a family of cell-surface glycoproteins called *major histocompatibility complex (MHC)* proteins. In humans, the MHC proteins are called *human leukocyte antigen (HLA)* molecules. As discussed in Chapter 2, 6 different families of HLA molecules have been identified:

- 3 class I MHC: HLA-A, -B, -C
- 3 class II MHC: HLA-DR, -DP, -DQ

A seventh category, HLA-D, does not exist as a specific molecule but instead represents a functional classification as determined by an in vitro assay. Class III MHC molecules and minor MHC antigens have also been identified, but they are not discussed here.

The important role MHC molecules play in immunologic function is discussed in Chapter 2; Table 5-1 gives a historical perspective linking MHC molecules and transplantation biology with immune response genes. HLAs are also considered to be human immune response genes, because the HLA type determines the capacity of the antigen-presenting cell (APC) to bind peptide fragments and thus determines T-lymphocyte immune responsiveness.

Allelic Variation

Many different alleles or polymorphic variants of each of the 6 HLA types exist within the population: more than 25 alleles for HLA-A, 50 for -B, 10 for -C, 100 for -DR, and so on. Because there are 6 major HLA types and each individual has a pair of each HLA type, or 1 *haplotype,* from each parent, an APC expresses 6 pairs of MHC molecules. Thus, with the exception of identical twins, only rarely will 2 individuals match all 12 potential haplotypes. Alleles and genetic variations are discussed in greater detail in BCSC Section 2, *Fundamentals and Principles of Ophthalmology,* Part III, Genetics.

Allelic diversity may be designed to provide protection through *population-wide immunity.* Each HLA haplotype theoretically covers a set of antigens to which a particular individual can respond adaptively. Thus, in theory, the presence of many different HLA alleles within a population should ensure that the adaptive immune system in at least some individuals in the whole group will be able to respond to a wide range of potential pathogens. The converse also holds true: Some individuals may be at increased risk for immunologic diseases. See Clinical Example 5-3.

Clinical detection and classification of different alleles

Traditionally, the different alleles of HLA-A, -B, -C, -DR, and -DQ have been detected by reacting lymphocytes with special antisera standardized by International HLA Workshops sponsored by the World Health Organization (WHO). HLA-DP and HLA-D typing requires specialized T-lymphocyte culture assays. Traditionally, provisional serotypes pending official recognition were often designated *workshop* (eg, DRw53). More recently, molecular techniques have been developed to characterize the nucleic acid sequence of various MHC alleles. HLA molecules are composed of 2 chains: α and β chains for class

Table 5-1 The Major Histocompatibility Complex Locus and the HLA System: A Short History

1940s	Skin autografts succeed, but allografts are rejected unless from a twin
1950s	Transfusion reactions noted against white blood cells among patients matched to RBC antigens, called *human leukocyte antigens (HLA)*
	Antibodies to disparate fetal HLA types noted among multiparous mothers
1960s	Immune response genes in mice control ability to respond to one antigen but not another
	Immune response genes probably code for mouse equivalent of HLA (immune antigen, or Ia)
	Allograft rejection is genetically determined by the major histocompatibility complex (MHC) locus
1970s	Ia in mice and HLA types in humans correlate with transplant rejection, giving rise to the concept that immune response genes are part of the MHC
	Prediction that Ia type in mice and HLA type in humans will correlate with propensity to autoimmunity on basis of immune responsiveness to environmental pathogens
	First HLA association with inflammatory disease (HLA-B27 and ankylosing spondylitis)
1980s	Mechanism of MHC function: HLA required on antigen-presenting cells to activate T lymphocytes—class I molecules present to CD8 T lymphocytes; class II molecules present to CD4 T lymphocytes
	T lymphocytes and B lymphocytes see antigen differently; B lymphocytes see the whole, natural antigen; T lymphocytes "see" antigens after they are chopped up into peptides
	Function of class I and II molecules confirmed—antigen fragments are placed within a groove formed by the tertiary structure of the molecule to allow presentation to the T-lymphocyte receptor
	Different HLA molecules have different capacities to bind different fragments, explaining role as immune response gene
	Mutations in the binding site within the groove of class I and II molecules may allow some individuals to bind and present certain environmental or self-peptides, thereby predisposing to autoimmunity
1990s	Molecular typing of HLA becoming more available and better than serotyping
	Molecular mechanism of antigen processing well characterized
	Complete sequencing of human genome by Human Genome Project
2000s–Present	MHC class III region on chromosome 6 identified and sequenced. This region encodes for other immune components, such as complement (eg, C2, C4, factor B) and some cytokines (eg, TNF-α)

II, an α chain and the β_2-microglobulin chain for class I. Because subtle differences in molecular structure can be easily missed during antisera-based assays, molecular genotyping is a more precise method to determine MHC types. Thus, the genotype specifies the chain, the major genetic type, and the specific minor molecular variant subtype. For example, genotype DRB1*0408 refers to the HLA-DR4 molecule β chain with the "–08" minor variant subtype.

New serotypes now must correspond to a specific genotype, and the provisional "w" label is rarely used. Nonetheless, haplotypes currently recognized as a single group will continue to be subdivided into new categories or new subtypes. For example, at least 2 different A29 subtypes and 8 different HLA-B27 subtypes have been recognized. Finally, some investigators have proposed that HLA classification based on similarities of peptide binding, rather than on serotyping or genetic typing, may reveal other disease associations.

CLINICAL EXAMPLE 5-3

HLA-B27–associated acute anterior uveitis Approximately 50% of patients with acute anterior uveitis (AAU) express the HLA-B27 haplotype, and many of these patients also experience other immunologic disorders, such as Reiter syndrome, ankylosing spondylitis, inflammatory bowel disease, and psoriatic arthritis (see Chapter 7). Although the immunopathogenesis remains unknown, various animal models permit some informed speculation. Many cases of uveitis or Reiter syndrome follow gram-negative bacillary dysentery or chlamydial infection. The possible role of bacterial lipopolysaccharide and innate mechanisms was discussed in Chapter 4. Experiments in rats and mice genetically altered to express human HLA-B27 molecules seem to suggest that bacterial infection of the gut predisposes rats to arthritis and a Reiter-like syndrome, although uveitis is uncommon.

It has been suggested that chronic intracellular chlamydial infection of a joint, and presumably the eye, might stimulate an adaptive immune response using the endogenous (class I) antigen-processing pathway of the B27 molecule, invoking a CD8 T-lymphocyte effector mechanism activated to kill the microbe but indirectly injuring the eye. Others have suggested that B27 amino acid sequences might present *Klebsiella* peptide antigens to CD8 T lymphocytes, but how a presumed exogenous bacterial antigen would be presented through the class I pathway is unknown. Another hypothesis posits that molecular mimicry may exist between bacterial antigens and some amino acid sequences of HLA-B27. Analysis of human AAU fluids and various animal models of AAU and arthritis suggests that anterior uveitis might be a CD4 Th1–mediated DH response, possibly in response to bacteria-derived antigens such as bacterial cell wall antigens or heat shock proteins trapped in the uvea or to endogenous autoantigens of the anterior uvea, possibly melanin-associated antigens, type I collagen, or myelin-associated proteins. How a CD4-predominant mechanism would relate to a class I immunogenetic association is unclear.

MHC and Transplantation

As indicated in Table 5-1, the failure of *allogeneic* transplanted tissue, from a genetically nonidentical donor, to remain viable was first recognized as an adaptive immune response in the 1940s. The association between transplantation antigens (ie, MHC antigens) and immune response genes was not recognized until decades later. How the immune system recognizes HLA haplotype differences as foreign antigens is not entirely clear. Intuitively, it seems that T lymphocytes from a recipient individual should simply ignore APCs from a donor individual bearing a different HLA haplotype. Short-term cell culture experiments (ie, 1–3 days) accordingly show that a recipient's T lymphocytes do fail to recognize exogenous foreign antigens presented by the donor APCs, even if the T lymphocytes have been previously sensitized. However, if the T-lymphocyte cultures and donor APCs are left to react over a longer term (ie, 5–7 days), a significant fraction of the recipient T lymphocytes unexpectedly become activated in response to the donor APC HLA molecules, especially class II differences. What remains unknown is whether this *mixed lymphocyte reaction*–induced activation process represents a direct interaction between the foreign HLA and the recipient's T-lymphocyte receptor, or if the foreign HLA molecule is processed as a foreign protein and presented by host APCs to host T lymphocytes. Both delayed hypersensitivity (DH) and cytotoxic T-lymphocyte effector responses are activated by this process, and both appear crucial in transplant rejection, including corneal allograft rejection.

Although antibodies to class I transplantation antigens can also occur in some cases of hyperacute rejection, this mechanism does not appear to be important in corneal graft rejection. In general, HLA matching, especially at DR loci, then at A and B loci, greatly reduces rejection for many types of organ allografts. Similar observations have not been confirmed for high-risk corneal allograft rejection.

Disease Associations

In 1973, the first association between HLA haplotype and ankylosing spondylitis was identified. Since then, more than 100 other disease associations have been made, including several for ocular inflammatory diseases (Table 5-2). In general, an HLA disease association is defined as the statistically increased frequency of an HLA haplotype in persons with that disease as compared to the frequency in a disease-free population. The ratio of these 2 frequencies is called *relative risk,* which is the simplest method for expressing the magnitude of an HLA disease association. Nevertheless, several caveats must be kept in mind.

- The association is only as strong as the clinical diagnosis. Diseases that are difficult to diagnose on clinical features may obscure real associations.
- The association depends on the validity of the haplotyping. Older literature often reflects associations based on HLA classifications (some provisional) that might have changed.
- The HLA association identifies individuals at risk and is not a diagnostic marker. The associated haplotype is not necessarily present in all people affected with the specific disease, and its presence in a person does not ensure the correct diagnosis.
- The concept of linkage disequilibrium proposes that if 2 genes are physically near on the chromosome, they may be inherited together rather than undergo genetic randomization in a population. Thus, HLA may be coinherited with an unrelated disease gene, and sometimes 2 HLA haplotypes can occur together more frequently than predicted by their independent frequencies in the population.

At least 4 theoretical explanations have been offered for HLA disease associations. The most direct theory postulates that HLA molecules act as peptide-binding molecules for etiologic antigens or infectious agents. Thus, individuals bearing a specific HLA molecule might be predisposed to processing certain antigens, such as an infectious agent that cross-reacts with a self-antigen, and other individuals, lacking that haplotype, would not be so predisposed. Specific variations or mutations in the peptide-binding region would greatly influence this mechanism; these variations can be detected only by molecular typing. Preliminary data in support of this theory have been provided for type 1 diabetes.

A second theory proposes molecular mimicry between bacterial antigens and an epitope of an HLA molecule (ie, an antigenic site on the molecule itself). An appropriate

Table 5-2 HLA Associations and Ocular Inflammatory Disease

Disease	HLA Association	Specific Relative Risk (RR) for Associated Subgroup
Acute anterior uveitis	HLA-B27	RR = 8
Reiter syndrome	HLA-B27	RR = 60
Juvenile rheumatoid arthritis/ juvenile idiopathic arthritis	HLA-DR4, -Dw2	Acute systemic disease
Adamantiades-Behçet syndrome	HLA-B51	Japanese and Middle Eastern descent RR = 4–6
Birdshot chorioretinitis	HLA-A29, -A29.2	RR = 80–100, for North Americans and Europeans
Intermediate uveitis	HLA-B8, -B51, -DR2 HLA-DR15	RR = 6, possibly the DRB1*1501 genotype
Sympathetic ophthalmia	HLA-DR4	
VKH syndrome	HLA-DR4	Japanese and North Americans
Sarcoidosis	HLA-B8 HLA-B13	Acute systemic disease Chronic systemic disease but not for eye
Multiple sclerosis	HLA-B7, -DR2	
Ocular histoplasmosis syndrome (OHS)	HLA-B7, -DR2	RR = 12
Retinal vasculitis	HLA-B44	Britons

antibacterial effector response might inappropriately initiate a cross-react effector response with an epitope of the HLA molecule. A third theory suggests that the T-lymphocyte antigen receptor (gene) is really the true susceptibility factor. Because a specific T-lymphocyte receptor uses a specific HLA haplotype, a strong correlation would exist between an HLA and the T-lymphocyte antigen receptor repertoire. A fourth theory implicates an innate cause unrelated to the role of HLAs in adaptive immunity. For example, transgenic mice genetically altered to express the HLA-B51 molecule, which is associated with Adamantiades-Behçet syndrome, develop neutrophils with enhanced activation and perhaps exaggerated innate effector function.

Immunotherapeutics

BCSC Section 2, *Fundamentals and Principles of Ophthalmology,* includes chapters on pharmacologic principles and ocular pharmacotherapeutics in Part V, Ocular Pharmacology. See also Chapter 6 of this volume, under Medical Management of Uveitis.

Jabs DA, Rosenbaum JT, Foster CS, et al. Guidelines for the use of immunomodulatory drugs in patients with ocular inflammatory disorders: recommendations of an expert panel. *Am J Ophthalmol.* 2000;130:492–513.

Solomon SD, Cunningham ET Jr. Use of corticosteroids and noncorticosteroid immunomodulatory agents in patients with uveitis. *Comprehensive Ophthalmology Update.* 2001;165:273–286.

Nonsteroidal Anti-Inflammatory Drugs

Nonsteroidal anti-inflammatory drugs (NSAIDs) are a family of drugs that inhibit the production of prostaglandins by acting on cyclooxygenase (COX). COX itself has a complex structure that includes a helical channel at the enzymatically active site that oxidizes arachidonic acid. Aspirin and most other NSAIDs act by various mechanisms to reversibly or irreversibly inhibit the arachidonic acid–binding site in the channel of both COX-1 and COX-2. COX-2–specified NSAIDs selectively block the inflammation mediated by COX-2 with concomitant reduction in the prevalence of the adverse effects of stomach mucosal erosions and renal toxicity compared to COX-1 inhibition. Topical or systemic NSAIDs are moderately effective at inhibiting COX in the eye but appear to have only mild anti-inflammatory efficacy for most types of acute ocular inflammation. Nevertheless, some authorities think that such agents can play an important supplementary role in the treatment of uveitis, and in particular preventing recurrences in patients who have experienced multiple recurrences of nongranulomatous anterior uveitis.

Glucocorticosteroids

The mainstay of uveitis therapy is topical, periocular, or systemic administration of glucocorticosteroids. Corticosteroids bind intracellular receptors that translocate into the nucleus, where the drug acts to alter DNA transcription into mRNA. Systemically administered, corticosteroids can alter the homing pattern of T lymphocytes and other effector cells to prevent recruitment into sites of inflammation. Local corticosteroids suppress inflammation through many cellular mechanisms, but the most potent is direct inhibition of most types of inflammatory mediator synthesis or release by effector cells, especially macrophages and neutrophils, as well as T lymphocytes.

Immunomodulatory Therapy

Immunomodulation may be accomplished through a wide variety of unrelated compounds, including some used in treating cancer (see further discussion in Chapter 6):

- alkylating agents such as cyclophosphamide (Cytoxan) and chlorambucil (Leukeran)
- antimetabolites such as methotrexate (Rheumatrex), azathioprine (Imuran), and mycophenolate mofetil (Cellcept)

Signal transduction inhibitors such as cyclosporine (Neoral), tacrolimus (Prograf), and sirolimus (Rapamune) are transported into the cytoplasm of T lymphocytes, particularly CD4 T lymphocytes, and inhibit the activation of the gene responsible for production of interleukin 2.

Alkylating agents cross-link DNA, thereby preventing cell division. These agents function to prevent the bone marrow from replenishing lymphocytes and other effector subpopulations that mediate inflammation. Methotrexate is a folate analog that inhibits folate metabolism to block pyrimidine ring biosynthesis, ultimately affecting pathways that require nucleotide precursors, such as DNA and mRNA synthesis. Thus, this drug will theoretically inhibit protein synthesis in nondividing effector cells, limit activation and differentiation of T lymphocytes within lymphoid tissue, and suppress effector cell expansion within bone marrow. Azathioprine and mycophenolate mofetil work by a similar mechanism on purine incorporation into DNA.

Signal transduction inhibitors, such as cyclosporine, tacrolimus, and sirolimus, inhibit intracellular signaling critical to interleukin production and so especially inhibit T-lymphocyte responses. Topical cyclosporine is now commercially available (Restasis)

Table 5-3 Biologic Response Modifiers

- Receptor antagonists
  Alefacept: binds to the CD2 receptor on T lymphocytes
  Efalizumab: binds to the CD11a receptor on T lymphocytes
  Anakinra: binds to the IL-1 receptor on macrophages
- Cytokine inhibitors
  Etanercept: binds to TNF-α
  Infliximab: binds to TNF-α
  Adalimumab: binds to TNF-α
- Cell-specific antibodies
  Rituximab: binds to the CD20 glycoprotein on B lymphocytes
  Daclizumab: binds to the CD25 glycoprotein on activated T lymphocytes
- Other
  Interferon α2a
  IV-Ig

for treating dry-eye disease associated with lacrimal gland dysfunction as a consequence of lymphocyte infiltration into the gland.

Biologic response modifiers (Table 5-3), such as infliximab, modify a biologic response by neutralizing a cytokine, such as TNF-α, or by occupying the receptor for that cytokine, thereby blocking the cytokine from binding to the receptor and so inhibiting the response that would have occurred had the cytokine attached to it. Cell-specific antibodies bind to and eliminate or inactivate specific cell types; thus, daclizumab attaches to the CD25 cell-surface glycoprotein that is expressed on activated—but not on resting—T lymphocytes and eliminates those activated T lymphocytes from the patient's T-lymphocyte repertoire. Rituximab attaches to the CD20 cell-surface glycoprotein, which is present on all B lymphocytes, and depletes all B lymphocytes from the patient treated with this monoclonal antibody, thus profoundly affecting immunologic reactions that are dependent on antibody. IV-Ig immunomodulates through a complex and incompletely understood set of mechanisms, at least one of which almost certainly is the Jerne idiotype-antiidiotype immunoregulatory network, which downregulates aberrant, inappropriate immune responses without immunomodulating the patient.

PART II

Intraocular Inflammation and Uveitis

CHAPTER 6

Clinical Approach to Uveitis

The uvea consists of the middle, pigmented, vascular structures of the eye and includes the iris, ciliary body, and choroid. *Uveitis* is broadly defined as inflammation (ie, *-itis*) of the uvea (from the Latin *uva,* meaning "grape"). The study of uveitis is complicated by myriad causes of inflammatory reaction of the inner eye that can be broadly categorized into infectious and noninfectious etiologies. In addition, processes that may only secondarily involve the uvea, such as ocular toxoplasmosis, a disease that primarily affects the retina, may cause a marked inflammatory spillover into the choroid and vitreous.

Because uveitis is frequently associated with systemic disease, a careful history and review of systems is an important first step in elucidating the cause of a patient's inflammatory disease. Next, a thorough examination must be done to determine the type of inflammation present. Each patient demonstrates only some of the possible symptoms and signs of uveitis. After the physician has used the information obtained from the history and physical examination to determine the *anatomical classification* of uveitis, he or she can use several *associated factors* to further subcategorize, which leads in turn to choosing the *laboratory studies.* Laboratory studies help determine the etiology of the intraocular inflammation, which then leads to the selection and administration of *therapeutic options.*

This text uses an etiologic division of uveitis entities into noninfectious (autoimmune) and infectious conditions. These conditions are then further subcategorized and described using the anatomical classification of uveitis.

Albert DM, Jakobiec FA, eds. *Principles and Practice of Ophthalmology.* 2nd ed. Philadelphia: Saunders; 1999.

Foster CS, Vitale AT. *Diagnosis and Treatment of Uveitis.* Philadelphia: Saunders; 2002.

Michelson JB. *Color Atlas of Uveitis.* 2nd ed. St Louis: Mosby; 1991.

Nussenblatt RB, Whitcup SM, Palestine AG. *Uveitis: Fundamentals and Clinical Practice.* 3rd ed. Philadelphia: Mosby; 2004.

Rao NA, Forster DJ, Augsburger JJ. *The Uvea: Uveitis and Intraocular Neoplasms.* New York: Gower; 1992.

Classification of Uveitis

Several uveitis classification schemes currently exist. These are based on anatomy (portion of the uvea involved), clinical course (acute, chronic, and recurrent), etiology (infectious and noninfectious), and histopathology (granulomatous or nongranulomatous). The rapid expansion of published clinical information on various uveitic entities from a myriad of global sources using different classification and grading systems and the undeniable need for multicenter randomized clinical trials to better understand the course, prognosis, and treatment of various uveitic entities, led the Standardization of Uveitis Nomenclature (SUN) Working Group, in 2005, to develop an anatomical classification system, descriptors, standardized grading systems, and terminology to use for following the activity of uveitis. This system was adopted by leading uveitis specialists from all over the world. Discussion in this book divides uveitis entities into etiologic categories (infectious, noninfectious) and then follows this basic anatomical classification into 4 uveitic groups (Table 6-1):

- anterior uveitis
- intermediate uveitis
- posterior uveitis
- panuveitis

The SUN group further refined this anatomical classification of uveitis by also defining descriptors based on clinical onset, duration, and course (Table 6-2).

In addition, the SUN working group recommended specific terminology for grading and following uveitic activity (Table 6-3).

Jabs DA, Nussenblatt RB, Rosenbaum JT, The Standardization of Uveitis Nomenclature (SUN) Working Group. Standardization of uveitis nomenclature for reporting clinical data. Results of the First International Workshop. *Am J Ophthalmol.* 2005;140:509–516.

Table 6-1   The SUN Working Group Anatomical Classification of Uveitis

Type	Primary Site of Inflammation	Includes
Anterior uveitis	Anterior chamber	Iritis Iridocyclitis Anterior cyclitis
Intermediate uveitis	Vitreous	Pars planitis Posterior cyclitis Hyalitis
Posterior uveitis	Retina or choroid	Focal, multifocal, or diffuse choroiditis Chorioretinitis Retinochoroiditis Retinitis Neuroretinitis
Panuveitis	Anterior chamber, vitreous, and retina or choroid	

The Standardization of Uveitis Nomenclature (SUN) Working Group. Standardization of nomenclature for reporting clinical data: results of the First International Workshop. *Am J Ophthalmol.* 2005;140:509–516: Table 1.

Table 6-2 The SUN Working Group Descriptors in Uveitis

Category	Descriptor	Comment
Onset	Sudden	
	Insidious	
Duration	Limited	≤3 months' duration
	Persistent	>3 months' duration
Course	Acute	Episode characterized by sudden onset and limited duration
	Recurrent	Repeated episodes separated by periods of inactivity without treatment ≥3 months' duration
	Chronic	Persistent uveitis with relapse in <3 months after discontinuing treatment

The Standardization of Uveitis Nomenclature (SUN) Working Group. Standardization of nomenclature for reporting clinical data: results of the First International Workshop. *Am J Ophthalmol.* 2005;140:509–516: Table 2.

Table 6-3 The SUN Working Group Activity of Uveitis Terminology

Term	Definition
Inactive	Grade 0 cells (anterior chamber)
Worsening activity	2-step increase in level of inflammation (eg, anterior chamber cells, vitreous haze) or increase from grade 3+ to 4+
Improved activity	2-step decrease in level of inflammation (eg, anterior chamber cells, vitreous haze) or decrease to grade 0
Remission	Inactive disease for ≥3 months after discontinuing all treatments for eye disease

The Standardization of Uveitis Nomenclature (SUN) Working Group. Standardization of nomenclature for reporting clinical data: results of the First International Workshop. *Am J Ophthalmol.* 2005;140:509–516: Table 5.

Anterior Uveitis

According to the SUN classification system, the anterior chamber is the primary site of inflammation in anterior uveitis. Anterior uveitis can have a range of presentations, from a quiet white eye with low-grade inflammatory reaction apparent only on close examination to a painful red eye with moderate or severe inflammation. Inflammation confined to the anterior chamber is called *iritis;* if it spills over into the retrolental space, it is called *iridocyclitis;* if it involves the cornea, it is called *keratouveitis;* and if the inflammatory reaction involves the sclera and uveal tract, it is called *sclerouveitis.*

By far, most types of anterior uveitis are sterile inflammatory reactions, whereas many of the posterior uveitic syndromes are infectious in origin. In contrast to endophthalmitis from an infectious source, only 2 noninfectious causes—typically the diseases associated with HLA-B27 and Adamantiades-Behçet syndrome—are associated with hypopyon. Many cases of anterior uveitis are isolated instances of unknown cause that often resolve within 6 weeks, such as idiopathic iritis. Other examples include glaucomatocyclitic crisis, which causes a moderately inflamed eye with elevated IOP that subsides quickly over a few weeks, and blunt trauma, a fairly common cause of a generally self-limiting uveitis.

The anterior uveitis associated with juvenile rheumatoid (idiopathic) arthritis (JRA/JIA)* can be deceptive, because, although the conjunctiva appears quiet externally, the anterior segment may be severely involved in a child without any symptomatic complaints. Another low-grade inflammation of the anterior portion of the eye is seen in Fuchs heterochromic iridocyclitis. Here the damage to the anterior segment is apparently minimal, but the eye needs continued observation because of the commonly occurring secondary complications of cataract and glaucoma. Chapter 7 discusses anterior uveitis in greater detail. See Table 6-4.

Intermediate Uveitis

The SUN working group defines intermediate uveitis as the subset of uveitis where the major site of inflammation is the vitreous. Inflammation of the middle portion (posterior ciliary body, pars plana) of the eye manifests primarily as floaters affecting vision; the eye frequently appears quiet externally. Visual loss is primarily a result of chronic CME or, less commonly, cataract formation. See Chapter 8 of this volume for discussion, as well as Table 6-4.

Posterior Uveitis

Posterior uveitis is defined by the SUN classification system as intraocular inflammation primarily involving the retina and/or choroid. Inflammatory cells may be observed diffusely throughout the vitreous cavity, overlying foci of active inflammation, or on the posterior vitreous face. Ocular examination reveals focal, multifocal, or diffuse areas of retinitis or choroiditis, with varying degrees of vitreous cellular activity, the clinical appearances of which may be similar for different entities. Certain posterior uveitic syndromes present either as a focal or multifocal retinitis, whereas others localize predominantly to the choroid in a similar distribution, involving the retina secondarily, with or without vitreous cells and/or involvement of the retinal vasculature (Tables 6-5, 6-6, 6-7, and 6-8). For example, cytomegalovirus causes a multifocal retinitis, typically with scant vitreous cells; toxoplasmosis characteristically produces a focal retinochoroiditis and heavy vitritis; and histoplasmosis presents as a multifocal chorioretinitis in the absence of vitreous involvement. Macular edema, retinal vasculitis, and retinal

---

*The term *juvenile rheumatoid arthritis (JRA)* refers to the most common type of juvenile arthritis associated with uveitis in children. In the European Union, the most commonly used term is *juvenile idiopathic arthritis (JIA)*. The extended oligoarticular subgroup of JIA would be called "JRA" in the United States. The term *JIA* has not been accepted by the American Rheumatism Association (ARA), although it has been accepted by the American College of Rheumatology. The combined term *JRA/JIA,* which we use throughout the text, reflects this situation.

Table 6-4 Flowchart for Evaluation of Uveitis Patients

Type of Inflammation	Associated Factors	Suspected Disease	Laboratory Tests
		Panuveitis	
	See entities described below: sarcoidosis, toxoplasmosis, toxocariasis, endophthalmitis, VKH syndrome, sympathetic ophthalmia, syphilis, cysticercosis		
		Anterior Uveitis	
Acute/sudden onset, severe with or without fibrin membrane or hypopyon	Arthritis, back pain, GI/GU symptoms	Seronegative spondyloarthropathies	HLA-B27, sacroiliac films
	Aphthous ulcers	Adamantiades-Behçet syndrome	HLA-B5, -B51
	Postsurgical, posttraumatic	Infectious endophthalmitis	Vitreous culture, vitrectomy
	None	Idiopathic	Possibly HLA-B27
Moderate severity (red, painful)	Shortness of breath, African descent	Sarcoidosis	Serum ACE, lysozyme; chest x-ray; gallium scan; biopsy
	Posttraumatic	Traumatic iritis	
	Increased IOP	Glaucomatocyclitic crisis, herpetic iritis	
	Poor response to steroids	Syphilis	RPR, VDRL (screening); FTA-ABS (confirmatory)
	Post-cataract extraction	Low-grade endophthalmitis, IOL-related iritis	Consider vitrectomy, culture
	None	Idiopathic	
Chronic; minimal redness, pain	Child, especially with arthritis	JRA/JIA-related iridocyclitis	ANA, ESR
	Heterochromia, diffuse KP, unilateral	Fuchs heterochromic iridocyclitis	None
	Postsurgical	Low-grade endophthalmitis (eg, *P acnes*); IOL-related	Consider vitrectomy, capsulectomy with culture
	None	Idiopathic	
		Intermediate Uveitis	
Mild to moderate	Shortness of breath, African descent	Sarcoidosis	As above
	Tick exposure, erythema chronicum migrans rash	Lyme disease	ELISA
	Neurologic symptoms	Multiple sclerosis	MRI of brain
	Over age 50	Intraocular lymphoma	Vitrectomy, cytology
	None	Pars planitis	

(Continued)

Table 6-4 (continued)

Type of Inflammation	Associated Factors	Suspected Disease	Laboratory Tests
		Posterior Uveitis	
Chorioretinitis *with* vitritis			
Focal	Adjacent scar; raw meat ingestion	Toxoplasmosis	ELISA
	Child; history of geophagia	Toxocariasis	ELISA
	HIV infection	CMV retinitis	As above
Multifocal	Shortness of breath	Sarcoidosis	PPD, chest x-ray
		Tuberculosis	
	Peripheral retinal necrosis	Acute retinal necrosis (ARN)	VZV, HSV titers (ELISA), possibly vitrectomy/retinal biopsy
		Progressive outer retinal necrosis (PORN, if immunocompromised)	
	AIDS	Syphilis, toxoplasmosis	As above
	IV drug use, hyperalimentation, immunosuppression	*Candida, Aspergillus*	Blood, vitreous cultures
	Visible intraocular parasite; from Africa or Central or South America	Cysticercosis	
		Onchocerciasis	
	Over age 50	Intraocular lymphoma	As above
	None	Birdshot choroidopathy	HLA-A29, fluorescein angiography (FA)
		Multifocal choroiditis with panuveitis	Rule out TB, sarcoidosis, syphilis
Diffuse	Dermatologic/CNS symptoms; serous RD	Vogt-Koyanagi-Harada syndrome (VKH)	FA, lumbar puncture to document CSF pleocytosis
	Postsurgical/traumatic, bilateral	Sympathetic ophthalmia	FA
	Postsurgical/traumatic, unilateral	Infectious endophthalmitis	As above
	Child; history of geophagia	Toxocariasis	As above
Chorioretinitis *without* vitritis			
Focal	None; history of carcinoma	Neoplastic	Metastatic workup
Multifocal	Ohio/Mississippi Valley	Ocular histoplasmosis	FA if macula involved
	Lesions confined to posterior pole	White dot syndromes (eg, APMPPE, MEWDS, PIC)	FA
	Geographic (maplike) pattern of scars	Serpiginous choroidopathy	FA
Diffuse	From Africa, Central/South America	Onchocerciasis	
Vasculitis			
	Aphthous ulcers, hypopyon	Adamantiades-Behçet syndrome	As above
	Malar rash, female, arthralgias	Systemic lupus erythematosus (SLE)	ANA

Table 6-5 **Posterior Uveitis With Retinitis**

Focal Retinitis	Multifocal Retinitis
Toxoplasmosis	Syphilis
Onchocerciasis	HSV
Cysticercosis	VZV
Masquerade syndromes	CMV
	DUSN
	Candida
	Sarcoidosis
	Cat-scratch disease
	Masquerade syndromes

CMV = cytomegalovirus, DUSN = diffuse unilateral subacute neuroretinitis, HSV = herpes simplex virus, VZV = varicella-zoster virus

Adapted from Foster CS, Vitale AT. *Diagnosis and Treatment of Uveitis*. Philadelphia: Saunders; 2002.

Table 6-6 **Posterior Uveitis With a Focal (Solitary) Chorioretinal Lesion**

With Vitreal Cells	Without Vitreal Cells
Toxocariasis	Tumor
Sarcoidosis	Serpiginous choroidopathy
Tuberculosis	
Nocardia	
Cat-scratch disease	

Adapted from Foster CS, Vitale AT. *Diagnosis and Treatment of Uveitis*. Philadelphia: Saunders; 2002.

Table 6-7 **Posterior Uveitis With Multifocal Chorioretinal Lesions**

With Vitreal Cells	Without Vitreal Cells
Birdshot retinochoroidopathy	OHS
MCP	PIC
SFU	PORT
Sympathetic ophthalmia	Acute retinal pigment epitheliitis
VKH	Subacute sclerosing panencephalitis
Sarcoidosis	Serpiginous*
West Nile virus	
Cat-scratch disease	
Malignant masquerade	
Rubella measles*	
MEWDS*	
APMPPE*	

* Usually.

APMPPE = acute posterior multifocal placoid pigment epitheliopathy, MCP = multifocal choroiditis and panuveitis, MEWDS = multiple evanescent white dot syndrome, OHS = ocular histoplasmosis syndrome, PIC = punctate inner choroiditis, PORT = punctate outer retinal toxoplasmosis, SFU = subretinal fibrosis and uveitis syndrome, VKH = Vogt-Koyanagi-Harada syndrome

Adapted from Foster CS, Vitale AT. *Diagnosis and Treatment of Uveitis*. Philadelphia: Saunders; 2002.

Table 6-8 **Posterior Uveitis With Retinal Vasculitis**

Primarily Arteritis	Primarily Phlebitis	Arteritis and Phlebitis
Systemic lupus erythematosus	Sarcoidosis	Toxoplasmosis
Polyarteritis nodosa	Multiple sclerosis	Relapsing polychondritis
Syphilis	Adamantiades-Behçet disease	Wegener granulomatosis
HSV (ARN/BARN)	Birdshot retinochoroidopathy	Crohn disease
VZV (PORN)	HIV paraviral syndrome	Frosted branch angiitis
IRVAN	Eales disease	
Churg-Strauss syndrome		

ARN = acute retinal necrosis; BARN = bilateral acute retinal necrosis; HIV = human immunodeficiency virus; HSV = herpes simplex virus; IRVAN = idiopathic retinal vasculitis, aneurysms, and neuroretinitis; PORN = progressive outer retinal necrosis; VZV = varicella-zoster virus

Adapted from Foster CS, Vitale AT. *Diagnosis and Treatment of Uveitis*. Philadelphia: Saunders; 2002.

or choroidal neovascularization, although not infrequent structural complications of certain uveitic entities, are not considered essential to the anatomical classification of posterior uveitis.

Panuveitis

The primary sites of inflammation in panuveitis (diffuse uveitis), according to the SUN classification system, are the anterior chamber, vitreous, and retina or choroid. Many systemic infectious and noninfectious diseases associated with uveitis may produce diffuse intraocular inflammation with concomitant iridocyclitis and posterior uveitis. These include tuberculosis (the "great imitator") and spirochetal diseases such as Lyme disease and syphilis (the "great masquerader"), as well as sarcoidosis, sympathetic ophthalmia, Vogt-Koyanagi-Harada (VKH) disease, and Adamantiades-Behçet's disease. Other uveitic entities, such as lens-induced uveitis and severe cases of toxoplasmosis or toxocariasis, may present initially as predominantly anterior or posterior segment inflammation only to evolve into panuveitis. Some patients with this condition follow a stormy course; others have a quiet-appearing eye that nonetheless follows a slowly debilitating course. Sarcoidosis and syphilis can cause a bilateral panuveitis, whereas postoperative endophthalmitis generally is a unilateral process. Chapters 7 and 8 discuss noninfectious and infectious panuveitis in greater depth, and Chapter 9 covers endophthalmitis. See also Table 6-4.

Symptoms of Uveitis

Symptoms produced by uveitis depend on which part of the uveal tract is inflamed, the rapidity of onset (sudden or insidious), the duration of the disease (limited or persistent), and the course of the disease (acute, recurrent, or chronic) (Table 6-9).

Acute-onset anterior uveitis (iridocyclitis) causes pain, photophobia, redness, and blurred vision. In contrast, chronic iridocyclitis in patients with JRA/JIA may not be associated with any symptoms at all. However, with chronic iridocyclitis, blurred vision

Table 6-9 Symptoms of Uveitis

Redness
Pain
Photophobia
Epiphora
Visual disturbances
    Diffuse blur, caused by:
        Myopic or hyperopic shift
        Inflammatory cells
        Cataract
    Scotoma (central or peripheral)
Floaters

may develop as a result of calcific band keratopathy, cataract, or cystoid macular edema (CME). Recurrent anterior uveitis is marked by periods of inactivity of 3 or more months off medications followed by a return of symptoms.

Intermediate uveitis produces symptoms of floaters and blurred vision. Floaters result from the shadows cast by vitreous cells and snowballs on the retina. Blurred vision may be due to CME or vitreous opacities in the visual axis.

Presenting symptoms in patients with posterior uveitis include painless decreased visual acuity, floaters, photopsias, metamorphopsia, scotomata, nyctalopia, or a combination of these. This blurred vision may be due to the primary effects of uveitis such as retinitis and/or choroiditis directly affecting macular function or to the complications of inflammation such as CME, epiretinal membrane, retinal ischemia, and choroidal neovascularization. Blurred vision may also result from refractive error such as a myopic or hyperopic shift associated with macular edema, hypotony, or a change in lens position. Other possible causes of blurred vision include opacities in the visual axis from inflammatory cells, fibrin, or protein in the anterior chamber; keratic precipitates (KPs); secondary cataract; vitreous debris; macular edema; and retinal atrophy.

The pain of uveitis usually results from the acute onset of inflammation in the region of the iris, as in acute iritis, or from secondary glaucoma. The pain associated with ciliary spasm in iritis may be a referred pain that seems to radiate over the larger area served by cranial nerve V *(trigeminal nerve)*. Epiphora and photophobia are usually present when inflammation involves the iris, cornea, or iris–ciliary body. Occasionally, uveitis is discovered on a routine ophthalmic examination in an asymptomatic patient.

Signs of Uveitis

Part I of this volume reviews the basic concepts of immunology, which can be used to understand the symptoms and signs of inflammation in uveitis. An inflammatory response to infectious, traumatic, neoplastic, or autoimmune processes produces the signs of uveitis (Table 6-10). Chemical mediators of the acute stage of inflammation include serotonin,

Table 6-10 Signs of Uveitis

Eyelid and skin
  Vitiligo
  Nodules
	Intraocular pressure
	  Hypotony
	  Secondary glaucoma

Conjunctiva
  Perilimbal or diffuse injection
  Nodules
	Vitreous
	  Inflammatory cells (single/clumped)
	  Traction bands

Corneal endothelium
  Keratic (cellular) precipitates (diffuse or
    gravitational)
  Fibrin
  Pigment (nonspecific)
	Pars plana
	  Snowbanking
	Retina
	  Inflammatory cells
	  Inflammatory cuffing of blood vessels

Anterior/posterior chamber
  Inflammatory cells
  Flare (proteinaceous influx)
  Pigment (nonspecific)
	Edema
	  Cystoid macular edema
	  RPE: hypertrophy/clumping/loss
	  Epiretinal membranes

Iris
  Nodules
  Posterior synechiae
  Atrophy
  Heterochromia
	Choroid
	  Inflammatory infiltrate
	  Atrophy
	  Neovascularization
	Optic Nerve
	  Edema (nonspecific)

Angle
  Peripheral anterior synechiae
  Nodules
  Vascularization
	Neovascularization

complement, and plasmin. Leukotrienes, kinins, and prostaglandins modify the second phase of the acute response through antagonism of vasoconstrictors. Activated complement is a leukotactic agent. Polymorphonuclear leukocytes, eosinophils, and mast cells may all contribute to signs of inflammation. However, the lymphocyte is, by far, the predominant inflammatory cell in the inner eye in uveitis. These chemical mediators result in vascular dilation *(ciliary flush),* increased vascular permeability *(aqueous flare),* and chemotaxis of inflammatory cells into the eye *(aqueous and vitreous cellular reaction).*

Anterior Segment

Signs of uveitis in the anterior portion of the eye include

- keratic precipitates (KPs) (Figs 6-1, 6-2)
- cells
- flare (Fig 6-3)
- fibrin
- hypopyon
- pigment dispersion
- pupillary miosis
- iris nodules (Fig 6-4)

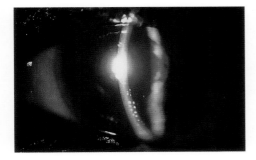

Figure 6-1 Keratic precipitates (medium and small) with broken posterior synechiae. *(Courtesy of H. Jane Blackman, MD.)*

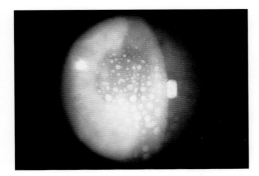

Figure 6-2 Large "mutton-fat" keratic precipitates in a patient with sarcoidosis. Large KPs such as these generally indicate a granulomatous disease process. *(Courtesy of David Forster, MD.)*

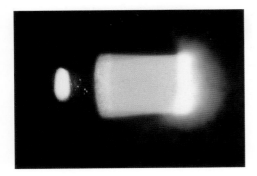

Figure 6-3 Aqueous flare (4+) in acute iritis.

- synechiae, both anterior and posterior (Fig 6-5)
- band keratopathy (seen with long-standing uveitis)

Keratic precipitates are collections of inflammatory cells on the corneal endothelium. When newly formed, they tend to be white and smoothly rounded, but they then become crenated (shrunken), pigmented, or glassy. Large, yellowish KPs are described as *mutton-fat KPs;* these are usually associated with granulomatous types of inflammation (see the discussion later in this section on the distinction between granulomatous and nongranulomatous inflammation). The SUN group (see Classification of Uveitis earlier in the chapter) is working to establish photographic guidelines for describing KPs.

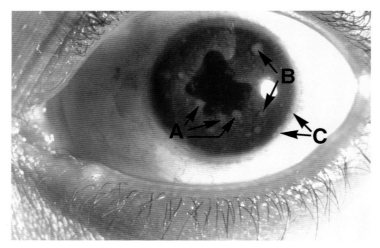

Figure 6-4 Posterior synechiae and iris nodules in a patient with sarcoidosis. Note the 3 types of iris nodules: *A*, Koeppe nodules (pupillary border); *B*, Busacca nodules (midiris); and *C*, Berlin nodules (iris angle). *(Courtesy of David Forster, MD.)*

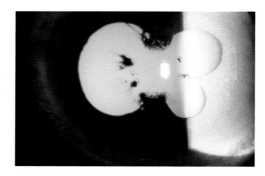

Figure 6-5 Multiple posterior synechiae preventing complete dilation of the pupil. *(Courtesy of David Forster, MD.)*

Perilimbal vascular engorgement (ciliary flush) or diffuse injection of the conjunctiva, episclera, or both is typical with acute anterior uveitis. With increased capillary permeability, the anterior chamber reaction can be described as

- serous (aqueous flare caused by protein influx)
- purulent (polymorphonuclear leukocytes and necrotic debris causing hypopyon)
- fibrinous (plasmoid, or intense fibrinous exudate)
- sanguinoid (inflammatory cells with erythrocytes manifested by hypopyon mixed with hyphema)

The SUN group also specifically developed an updated method of grading anterior chamber cell and flare. The intensity of the cellular reaction in the anterior chamber is graded according to the number of inflammatory cells seen in a 1 × 1-mm high-powered beam at full intensity at a 45°–60° angle (Table 6-11).

Flare may also be graded similarly, and the SUN group described flare intensity as it had been described previously by Hogan and Kimura (Table 6-12).

Hogan MJ, Kimura SJ, Thygeson P. Signs and symptoms of uveitis. I. Anterior uveitis. *Am J Ophthalmol.* 1959;47:155–170.

Table 6-11 The SUN Working Group Grading Scheme for Anterior Chamber Cells

Grade	Cells in Field (high-intensity 1 × 1-mm slit beam)
0	<1
0.5+	1–5
1+	6–15
2+	16–25
3+	26–50
4+	>50

The Standardization of Uveitis Nomenclature (SUN) Working Group. Standardization of nomenclature for reporting clinical data: results of the First International Workshop. *Am J Ophthalmol.* 2005;140:509–516: Table 3.

Table 6-12 The SUN Working Group Grading System for Anterior Chamber Flare

Grade	Description
0	None
1+	Faint
2+	Moderate (iris and lens details clear)
3+	Marked (iris and lens details hazy)
4+	Intense (fibrin or plasmoid aqueous)

The Standardization of Uveitis Nomenclature (SUN) Working Group. Standardization of nomenclature for reporting clinical data: results of the First International Workshop. *Am J Ophthalmol.* 2005;140:509–516: Table 4.

Iris involvement may manifest as either anterior or posterior synechiae, iris nodules (Koeppe nodules at the pupillary border, Busacca nodules within the iris stroma, and Berlin nodules in the angle; see Fig 6-4), iris granulomas, heterochromia (eg, Fuchs heterochromic iridocyclitis), or stromal atrophy (eg, herpetic uveitis).

With uveitic involvement of the ciliary body and trabecular meshwork, IOP often is low secondary to decreased aqueous production or increased alternative outflow, but IOP may increase precipitously if the meshwork becomes clogged by inflammatory cells or debris or if the trabecular meshwork itself is the site of inflammation *(trabeculitis)*. Pupillary block with iris bombé and secondary angle closure may also lead to an acute rise in IOP.

Intermediate Segment

Signs in the intermediate anatomical area of the eye include

- vitreal inflammatory cells, which are graded from 0 to 4+ in density:

Grade	Number of cells
0	No cells
0.5+	1–10
1+	10–20
2+	20–30
3+	30–100
4+	>100

The SUN group did not achieve consensus regarding a grading system for vitreous cells. However, the NIH grading system for vitreous haze, which has now been adopted by the SUN group, grades both vitreous cell and flare and may be a better indicator of disease activity than cell counts alone. With this method, standardized photographs are used for comparison to ultimately arrive at the level of vitreous haze.

- *snowball opacities,* which are common with sarcoidosis or intermediate uveitis
- exudates over the pars plana *(snowbank).* Active snowbanks have a fluffy or shaggy appearance. If pars planitis becomes inactive, the pars plana appears gliotic or fibrotic and smooth; thus, these changes are not referred to as "snowbanks."
- vitreal strands

Chronic uveitis may be associated with cyclitic membrane formation, with secondary ciliary body detachment and hypotony.

Posterior Segment

Signs in the posterior segment of the eye include

- retinal or choroidal inflammatory infiltrates
- inflammatory sheathing of arteries or veins
- perivascular inflammatory cuffing
- retinal pigment epithelial hypertrophy or atrophy
- atrophy or swelling of the retina, choroid, or optic nerve head
- pre- or subretinal fibrosis
- exudative, tractional, or rhegmatogenous retinal detachment
- retinal or choroidal neovascularization

Retinal and choroidal signs may be unifocal, multifocal, or diffuse. The uveitis can be diffuse throughout the eye *(panuveitis)* or appear dispersed with spillover from 1 area to another, as with toxoplasmosis primarily involving the retina but showing anterior chamber inflammation as well.

Review of the Patient's Health and Other Associated Factors

Many historical factors other than ocular symptoms and signs can help in the classification or identification of uveitis (Table 6-13). A comprehensive history and review of systems is of paramount importance in helping to elucidate the cause of uveitis. In this regard, a uveitis survey such as that shown at the end of this chapter can be very helpful.

Determining whether the onset was sudden or insidious may help the clinician narrow the range of diagnostic possibilities. Uveitis may be subcategorized as acute, chronic, and recurrent: *acute* is generally the term used to describe episodes of sudden onset and limited duration that usually resolve within a few weeks to months, whereas *chronic* uveitis is persistent, with relapse in less than 3 months after discontinuing treatment. Recurrent uveitis is characterized by repeated episodes separated by periods of inactivity without treatment 3 months or longer in duration.

Table 6-13 Historical Factors in Diagnosis of Uveitis

Modifying Factors	Associated Factors Suggesting Systemic Conditions
Time course of disease	Immune system status
Acute	Systemic medications
Recurrent	Trauma history
Chronic	Travel history
Severity	Social history
Severe	Eating habits
Inactive	Pets
Distribution of uveitis	Sexual practices
Unilateral	Occupation
Bilateral	Drug use
Alternating	
Focal	
Multifocal	
Diffuse	
Patient's sex	
Patient's age	
Patient's race	

Whether the inflammation is severe or low grade can influence categorization and prognosis. The inflammatory process may occur in 1 or both eyes, or it may alternate between them. The distribution of ocular involvement—focal, multifocal, or diffuse—is also helpful to note when classifying uveitis. The age, gender, sexual practices, and racial background of the patient are important findings in some uveitic syndromes.

Chronic uveitis can be further characterized histopathologically as being either granulomatous or nongranulomatous. *Nongranulomatous* inflammation typically has a lymphocytic and plasma cell infiltrate, whereas *granulomatous* reactions also include epithelioid and giant cells. Discrete granulomas are characteristic of sarcoidosis; diffuse granulomatous inflammation appears in VKH disease and sympathetic ophthalmia. Zonal granulomatous disease can be seen with lens-induced uveitis. However, the physician should be aware that the *clinical* appearance of uveitis as granulomatous or nongranulomatous may not necessarily correlate with the *histopathologic* description and may instead be related to the stage in which the disease is first seen, the amount of presenting antigen, or the host's state of immunocompromise (eg, a patient being treated with corticosteroids).

Although ocular inflammation may be an isolated process involving only the eye, it can also be associated with a systemic condition. However, ocular inflammation frequently does not correlate with the inflammatory activity elsewhere in the body, so it is important for the clinician to carefully review systems. In some cases, the uveitis may actually precede the development of inflammation at other body sites. The presence of immunocompromise, use of intravenous drugs, hyperalimentation, and the patient's occupation are just a few risk factors that can direct the investigation of uveitis. Neoplastic disease can masquerade as inflammatory disease. Large cell lymphoma (previously called *reticulum cell sarcoma*), retinoblastoma, leukemia, and malignant melanoma may all be mistaken for uveitis. In addition, juvenile xanthogranuloma, pigment dispersion syndrome, retinal detachment, retinitis pigmentosa, and ischemia all must be considered in the differential diagnosis of uveitis.

The chapters that follow describe discrete uveitis entities. However, many patients do not present with the classic signs and symptoms of a particular disease. Some patients require monitoring through follow-up visits, and laboratory tests may need to be repeated at a later date, as the clinical appearance may be unclear or change with time and treatment. The presentation of disease can also be modified by prior therapy or by a delay in seeing the physician.

Differential Diagnosis of Uveitic Entities

The differential diagnosis is broad and includes infectious agents (viruses, bacteria, fungi, protozoa, and helminths), noninfectious entities of presumed immunologic or allergic origin, masquerade syndromes such as endophthalmitis and neoplasms, and unknown or idiopathic causes. Although pattern recognition alone is frequently sufficient to establish a definitive diagnosis, an accurate biomicroscopic and funduscopic description of posterior segment inflammatory conditions is extremely helpful in narrowing the differential and in conceptualizing individual entities, because their distribution and evolution may be quite characteristic.

Once a comprehensive history has been taken and a physical examination performed, the most likely causes are ranked in a list based on how well the individual patient's type of uveitis "fits" with the various known uveitic entities. This *naming-meshing system* first names the type of uveitis based on anatomical criteria and associated factors (eg, acute versus chronic, unilateral versus bilateral) and then matches the pattern of uveitis exhibited by the patient with a list of potential uveitic entities that share similar characteristics. One such system for helping to identify a possible cause for a particular patient's uveitis is outlined in Table 6-4.

Epidemiology of Uveitis

A knowledge of the prevalence of the various causes seen in uveitis survey populations is also helpful in determining the most probable cause of the uveitis. Numerous studies have been performed to determine the prevalence of various types of uveitis, but the data often vary from one study to another, depending on whether the study was performed at a tertiary referral center or was community-based. The location of the study population also produces differing results. For example, the prevalence of cytomegalovirus retinitis would be expected to be much higher in large urban areas with higher rates of AIDS, whereas ocular histoplasmosis would be more prevalent in rural areas in the midwestern United States. Certain types of uveitis also show large, worldwide variations. For example, entities such as Adamantiades-Behçet syndrome and VKH disease are much more common in Japan than in Europe or the United States. Recent observations made in an epidemiologic study of uveitis in northern California, utilizing a large health maintenance organization in 6 target communities with a combined population of nearly 732,000, suggest an incidence rate of 52.4/100,000 person-years, a 3-fold higher incidence of uveitis than previously reported in studies from the United States. In addition, the incidence and prevalence were lowest in the pediatric age groups and highest in those over age 65. Further, although the prevalence of affected women was greater than that of men in northern California, the incidence rates were similar for women and men.

Table 6-14 summarizes the data from several surveys, comparing the prevalence of various types of uveitis in both university/referral-based and community-based populations from around the world. The anatomical distribution of uveitis is similar to that reported in the United States, with a higher prevalence of anterior involvement followed by panuveitis, then posterior uveitis, and finally intermediate uveitis. Also, most university/referral-based studies probably overestimate the prevalence of intermediate and posterior uveitis compared to cases actually seen in the community.

The etiologic distribution of uveitis varies around the globe. In general, the data demonstrate that idiopathic causes are frequently found in anterior uveitis and that infectious causes are more common in posterior uveitis. Adamantiades-Behçet syndrome seems highly prevalent in Turkey and in China, whereas birdshot retinochoroidopathy is more common in western Europe. Vogt-Koyanagi-Harada disease is clearly more prevalent in China. Tuberculosis remains the main etiology of infectious uveitis in India. Viral uveitis is predominant in the Middle East and in France, followed by toxoplasmosis.

Bodaghi B, Cassoux N, Wechsler B, et al. Chronic severe uveitis: etiology and visual outcome in 927 patients from a single center. *Medicine (Baltimore)*. 2001;80:263–270.

Gritz DC, Wong IG. The incidence and prevalence of uveitis in northern California. The Northern California Epidemiology of Uveitis Study. *Ophthalmology*. 2004;111:491–500.

Islam SM, Tabbara KF. Causes of uveitis at The Eye Center in Saudi Arabia: a retrospective review. *Ophthalmic Epidemiol*. 2002;9:239–249.

McCannel CA, Holland GN, Helm CJ, Cornell PJ, Winston JV, Rimmer TG. Causes of uveitis in the general practice of ophthalmology. UCLA Community-Based Uveitis Study Group. *Am J Ophthalmol*. 1996;121:35–46.

Rodriguez A, Calonge M, Pedroza-Seres M, et al. Referral patterns of uveitis in a tertiary eye care center. *Arch Ophthalmol*. 1996;114:593–599.

Sengun A, Karadag R, Karakurt A, Saricaoglu MS, Abdik O, Hasiripi H. Causes of uveitis in a referral hospital in Ankara, Turkey. *Ocul Immunol Inflamm*. 2005;13:45–50.

Singh R, Gupta V, Gupta A. Patterns of uveitis in a referral eye clinic in north India. *Indian J Ophthalmol*. 2004;52:121–125.

Yang P, Zhang Z, Zhou H, et al. Clinical patterns and characteristics of uveitis in a tertiary center for uveitis in China. *Curr Eye Res*. 2005;30:943–948.

Laboratory and Medical Evaluation

The diagnosis may require laboratory and medical evaluation guided by the history and physical examination. *There is no one standardized battery of tests that needs to be ordered for all patients with uveitis.* Rather, a tailored approach should be taken based on the most likely causes for each patient. Once a list of differential diagnoses is compiled, appropriate laboratory tests can be ordered, if necessary. Many patients require only 1 or a few

Table 6-14 Most Common Causes of Uveitis

	Bodaghi (2001) France (n = 927)	Yang (2005) China (n = 1752)	Gritz (2004) U.S. (n = 382, new cases only)	Islam (2002) Saudi Arabia (n = 200)	Singh (2004) India (n = 1233)	Sengun (2005) Turkey (n = 300)
Anterior						
Idiopathic	28.5%	45.6%	70.2%	59.5%	49.2%	43.6%
HLA-B27 +/seronegative spondyloarthropathies	3.9	27		29	30.2	17
JRA/JIA-associated	5	4.6		4	6.4	1.7
Herpes simplex/zoster	2.7	2			1.6	1.7
Fuchs heterochromic	8.8	1.5		15	0.9	3
Intraocular lens–related	2.7	5.7		3.5	2.5	2.7
Sarcoidosis		1				
Traumatic	1.9	0.1		0	1.9	0.6
Intermediate						
Idiopathic	15%	6.1%	2.9%	6.5%	16.1%	9%
Sarcoidosis	11.3	6.1		4.5	14.7	7.3
Multiple sclerosis	0.4	0		0.5	0.6	0
Posterior						
Toxoplasmosis	21.6%	6.8%	2.1%	13.5%	20.2%	26.6%
Retinal vasculitis	8.4	0.1		6.5	1.7	7.3
Idiopathic	3.5	0.05			4.9	0.6
Ocular histoplasmosis		5.6				4.7
Toxocariasis						
Cytomegalovirus retinitis		0.2			0.2	
Serpiginous choroidopathy		0.3			5	0.3
Acute multifocal placoid pigment epitheliopathy						
Necrotizing herpetic retinopathy (ARN/PORN)	1.5	0.1			0.3	0.3
Birdshot retinochoroidopathy	4.4				0.6	0.3
Sarcoidosis	0.3					0.7
Panuveitis						
Idiopathic	35%	41.5%	5.0%	20.5%	14.7%	20.6%
Sarcoidosis	13.1	6.2		6.5	1.4	5
Vogt-Koyanagi-Harada	3.7	0.1		3	1.4	1
Multifocal choroiditis with panuveitis	2	15.9		2.5	3.6	1
Adamantiades-Behçet syndrome	5.9	16.5		6.5	1.8	1.3
Tuberculosis	4	0.74		10.5	10.1	26
Indeterminate location			18.8%			1.3

diagnostic tests. When the history and physical examination do not clearly indicate the cause, most uveitis specialists recommend a subset of core tests, including complete blood count, erythrocyte sedimentation rate (ESR), angiotensin-converting enzyme (ACE), lysozyme, syphilis serologic profile, and chest radiographs. Risk factors may also indicate testing for tuberculosis and Lyme disease. Table 6-4 lists some of the laboratory tests that may be useful for particular presentations of uveitis. These laboratory tests are discussed further in the chapters that follow, covering the various types of uveitis.

In the evaluation of patients with certain types of uveitis, ancillary testing can be extremely helpful:

- *Fluorescein angiography (FA)* is an essential imaging modality in evaluating eyes with chorioretinal disease and structural complications of posterior uveitis. It frequently provides critical information not obtainable from biomicroscopic or fundus examination and is useful both diagnostically and in monitoring a patient's response to therapy. Cystoid macular edema (Fig 6-6); retinal vasculitis; secondary choroidal or retinal neovascularization; and areas of optic nerve, retinal, and choroidal inflammation can all be detected angiographically. Several of the retinochoroidopathies, or white dot syndromes, have characteristic appearances on FA.

- *Indocyanine green (ICG) angiography* may show 2 patterns of hypofluorescence in the presence of inflammatory choroidal vasculopathies. Type 1, which represents more selective inflammatory choriocapillaropathies, demonstrates early and late multifocal areas of hypofluorescence and may be seen in multiple evanescent white dot syndrome (MEWDS). Type 2 represents stromal inflammatory vasculopathies of the choroids and demonstrates areas of early hypofluorescence and late hyperfluorescence and may be seen in sarcoidosis, sympathetic ophthalmia, birdshot chorioretinopathy, and VKH syndrome.

- *Ultrasonography* can be useful in demonstrating vitreous opacities, choroidal thickening, retinal detachment, or cyclitic membrane formation, particularly if media opacities preclude a view of the posterior segment.

- *Optical coherence tomography (OCT),* a cross-sectional imaging method using coherent light to develop a low-coherence interferometric image of the retina, has become a standard of care for the objective measurement of uveitic CME (Fig 6-7),

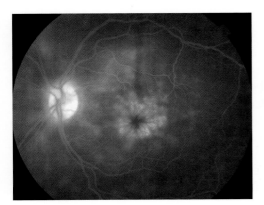

Figure 6-6 Late transit phase fluorescein angiogram of the left eye of a patient with sarcoid-associated anterior uveitis and cystoid macular edema (CME). *(Courtesy of Ramana S. Moorthy, MD.)*

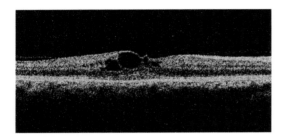

Figure 6-7 OCT image of the macula of the same eye as in Figure 6-6, showing cystoid spaces in the parafoveal outer plexiform layer. *(Courtesy of Ramana S. Moorthy, MD.)*

retinal thickening, subretinal fluid associated with choroidal neovascularization, and serous retinal detachments. It can be useful in eyes with smaller pupils but can be limited by media opacities. OCT can be invaluable in following patients with uveitic glaucoma. Nerve fiber layer defects and visual field defects correlate well to changes seen on OCT imaging of the optic nerve head.

- *Anterior chamber paracentesis:* Aqueous humor may be analyzed following anterior chamber paracentesis. Compared with diagnostic vitrectomy, this procedure is more frequently used in Europe, in patients presenting with atypical features of infectious uveitis or a suspicion of primary intraocular lymphoma. Evaluation of local antibody production based on the Goldmann-Witmer (GW) coefficient is considered the gold standard for the diagnosis of toxoplasmosis in Europe. PCR technology is a valuable tool in cases of viral uveitis or retinitis but is less sensitive in diagnosing parasitic conditions. Diagnostic yield is increased when PCR and the GW coefficient are combined, especially in viral infections. New technological developments, such as real-time PCR, have improved the sensitivity and specificity of the method, even though results should be interpreted with care. The surgical technique is discussed at the end of this chapter.

- *Vitreous biopsy* may be necessary for a diagnostic evaluation in suspected cases of primary intraocular lymphoma (formerly called *reticulum cell sarcoma*) or bacterial or fungal endophthalmitis. Cytologic, cytofluorographic, and microbiologic examination of vitreous fluid may be performed. Bacterial and fungal cultures of vitreous and aqueous specimens may also be performed in cases when infections are suspected. Carefully planned testing in selected patients can be an effective means of confirming clinical diagnoses in intraocular lymphoma, chronic ocular infections, and atypical chorioretinitis. Fluid may also be analyzed by PCR to determine the cause of certain cases. Specific primers for *Toxoplasma gondii,* herpes simplex virus, varicella-zoster virus, and cytomegalovirus are readily available. Combined with the clinical picture, evaluating for the presence of DNA from specific pathogens can be moderately sensitive and specific in establishing an etiologic diagnosis. Surgical management is discussed later in this chapter and in Chapter 11. Aqueous specimens may also be evaluated in a similar manner in some cases.

- *Chorioretinal biopsy* may be useful when the diagnosis cannot be confirmed on the basis of clinical appearance or other laboratory investigations (eg, certain cases of necrotizing retinitis in patients with AIDS or suspected cases of primarily subretinal intraocular lymphoma). Surgical management is further discussed later in this chapter.

Ciardella AP, Prall FR, Borodoker N, Cunningham ET Jr. Imaging techniques for posterior uveitis. *Curr Opin Ophthalmol.* 2004;15:519–530.

Davis JL, Miller DM, Ruiz P. Diagnostic testing of vitrectomy specimens. *Am J Ophthalmol.* 2005;140:822–829.

de Groot-Mijnes JD, Rothova A, van Loon AM, et al. Polymerase chain reaction and Goldmann-Witmer coefficient analysis are complementary for the diagnosis of infectious uveitis. *Am J Ophthalmol.* 2006;141:313–318.

Quentin CD, Reiber H. Fuchs heterochromic cyclitis: rubella virus antibodies and genome in aqueous humor. *Am J Ophthalmol.* 2004;138:46–54.

Therapy

Many patients with mild, self-limiting uveitis need no referral to a uveitis specialist. However, in uveitis with a chronic or downwardly spiraling course, referring the patient to a uveitis specialist may be helpful not only in eliciting the cause and determining the therapeutic regimen but also in reassuring the patient that all avenues are being explored. Evaluation of vision-threatening uveitis may require coordination with other medical or surgical consultants (eg, in pursuing the diagnosis of HIV-related diseases or in kidney transplant patients on immunomodulatory therapy). Discussion with the patient and other specialists about the prognosis and complications of uveitis helps to determine the appropriate therapy. Therapy for uveitis ranges from simple observation to medical or surgical intervention (Table 6-15).

Medical Management of Uveitis

Generally, medical therapy includes topical cycloplegics, topical or systemic nonsteroidal anti-inflammatory drugs (NSAIDs), and topical or systemic corticosteroids. Immunomodulatory therapy may be required in patients with uveitis unresponsive to corticosteroid therapy, in patients with corticosteroid-induced complications, and in patients with disorders shown to be associated with poor long-term outcomes when corticosteroids have been the sole therapeutic modality. The choice of therapeutic approach depends on the relative risk of complications of uveitis, of which the most common are cataracts, glaucoma, CME, and hypotony. Treatment should be tailored as specifically as possible to the individual patient and adjusted according to response. The physician should consider the patient's systemic involvement and other factors, such as age, immune status, and tolerance for side effects. See also Immunotherapeutics in Chapter 5.

Mydriatic and Cycloplegic Agents

Topical mydriatic and cycloplegic agents are beneficial for breaking or preventing the formation of posterior synechiae and for relieving photophobia secondary to ciliary spasm.

Table 6-15 Therapy for Uveitis

Observation
  For development of complications
  For change in the appearance/severity/progression

Medical therapy
Cycloplegics
  To relieve pain
  To break posterior synechiae/pupillary block
Corticosteroids
  Topical drops/ointment
  Sub-Tenon's or retroseptal injection
  Oral or intravenous injection
  Intravitreal injection of triamcinolone
  Intravitreal fluocinolone implant (surgically placed)
Immunomodulators
  Alkylating agents
  Antimetabolites
  T-lymphocyte modulators
  Biologic response modifiers

Surgical therapy
Diagnostic procedures
  Aqueous paracentesis
  Vitreous biopsy
  Chorioretinal biopsy
Reparative procedures
  Cataract extraction
  Pupillary reconstruction
  Glaucoma surgery
  Epiretinal membrane peeling
  Scleral buckle
  Pars plana vitrectomy

The stronger the inflammatory reaction, the stronger or more frequent the dosage of cycloplegic. Short-acting drops such as cyclopentolate hydrochloride (Cyclogyl) or long-acting drops such as atropine may be used. Most cases of acute anterior uveitis require only short-acting cycloplegics; these allow the pupil to remain mobile and permit rapid recovery when they are discontinued. Patients with chronic uveitis and moderate flare in the anterior chamber (eg, JRA/JIA-associated iritis) may need to be maintained on short-acting agents (eg, tropicamide) for the long term to prevent posterior synechiae.

NSAIDs

Nonsteroidal anti-inflammatory drugs (NSAIDs) work by inhibiting cyclooxygenase (isoforms 1 and 2 or 2 alone) and reduce the synthesis of prostaglandins that mediate inflammation. Topical NSAIDs may be useful in the treatment of postoperative inflammation and CME, but their usefulness in treating endogenous anterior uveitis has not been proven. Several studies have shown that systemic NSAIDs may be efficacious in the treatment of chronic iridocyclitis (eg, JRA/JIA-associated iridocyclitis) and possibly CME; NSAIDs may allow the practitioner to maintain the patient on a lower dose of topical corticosteroids. Potential complications of prolonged systemic NSAID use include gastric ulceration, GI bleeding, nephrotoxicity, and hepatotoxicity. See also BCSC Section 1, *Update on General Medicine,* Chapter 8.

Corticosteroids

Corticosteroids are the mainstay of uveitis therapy (Table 6-16). Because of their potential side effects, however, they should be reserved for specific indications:

- treatment of active inflammation in the eye
- prevention or treatment of complications such as CME
- reduction of inflammatory infiltration of the retina, choroid, or optic nerve

Table 6-16 Corticosteroids Frequently Used in Uveitis Therapy and Their Complications

Route of Administration		Complications
Topical (relative anti-inflammatory activity compared to hydrocortisone)		
Prednisolone acetate 1%	(2.3)*	Cataract formation
Prednisolone sodium phosphate 1%	(2.3)	Elevation of IOP
Fluorometholone 0.1%	(21)	Worsening of external infection
Dexamethasone phosphate 0.1%	(24)	Corneal/scleral thinning or perforation
Rimexolone 1%		
Loteprednol etabonate 0.5% or 0.2%		
Periocular		Same complications as topical above and
Long-acting		Ptosis
Methylprednisolone acetate (Depo-Medrol)	(5.0)	Scarring of conjunctiva/Tenon's capsule
Triamcinolone acetonide (Kenalog)	(5.0)	Worsening of infectious uveitis
Triamcinolone diacetate (Aristocort)	(5.0)	Scleral perforation
Short-acting		Hemorrhage
Hydrocortisone sodium succinate (Solu-Cortef)	(1.0)	
Betamethasone (Celestone)	(25)	
Systemic		Same complications as topical above and
Prednisone	(4.0)	Increased appetite
Triamcinolone	(5.0)	Weight gain
Dexamethasone	(25)	Peptic ulcers
Methylprednisolone	(5.0)	Sodium and fluid retention
		Osteoporosis/bone fractures
		Aseptic necrosis of hip
		Hypertension
		Diabetes mellitus
		Menstrual irregularities
		Mental status changes
		Exacerbation of systemic infections
		Impaired wound healing
		Acne
		Others

* Numbers in parentheses represent relative anti-inflammatory activity compared to that of hydrocortisone.

Complications of corticosteroid therapy are numerous and can be seen with any mode of administration. Therefore, these agents should be used only when the benefits of therapy outweigh the risks of the medications themselves. Corticosteroids are not always indicated in patients with chronic flare or in the therapy of specific diseases such as Fuchs heterochromic iridocyclitis or pars planitis without macular edema or with a peripheral lesion of toxoplasmosis (ie, a lesion that does not threaten the optic disc or macula).

The amount and duration of corticosteroid therapy must be individualized. It is generally preferable to begin therapy with a high dose of corticosteroids (topical or systemic) and taper the dose as the inflammation subsides, rather than beginning with a low dose that may have to be progressively increased to control the inflammation. To minimize complications of therapy, patients should be maintained on the minimal amount of corticosteroid needed to control the inflammation. If corticosteroid therapy is needed for longer than 2–3 weeks, the dosage should be tapered before discontinuation. The dosage may need to be increased if surgical intervention is required to prevent postoperative exacerbation of the uveitis. The relative potencies of various corticosteroid preparations are summarized in Table 6-16 and in BCSC 2, *Fundamentals and Principles of Ophthalmology*, Chapter 18, Table 18-8.

Topical administration

Topical corticosteroid drops are effective primarily for anterior uveitis, although they may have beneficial effects on vitritis or macular edema in patients who are pseudophakic or aphakic. These drops are given in time intervals ranging from once daily to hourly. They can also be given in an ointment form for nighttime use or if preservatives in the eyedrops are not well tolerated. Of the topical preparations, rimexolone, loteprednol, and fluorometholone have been shown to have less of an ocular hypertensive effect than other medications and may be particularly useful in patients who are corticosteroid responders. However, these agents are not as effective as prednisolone in controlling uveitis that is more intense than mild to moderate. Some generic forms of prednisolone, though, may have less of an anti-inflammatory effect than brand-name products; this should be considered when patients do not respond adequately to topical corticosteroid therapy. A difference in efficacy may be due to differences in particle size among various suspensions and may necessitate more vigorous agitation before instillation.

Periocular administration

Periocular corticosteroids are generally given as depot injections when a more posterior effect is needed or when a patient is noncompliant or poorly responsive to topical or systemic administration. They are often preferred for patients with intermediate or posterior uveitis or for those with CME, because they deliver a therapeutic dose of medication close to the site of inflammation and have few if any systemic side effects in adults. Triamcinolone acetonide (40 mg) and methylprednisolone acetate (40–80 mg) are the most commonly used agents.

Periocular injections can be performed using either a transseptal or a sub-Tenon's (Nozik technique) approach (Fig 6-8). With a sub-Tenon's injection, a 25-gauge, ⅝-in. needle is used. If the injection is given in the superotemporal quadrant (the preferred location), the upper eyelid is retracted and the patient is instructed to look down and nasally. After anesthesia is applied with a cotton swab soaked in proparacaine or tetra-

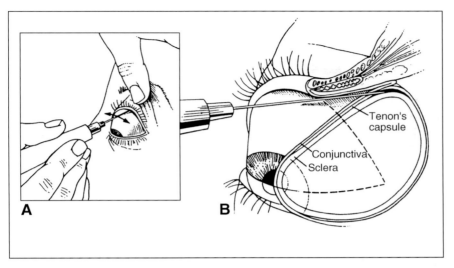

Figure 6-8 Posterior sub-Tenon's injection. **A,** The correct position of the operator's hands and the needle. The *arrows* indicate the direction of the side-to-side circumferential motion (here exaggerated for emphasis). **B,** The positioning of the tip of the needle in its ideal location between Tenon's capsule and the sclera. *(Reproduced with permission from Smith RE, Nozik RA.* Uveitis: A Clinical Approach to Diagnosis and Management. *2nd ed. Baltimore: Williams & Wilkins; 1989.)*

caine, the needle is placed bevel-down against the sclera and advanced through the conjunctiva and Tenon's capsule using a side-to-side movement, which allows the physician to determine whether the needle has entered the sclera or not. As long as the globe does not torque with the side-to-side movement of the needle, the physician can be reasonably sure that the needle has not penetrated the sclera. Once the needle has been advanced to the hub, the corticosteroid is injected into the sub-Tenon's space. Complications of the superotemporal approach include upper lid ptosis, periorbital hemorrhage, and globe perforation.

Although sub-Tenon's injections are typically given in the superotemporal quadrant, the inferotemporal approach can also be performed in a similar fashion. Generally, however, the inferior approach using the Nozik technique can be awkward to perform. The transseptal route of delivery is preferred for the inferior approach and is performed by using a short 27-gauge needle usually on a 3-cc syringe containing the drug (Fig 6-9). The index finger may be used to push the temporal lower lid posteriorly and locate the equator of the globe. The needle is inserted inferior to the globe through the skin of the eyelid, directed straight posteriorly through the orbital septum into the orbital fat to the hub of the needle. The needle is aspirated, and if there is no blood reflux, the corticosteroid is injected. Complications of the inferior approach can include periorbital and retrobulbar hemorrhage, lower lid retractor ptosis, orbital fat prolapse with periorbital festoon formation, orbital fat atrophy, and skin discoloration. This transseptal approach can be more painful to perform than the sub-Tenon's injection if a 25-gauge needle is used; pain can be minimized with a 27-gauge needle.

Periocular injections should not be used in cases of infectious uveitis (eg, toxoplasmosis) and should also be avoided in patients with necrotizing scleritis, because scleral

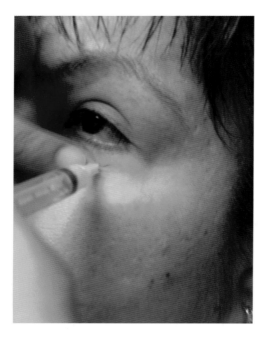

Figure 6-9 Inferior transseptal injection of triamcinolone acetonide (Kenalog) in the left eye of a patient with HLA-B27–associated anterior uveitis. A 27-gauge, ¹/₂″ needle on a 3-mL syringe is inserted through the skin of the lower eyelid and the inferior orbital septum. (The finger position was changed for photographic purposes.) By using the index finger of the opposite hand, the physician can determine the location of the equator of the globe to prevent perforation and to place the depot corticosteroid as posteriorly as possible. *(Courtesy of Ramana S. Moorthy, MD.)*

thinning and possible perforation may result. The physician should be aware that periocular corticosteroid injections have the potential to raise the IOP precipitously or for a long time, particularly with the longer-acting agents (triamcinolone or methylprednisolone).

Systemic administration

Oral or *intravenous* therapy may supplement or replace other routes of administration. Systemic corticosteroids are used for vision-threatening chronic uveitis when topical corticosteroids are insufficient or when the systemic disease also requires therapy. Many oral corticosteroid formulations are available; prednisone is the most commonly used. If systemic corticosteroids are used, the dosing and taper must be appropriate. The readily available dose packages of methylprednisolone that are used over a period of 1 week or less have little or no role in the treatment of uveitis. Duration of treatment with corticosteroids may last for 3 months. If corticosteroid therapy is required for longer than 3 months, immunomodulatory therapy is indicated.

Most patients require 1–2 mg/kg/day of oral prednisone, which is tapered in a gradual fashion every 1 to 2 weeks until the disease is quiescent. The lowest possible dose that will control the ocular inflammation and minimize side effects is desired. This dose should be 5–10 mg or less per day. If a dose greater than 10 mg/day is required, corticosteroid-sparing immunomodulatory therapy must be used.

In cases of an explosive onset of severe noninfectious posterior uveitis or panuveitis, intravenous, high-dose, pulse methylprednisolone (1 gm/day infused over 1 hour) therapy may be administered for 3 days, followed by a gradual taper of oral prednisone starting at 1.0–1.5 mg/kg day. Although this approach may control intraocular inflammation, side effects are numerous and can be life-threatening. These include psychological disturbances, hypertension, and elevated glucose levels. This form of therapy should be performed in a hospital setting by those experienced with this approach and its side effects.

Reed JB, Morse LS, Schwab IR. High-dose intravenous pulse methylprednisolone hemisuc-cinate in acute Behçet retinitis. *Am J Ophthalmol.* 1998;125:409–411.

Sasamoto Y, Ohno S, Matsuda H. Studies on corticosteroid therapy in Vogt-Koyanagi-Harada disease. *Ophthalmologica.* 1990;201:162–167.

Wakefield D, Jennings A, McCluskey PJ. Intravenous pulse methylprednisolone in the treatment of uveitis associated with multiple sclerosis. *Clin Experiment Ophthalmol.* 2000;28:103–106.

Wakefield D, McCluskey P, Penny R. Intravenous pulse methylprednisolone therapy in severe inflammatory eye disease. *Arch Ophthalmol.* 1986;104:847–851.

The many side effects of both short- and long-term corticosteroids must be discussed with patients, and their general health must be closely monitored, often with the assistance of an internist. Patients with a propensity toward or who have manifest diabetes mellitus; patients with hypertension, peptic ulcer, or gastroesophageal reflux disease; patients who are immunocompromised (from acquired or congenital causes); and patients with psychiatric conditions are at high risk for corticosteroid-induced exacerbations of their systemic conditions. Corticosteroids should be avoided, if at all possible, in these patients.

Patients on high-dose oral corticosteroids should be placed on histamine-2 receptor blockers or proton pump inhibitors to prevent gastric and peptic ulcer. The risk of gastric ulcer is particularly high in patients who are concomitantly taking systemic nonsteroidal anti-inflammatory medications. Patients maintained on long-term corticosteroid therapy, particularly elderly patients and postmenopausal women, should supplement their diet with calcium and vitamin D to lessen the chances of osteoporosis. The following tests may be used to evaluate patients at risk for corticosteroid-induced bone loss:

- serial height measurements
- serum calcium and phosphorus levels
- serum 25-hydroxycholecalciferol levels (if vitamin D stores are uncertain)
- follicle-stimulating hormone and testosterone levels (if gonadal status is uncertain)
- bone mineral density screening for anyone receiving corticosteroid therapy for more than 3 months

The FDA has approved the use of alendronate for prevention and treatment of corticosteroid-induced osteoporosis in men and women. This may be administered to at-risk patients receiving 7.5 mg or more of daily prednisone equivalent.

Niewoehner CB, Niewoehner DE. Steroid-induced osteoporosis. Are your asthmatic patients at risk? *Postgrad Med.* 1999;105:79–83, 87–88, 91. (Accessed online.)

Intravitreal administration

A more recent mode of therapy is the use of intravitreal corticosteroids. These can be administered by injection or by implantation of a sustained-release device.

Intravitreal injections of triamcinolone acetonide (Kenalog) have been used extensively in the treatment of uveitic conditions. Published literature on intravitreal triamcinolone suggests a definite treatment benefit, although of limited duration, for recalcitrant uveitic CME. Little is known about the efficacy of intravitreal triamcinolone injections for the treatment of chronic uveitis.

Single trans–pars plana intravitreal injections of 4 mg (0.1 cc) of triamcinolone may produce sustained visual acuity improvements for 6 months or more. Cystoid macular edema may relapse after 3 to 6 months. Multiple injections increase the risk of cataract formation in phakic patients, and intraocular pressure elevation may occur transiently in more than one half of patients. Up to 25% of patients may require topical medications to control IOP, and 1%–2% may require filtering surgery. Complications such as sterile "endophthalmitis" may occur in up to 1% of patients and require intensive corticosteroid therapy. Infectious endophthalmitis and rhegmatogenous retinal detachment may occur, but these are rare when proper technique is used. Long-term clinical efficacy and outcome studies are under way. This method of treatment is not curative of chronic uveitic conditions and should be used judiciously as its effects are relatively short-lived.

The sustained-release fluocinolone implant has been approved by the FDA for the treatment of chronic noninfectious posterior uveitis. Two phase 3 studies have shown that the 0.59-mg implant or the 2.1-mg implant releases drug for a median period of 30 months. Inflammation was well controlled in nearly all eyes, with no recurrences in any of the eyes in the pilot trial. The pilot study demonstrated that nearly 70% of implanted eyes required less local and systemic corticosteroid and immunomodulatory therapy. However, nearly all phakic eyes developed cataract within the first 2 years after implantation. Glaucoma necessitating topical therapy developed in nearly 60% of patients after 2 years, and 30% required filtering surgery. Complications such as endophthalmitis, wound leaks, hypotony, vitreous hemorrhage, and retinal detachments have been reported. Again, this method of treatment provides control of inflammation for 2–3 years but is not curative of chronic uveitis.

A new biodegradable intraocular implant containing 350 or 700 mcg of dexamethasone is currently under active investigation for the treatment of uveitis. The duration of action of this implant is about 6 months, and it can be implanted without the need for vitrectomy.

Androudi S, Letko E, Meniconi M, Papadaki T, Ahmed M, Foster CS. Safety and efficacy of intravitreal triamcinolone acetonide for uveitic macular edema. *Ocul Immunol Inflamm.* 2005;13:205–212.

Antcliff RJ, Spalton DJ, Stanford MR, Graham EM, ffytche TJ, Marshall J. Intravitreal triamcinolone for uveitic cystoid macular edema: an optical coherence tomography study. *Ophthalmology.* 2001;108:765–772.

Jaffe GJ, McCallum RM, Branchaud B, Skalak C, Butuner Z, Ashton P. Long-term follow-up results of a pilot trial of a fluocinolone acetonide implant to treat posterior uveitis. *Ophthalmology.* 2005;112:1192–1198.

Immunomodulatory Agents

Immunomodulatory medications

The addition of immunomodulatory (sometimes referred to as "immunosuppressive") medications may greatly benefit patients with severe sight-threatening uveitis or patients who are resistant to or intolerant of corticosteroids. These agents are thought to work by killing the rapidly dividing clones of lymphocytes that are responsible for the inflammation (see Part I, Immunology). As more evidence accumulates about the complications of long-term systemic corticosteroid use, immunomodulatory agents are being used with increasing frequency as corticosteroid-sparing agents. Although the early use of immuno-modulatory agents is indicated in certain diseases (see the following section), these drugs should also be considered in patients who require chronic corticosteroid therapy (longer than 3 months) at doses greater than 5–10 mg/day. The use of immunomodulatory agents can also be considered in patients with chronic topical corticosteroid dependence and patients requiring multiple periocular corticosteroid injections.

Indications The following indications generally apply to the therapeutic use of immuno-modulatory agents in uveitis:

- vision-threatening intraocular inflammation
- reversibility of the disease process
- inadequate response to corticosteroid treatment
  —failure of therapy
- contraindication of corticosteroid treatment because of systemic problems or intol-erable side effects
  —unacceptable corticosteroid side effects
  —chronic corticosteroid dependence

Corticosteroids are the mainstay of initial therapy, but certain specific uveitis enti-ties also warrant the early use of immunomodulatory agents for treatment of intraocular inflammation, including Adamantiades-Behçet syndrome, sympathetic ophthalmia, VKH disease, and necrotizing sclerouveitis. Although these disorders may initially respond well to corticosteroids, the initial treatment of these entities with immunomodulatory agents has been shown to improve the long-term prognosis and to lessen visual morbidity.

Relative indications for these agents include conditions that are initially treated with corticosteroids but do not respond adequately and patients who develop serious cortico-steroid-induced side effects. Examples in this category include intermediate uveitis (pars planitis), retinal vasculitis, panuveitis, and chronic iridocyclitis.

Treatment Before initiating therapy with any immunomodulatory agent, the physician should ensure that there is

- absence of infection
- absence of hepatic and hematologic contraindications
- meticulous follow-up by a physician who is, by virtue of training and experience, qualified to prescribe and safety monitor such medications and personally manage their potential toxicities
- objective longitudinal evaluation of the disease process
- informed consent

Several classes of immunomodulatory medications exist. These include antimetabo-lites, inhibitors of T-lymphocyte signaling, alkylating agents, and biologic response modi-fiers. These agents are listed in Table 6-17, along with their mechanisms of action, dosages, and potential complications. It should be noted that no therapeutic response may occur for several weeks after initiation of immunomodulatory therapy; therefore, most patients

Table 6-17 Immunomodulatory Medications in the Treatment of Uveitis

Medication	Mechanism of Action	Dosage	Potential Complications
Antimetabolites			
Methotrexate	Folate analog; inhibits dihydrofolate reductase	7.5–25.0 µg/wk PO or SQ	GI upset, fatigue, hepatotoxicity, pneumonitis
Azathioprine	Alters purine metabolism	100–250 mg/d PO	GI upset, hepatotoxicity
Mycophenolate mofetil	Inhibits purine synthesis	1–3 g/d PO	Diarrhea, nausea, GI ulceration
Alkylating agents			
Cyclophosphamide	Cross-links DNA	1–2 mg/d PO	Hemorrhagic cystitis, sterility, increased risk of malignancy
Chlorambucil	Cross-links DNA	2–12 mg/d PO	Sterility, increased risk of malignancy
Inhibitors of T-lymphocyte signaling			
Cyclosporine	Inhibits NF-AT (nuclear factor of activated T lymphocytes) activation	2.5–5.0 mg/kg/d PO	Nephrotoxicity, hypertension, gingival hyperplasia, GI upset, paresthesias
Tacrolimus	Inhibits NF-AT activation	0.1–0.2 mg/kg/d PO	Nephrotoxicity, hypertension, diabetes mellitus
Sirolimus*	Inhibits T-lymphocyte activation in G1 Blunts T- and B- lymphocyte responses to lymphokines	6 mg loading dose IV and then 4 mg/d IV increasing by 2-mg increments	Gastrointestinal, cutaneous at trough levels of >25 ng/mL
Biologic response modifiers			
Etanercept	TNF-α receptor blocker	0.4 mg/kg twice weekly SQ given 72–96 hours apart (max dose 25 mg)	Injection site reactions, infections (upper respiratory) Malignancies
Infliximab	TNF-α inhibitor	3 mg/kg IV week 0, 2, 6 and then q 6–8 weeks	Infusion reactions, infections (TB reactivation) Malignancy/ lymphoproliferative diseases Autoantibodies/lupuslike syndrome Congestive heart failure
Adalimumab*	TNF-α inhibitor	40 mg q 1 week or q 2 weeks	Headache, nausea, rash, stomach upset
Daclizumab*	Binds the alpha subunit of IL-2 receptor	1.0 mg/kg IV q 2 weeks × 5 doses	Rare if any; efficacy in uveitis not well studied
Efalizumab*	Binds CD11a, the alpha subunit of LFA-1	0.7 mg/kg SQ q week and then 1 mg/kg weekly (to max 200 mg) SQ	Headaches, fever, nausea, vomiting
Alefacept*	Binds to CD2 on T lymphocytes	15 mg IM or IV q week	Flulike symptoms

* Still under investigation.

need to be maintained on corticosteroid therapy until the immunomodulatory agent begins to take effect, at which time the corticosteroid dose may be gradually tapered.

Because of the potentially serious complications associated with the use of immunomodulatory medications, patients must be monitored closely by a practitioner who is experienced with them. Regular blood monitoring, including complete blood count and liver and renal function tests, should be performed. Serious complications include renal and hepatic toxicity, bone marrow suppression, and increased susceptibility to infection. In addition, the alkylating agents may cause sterility and have been associated with an increased risk of future malignancies such as leukemia or lymphoma. Trimethoprim/sulfamethoxazole prophylaxis against *Pneumocystis carinii* should be considered in patients receiving alkylating agents. The physician should obtain informed consent prior to beginning therapy.

Although these agents may be associated with serious life-threatening complications, they can be extremely effective in the treatment of ocular inflammatory disease in patients unresponsive to, or intolerant of, systemic corticosteroids. All of these agents are potentially teratogenic, and patients should be advised to refrain from becoming pregnant while on them. Again, the physician should obtain informed consent prior to beginning therapy.

Antimetabolites The antimetabolites include azathioprine, methotrexate, and mycophenolate mofetil. *Azathioprine (AZA),* a purine nucleoside analog, interferes with DNA replication and RNA transcription. It is well absorbed orally and, in a randomized, placebo-controlled trial, has been shown to be effective in preventing ocular involvement among those without eye disease and in decreasing the occurrence of contralateral eye involvement among those with unilateral Adamantiades-Behçet uveitis. It has also been found beneficial in patients with intermediate uveitis, VKH disease, sympathetic ophthalmia, and necrotizing scleritis. It is administered at a dose of 2 mg/kg/day. Many clinicians start administering the drug at 50 mg/day for 1 week to see if the patient develops any gastrointestinal side effects such as nausea, upset stomach, and vomiting before escalating the dose. These symptoms are common and may occur in up to 25% of patients, necessitating a discontinuation. Bone marrow suppression is unusual in doses used to treat uveitis. Reversible hepatic toxicity occurs in less than 2% of patients. Dose reduction may remedy mild hepatotoxicity. Complete blood counts and liver function tests must be obtained every 4–6 weeks. The variability of clinical response to azathioprine among patients is probably due to genetic variability in the activity of thiopurine S-methyltransferase (TPMT), an enzyme responsible for the metabolism of 6-mercaptopurine (6-MP). A genotypic test is now becoming available that can help determine patient candidacy for AZA/6-MP therapy before treatment and can help clinicians individualize patient dose. Evaluation of TPMT activity has revealed 3 groups of patients:

1. low/no TPMT enzyme activity (0.3% of patients); azathioprine therapy not recommended
2. intermediate TPMT enzyme activity (11% of patients); azathioprine therapy at reduced dosage

3. normal/high TPMT enzyme activity (89% of patients); azathioprine therapy at higher doses than in patients with intermediate TPMT activity

Methotrexate, a folic acid analog and inhibitor of dihydrofolate reductase, inhibits DNA replication. Numerous studies have shown methotrexate to be effective in treating various types of uveitis, including JRA/JIA-associated iridocyclitis, sarcoidosis, panuveitis, and scleritis. Treatment with this medication is unique in that it is given as a *weekly* dose, usually starting at 7.5–10.0 mg/week and gradually increasing to a maintenance dose of 15–25 mg/week. Methotrexate can be given orally, subcutaneously, intramuscularly, or intravenously and is usually well tolerated. It has greater bioavailability when given parenterally. Folate is given concurrently at a dose of 1 mg/day to reduce side effects. The full effect of methotrexate on controlling intraocular inflammation may take 6–8 weeks or longer. Gastrointestinal distress and anorexia may occur in 10% of patients. Reversible hepatotoxicity occurs in up to 15% of patients, and cirrhosis occurs in less than 0.1% of patients receiving long-term methotrexate. Methotrexate is teratogenic, and complete blood counts and liver function tests should be obtained every 4–6 weeks to monitor for side effects. The drug has a long record of success in the treatment of children with JRA/JIA. For that reason, it has been a first-line choice for immunomodulation in children. Uncontrolled clinical trials have shown that it can be corticosteroid-sparing in two thirds of patients with chronic ocular inflammatory disorders.

Mycophenolate mofetil inhibits both inosine monophosphate dehydrogenase and DNA replication. It has good oral bioavailability and is given at a dose of 1 gm twice daily. Reversible gastrointestinal distress and diarrhea are common side effects, although less than 20% of patients receiving mycophenolate do have side effects. These can usually be managed by dose reduction. Very few patients find the drug intolerable. Complete blood counts should be performed every week for 1 month, then every 2 weeks for 2 months, and then monthly. Mycophenolate mofetil has been found in uncontrolled studies to be an effective corticosteroid-sparing agent in up to two thirds of patients with chronic uveitis. Its side effect profile makes it a reasonable first choice for immunomodulation.

Inhibitors of T-lymphocyte signaling The T-lymphocyte inhibitors include cyclosporine, tacrolimus, and sirolimus. *Cyclosporine,* a macrolide product of the fungus *Hypocladium inflatum gams,* inhibits T-lymphocyte proliferation by blocking production of cytokines, especially interleukin-2 (IL-2). The most likely mechanism for this inhibition is interference with signaling from the T-lymphocyte receptor to genes that code for the various lymphokines and other substances (such as IL-2) that are necessary for T-lymphocyte activation. Cyclosporine preferentially inhibits the T helper-inducer and cytotoxic subsets, with minimal effects on regulatory (suppressor) T lymphocytes. It is available in 2 oral preparations. One is a microemulsion (Neoral), with better bioavailability than the other, gel capsules (Sandimmune). These 2 drugs are not bioequivalent formulations. Neoral is begun at 2 mg/kg/day and Sandimmune at 2.5 mg/kg/day. The dose is adjusted based on toxicity and clinical response between a range of 1 mg/kg/day and 5 mg/kg/day. The main potential toxicities are systemic hypertension and nephrotoxicity. Additional side effects include paresthesia, gastrointestinal upset, fatigue, hypertrichosis, and gingival hyperplasia. Monthly blood pressure, serum creatinine levels, and complete blood counts are used to monitor patients on cyclosporine. If the serum creatinine rises by 30%, dose adjustment is required. Sustained elevation of serum creatinine levels will require a drug holiday until creatinine levels return to baseline. It is usually not necessary to check drug levels unless there is a concern about compliance or absorption. Patients with psoriasis who are treated with cyclosporine appear to be at greater risk of primary skin cancers. Cyclosporine has been shown to be effective in randomized, controlled clinical trials for the treatment of Adamantiades-Behçet uveitis, with control of inflammation in 50% of patients. However, the dose used in this study was 10 mg/kg/day, substantially higher than what is used now (5 mg/kg/day), and led to substantial nephrotoxicity. Cyclosporine has also been shown to be effective in the treatment of intermediate uveitis and several types of posterior uveitis, including Adamantiades-Behçet syndrome and VKH disease.

Tacrolimus is a close relative of cyclosporine. It is a 10-amino-acid polypeptide immunomodulatory product of *Streptomyces tsukubaensis*. It is also a potent cytokine inhibitor and directly interferes with helper T-lymphocyte proliferation. It is given in oral doses of 0.10–0.15 mg/kg/day. Because of its lower dose and increased potency, its main side effect, nephrotoxicity, is less common than it is with cyclosporine. Serum creatinine and complete blood counts are monitored monthly. A prospective trial of cyclosporine and tacrolimus suggested equal efficacy in controlling chronic posterior and intermediate uveitis, with tacrolimus demonstrating greater safety with less risk of hypertension.

Sirolimus, also a macrolide antibiotic, was discovered in the soil of Easter Island; it is an antifungal agent produced by *Streptomyces hygroscopicus*. Despite its similarities to tacrolimus, its mechanism of action is different. Sirolimus blunts the responses of both T lymphocytes and B lymphocytes to specific lymphokines in the G1 phase of the cell cycle rather than inhibiting their production. Synergistic effects among sirolimus, tacrolimus, and cyclosporine A are found in animal models. Such effects may provide an avenue of highly effective treatment while minimizing dose-related toxicity. In 1 open-label prospective study, sirolimus was found to be effective in reducing or eliminating the need for systemic corticosteroids in patients with refractory noninfectious uveitis. Gastrointestinal and cutaneous side effects were common and dose-dependent. Most cases occurred at trough blood levels above 25 ng/mL. The drug is still under active investigation for the treatment of uveitis.

Alkylating agents Alkylating agents include cyclophosphamide and chlorambucil. Alkylating agents are at the top of the therapeutic stepladder and are used if the other immunomodulators fail to control uveitis; they are also used as first-line therapy for necrotizing scleritis associated with systemic vasculitides such as Wegener granulomatosis or relapsing polychondritis. They have been found beneficial as well in patients with intermediate uveitis, VKH disease, sympathetic ophthalmia, and Adamantiades-Behçet disease. The most worrisome side effect of alkylating agents is an increased risk of malignancy. In the doses used for the treatment of uveitis, the risk is probably low, but this is controversial. Patients with polycythemia rubra vera treated with chlorambucil had a 13.5-fold greater risk of leukemia. Patients with Wegener granulomatosis treated with cyclophosphamide had a 2.4-fold increased risk of cancer and a 33-fold increased risk of bladder cancer.

Therefore, these drugs should be used with great caution and only by those experienced in the management of their dosing and potential toxicity. Patients may wish to consider sperm or embryo banking prior to beginning cyclophosphamide or chlorambucil therapy because of the high rate of sterility if the cumulative dose exceeds certain limits.

Cyclophosphamide is an alkylating agent whose active metabolites alkylate purines in DNA and RNA, resulting in impaired DNA replication and cell death. Cyclophosphamide is cytotoxic to resting and actively dividing lymphocytes. It is absorbed orally and hepatically metabolized in the liver into its active metabolites. It is probably more effective in controlling ocular inflammation when given orally at a dose of 2 mg/kg/day than when given as intermittent intravenous pulses. Most patients are treated for 1 year and the dose is adjusted to maintain the leukocyte counts between 3000 and 4000 cells/μL after the patient has been tapered off corticosteroids. After 1 year of disease quiescence, cyclophosphamide is slowly tapered off. Myelosuppression and hemorrhagic cystitis are the most common side effects. Hemorrhagic cystitis is more common when cyclophosphamide is administered orally. Patients must be encouraged to drink more than 2 liters of fluid per day while on this regimen. Complete blood count and urinalysis are monitored weekly to monthly. Microscopic hematuria is a warning to increase hydration. Gross hematuria is an indication to discontinue therapy. If white cell counts fall below 2500/μL, cyclophosphamide should be discontinued until the counts recover. Other toxicities include teratogenicity, sterility, and reversible alopecia. Oppportunistic infections such as pneumocystis pneumonia occur more commonly in patients who are receiving cyclophosphamide. Trimethoprim-sulfamethoxazole prophylaxis is recommended for these patients. Cyclophosphamide has been shown to be effective in treating necrotizing scleritis and retinal vasculitis and other uveitic conditions in uncontrolled case series.

Chlorambucil is a very long acting alkylating agent that also interferes with DNA replication. It is absorbed well when administered orally. The drug is traditionally given as a single daily dose of 0.1–0.2 mg/kg. It may also be administered as short-term high-dose therapy, with an initial dose of 2 mg/day for 1 week, followed by an increase to 2 mg/day for each subsequent week until the inflammation is suppressed or the leukocyte count falls to below 2000 cells/μL, or the platelet count drops below 100,000/μL. Short-term therapy is continued for 3–6 months. Concurrent oral corticosteroids may be tapered and discontinued once ocular inflammation becomes inactive. Because it is myelosuppressive, complete blood counts should be obtained weekly. Chlorambucil is also teratogenic and causes sterility. Uncontrolled case series suggest that chlorambucil is effective in providing long-term drug-free remissions in 66%–75% of patients with sympathetic ophthalmia, Adamantiades-Behçet syndrome, and other sight-threatening uveitis syndromes.

Biologic response modifiers Inflammation is driven by a complex series of cell–cell and cell–cytokine interactions. Inhibitors of various cytokines may play an important therapeutic role in the future management of uveitis patients, as these drugs result in targeted immunomodulation, thereby theoretically reducing systemic side effects that are common with the previously discussed immunomodulatory agents. Drugs that inhibit cytokines have been labeled *biologic response modifiers*. Etanercept and infliximab are biologics that inhibit the action of tumor necrosis factor α (TNF-α) and have changed the management of some uveitis entities. TNF-α is believed to play a major role in the pathogenesis of

JRA/JIA, ankylosing spondylitis, and other spondyloarthropathies. Another biologic, daclizumab, is a humanized monoclonal antibody to the IL-2 receptor. It has been used for prevention of transplant rejection and for treatment of recalcitrant uveitis.

Etanercept, a dimeric fusion protein with the extracellular ligand-binding portion of the human 75 kDa (p75) TNF receptor linked to the Fc portions of human IgG1, thus allowing it to function as a TNF receptor blocker, has been proven effective in controlling joint inflammation in polyarticular JRA/JIA and adult rheumatoid arthritis. It appears to have mixed results in the treatment of iridocyclitis associated with these conditions. Some reports show a positive treatment effect, whereas 2 double-masked, placebo-controlled trials showed no effect in controlling active inflammation or in allowing the taper of other immunomodulators in previously well-controlled patients.

Infliximab, a monoclonal IgG1κ antibody directed against TNF-α, appears more promising. Initial and subsequent reports of its use in Adamantiades-Behçet uveitis suggest that it is effective in modulating current inflammation and decreasing the likelihood of future attacks. It has a corticosteroid-sparing effect and appears to have a favorable effect on the visual prognosis of patients with recalcitrant Adamantiades-Behçet uveitis. Similar favorable effects have been reported in patients with HLA-B27–associated anterior uveitis who have been treated with infliximab. However, in one recent study, although 78% of patients achieved successful control of inflammation at 10 weeks, nearly half of patients could not complete the 50 weeks of therapy due to drug-induced toxicity, such as drug-induced lupus, systemic vascular thromboses, congestive heart failure, new malignancy, and vitreous hemorrhage. As many as 75% of patients receiving more than 3 infusions developed antinuclear antibodies. It is unclear how many of these side effects are directly related to infliximab. Low-dose methotrexate (5–7.5 mg/week) may be administered concomitantly to reduce the risk of drug-induced lupus syndrome. Also, reports have clearly shown that some patients with unknown, inactive, post-primary tuberculosis treated with infliximab subsequently developed disseminated tuberculosis. Thus, a positive purified protein derivative (PPD) skin test is considered a contraindication for infliximab therapy.

Daclizumab has been shown in uncontrolled studies to be effective in controlling active chronic uveitis and in enabling discontinuation of other immunomodulators.

Efalizumab is a humanized, monoclonal antibody to CD11a, the alpha subunit of LFA-1. LFA-1 is a protein that functions in antigen presentation and in the adhesion of T lymphocytes to vascular endothelial cells as well as to keratinocytes—in this latter case, through the ability of LFA-1 to bind to the protein ICAM-1, which is present on the surface. It is still under investigation for treatment of uveitis.

Alefacept is a recombinant, fully human LFA-3/IgG1 fusion protein that binds to CD2 on T lymphocytes and functions to block the CD2/LFA-3 costimulatory signal for CD45 RO[+] memory effector T-lymphocyte activation. Alefacept also depletes the pool of activated T lymphocytes by enabling natural killer cells to bind to them, an interaction mediated by the Fc region of the bound fusion protein. It is this T-lymphocyte–depleting activity that explains the remittent function of Alefacept—namely, that patients continue to experience clinical improvement after therapy has ended. Alefacept has been shown to have efficacy against psoriatic arthritis. It is under active investigation as a possible treatment for uveitis.

Adalimumab, a fully human monoclonal antibody directed against TNF-α, has recently been shown to be effective in the treatment of psoriatic arthritis. It is also under active investigation for the treatment of uveitis.

These biologics should be used only when other immunomodulators have failed or are not well tolerated. Etanercept is usually administered at home in weekly or biweekly subcutaneous injections. Infliximab is administered in the form of intravenous infusions every 4–8 weeks in an office or hospital setting. Infusions are given on day 0, at 2 weeks, at 6 weeks, and then every 6–8 weeks thereafter. These therapies should be initiated with the help of a rheumatologist or internist.

Small studies have shown interferon α-2a and b (IFN-α2a/b) and intravenous immuno-globulin to be beneficial in some patients with uveitis. IFN-α2a seems to be an alternative to anti-TNF drugs. It has antiviral, immunomodulatory, and antiangiogenic effects. Recent reports in the European literature seem to emphasize the efficacy and good tolerance of IFN-α2a in patients with Adamantiades-Behçet disease. Initial dosage (doses ranging from 3 to 6 million units per injection and daily vs 3 times-a-week regimen), as well as the duration of IFN-α2a administration need to be better determined. Efficacy usually becomes obvious from 3 to 8 weeks after initiation. A flulike syndrome has been observed most frequently during the first weeks of therapy but may be improved by prophylactic administration of acetominophen. Despite the use of low interferon doses, leukopenia or thrombocytopenia may occur. Depression is another important side effect of interferon therapy.

Braun J, Baraliakos X, Listing J, Sieper J. Decreased incidence of anterior uveitis in patients with ankylosing spondylitis treated with the anti-tumor necrosis factor agents infliximab and etanercept. *Arthritis Rheum.* 2005;52:2447–2451.

Feron EJ, Rothova A, van Hagen PM, Baarsma GS, Suttorp-Schulten MS. Interferon-alpha 2b for refractory ocular Behçet's disease. *Lancet.* 1994;343:1428.

Foster CS, Tufail F, Waheed NK, et al. Efficacy of etanercept in preventing relapse of uveitis controlled by methotrexate. *Arch Ophthalmol.* 2003;121:437–440.

Goldstein DA, Fontanilla FA, Kaul S, Sahin O, Tessler HH. Long-term follow-up of patients treated with short-term high-dose chlorambucil for sight-threatening ocular inflammation. *Ophthalmology.* 2002;109:370–377.

Jabs DA, Akpek EK. Immunosuppression for posterior uveitis. *Retina.* 2005;25:1–18.

Jabs DA, Rosenbaum JT, Foster CS, et al. Guidelines for the use of immunosuppressive drugs in patients with ocular inflammatory disorders: recommendations of an expert panel. *Am J Ophthalmol.* 2000;130:492–513.

Kotter I, Zierhut M, Eckstein AK, et al. Human recombinant interferon alfa-2a for the treatment of Behçet's disease with sight threatening posterior or panuveitis. *Br J Ophthalmol.* 2003;87:423–431.

Malik AR, Pavesio C. The use of low dose methotrexate in children with chronic anterior and intermediate uveitis. *Br J Ophthalmol.* 2005;89:806–808.

Miserocchi E, Baltatzis S, Ekong A, Roque M, Foster CS. Efficacy and safety of chlorambucil in intractable noninfectious uveitis: the Massachusetts Eye and Ear Infirmary experience. *Ophthalmology.* 2002;109:137–142.

Murphy CC, Greiner K, Plskova J, et al. Cyclosporine vs tacrolimus therapy for posterior and intermediate uveitis. *Arch Ophthalmol.* 2005;123:634–641.

Papaliodis GN, Chu D, Foster CS. Treatment of ocular inflammatory disorders with daclizumab. *Ophthalmology.* 2003;110:786–789.

Reiff A, Takei S, Sadeghi S, et al. Etanercept therapy in children with treatment-resistant uveitis. *Arthritis Rheum.* 2001;44:1411–1415.

Samson CM, Waheed N, Baltatzis S, Foster CS. Methotrexate therapy for chronic noninfectious uveitis: analysis of a case series of 160 patients. *Ophthalmology.* 2001;108:1134–1139.

Schmeling H, Horneff G. Etanercept and uveitis in patients with juvenile idiopathic arthritis. *Rheumatology (Oxford).* 2005;44:1008–1011.

Sfikakis PP, Theodossiadis PG, Katsiari CG, Kaklamanis P, Markomichelakis NN. Effect of infliximab on sight-threatening panuveitis in Behçet's disease. *Lancet.* 2001;358:295–296.

Shanmuganathan VA, Casely EM, Raj D, et al. The efficacy of sirolimus in the treatment of patients with refractory uveitis. *Br J Ophthalmol.* 2005;89:666–669.

Smith JA, Thompson DJ, Whitcup SM, et al. A randomized, placebo-controlled, double-masked clinical trial of etanercept for the treatment of uveitis associated with juvenile idiopathic arthritis. *Arthritis Rheum.* 2005;53:18–23.

Smith JR, Levinson RD, Holland GN, et al. Differential efficacy of tumor necrosis factor inhibition in the management of inflammatory eye disease and associated rheumatic disease. *Arthritis Rheum.* 2001;45:252–257.

Smith JR, Rosenbaum JT. Management of uveitis: a rheumatologic perspective. *Arthritis Rheum.* 2002;46:309–318.

Suhler EB, Smith JR, Wertheim MS, et al. A prospective trial of infliximab therapy for refractory uveitis. Preliminary safety and efficacy outcomes. *Arch Ophthalmol.* 2005;123:903–912.

Thorne JE, Jabs DA, Qazi FA, Nguyen QD, Kempen JH, Dunn JP. Mycophenolate mofetil therapy for inflammatory eye disease. *Ophthalmology.* 2005;112:1472–1477.

Tugal-Tutkun I, Mudun A, Urgancioglu M, et al. Efficacy of infliximab in the treatment of uveitis that is resistant to treatment with the combination of azathioprine, cyclosporine, and corticosteroids in Behçet's disease: an open-label trial. *Arthritis Rheum.* 2005;52:2478–2484.

Vitale AT, Rodriguez A, Foster CS. Low-dose cyclosporin A therapy in treating chronic, noninfectious uveitis. *Ophthalmology.* 1996;103:365–373.

Surgical Management of Uveitis

Surgery is performed in uveitis patients for diagnostic and/or therapeutic reasons. Examination of intraocular fluids and tissues using microbiologic, histologic, and molecular techniques can be helpful in determining the etiology of uveitis. In fact, anytime a surgical procedure is performed on a uveitic eye, intraocular fluid and/or tissue samples should be obtained, especially if the etiology is unknown. Diagnostic procedures include paracentesis or vitreous and/or chorioretinal biopsy to rule out neoplastic or acute infectious processes. Therapeutic surgical procedures for complications of uveitis are discussed in Chapter 11. Therapeutic vitrectomy may be beneficial in cases of recalcitrant, visually significant vitritis or CME (or both) that have not responded to medical therapy. In addition, implantation of a sustained-release delivery system containing a corticosteroid or other immunomodulatory agent also requires limited pars plana vitrectomy in some cases.

Aqueous Paracentesis

Aqueous samples may be obtained for diagnostic purposes. Anterior chamber paracentesis may be performed using sterile techniques at the slit lamp or with the patient supine on a treatment gurney or chair. Topical anesthetic drops may be instilled. The eye is prepared with topical betadine solution, and a lid speculum is placed if the patient is supine. A tuberculin or 3-mL syringe is attached to a sterile 30-gauge needle, which is then advanced under direct or slit-lamp visualization into the anterior chamber through the temporal limbus or clear cornea parallel to the iris plane. As much aqueous is aspirated as is safely possible (usually 0.1–0.2 cc), avoiding the iris and lens. The needle is then withdrawn, and topical antibiotic drops are instilled.

The aqueous specimen may be processed for microbiologic evaluation, such as with a Gram stain, if infection is suspected. Histopathologic evaluation may be useful if leukemia/lymphoma is suspected, as in the case of a hypopyon/hyphema combination that may occur in acute myelogenous leukemic infiltration of the uveal tract. PCR evaluation may be useful if specific entities are suspected. Based on the available sample volume, the clinical appearance of the uveitis can often narrow the field of etiologies for which to test, making PCR testing highly specific. In Europe, aqueous and serum antibody levels may also be compared to generate Desmontes numbers (the ratio of aqueous to serum antibody levels). These ratios are used to confirm the suspected etiology of the uveitis.

The complications of aqueous paracentesis may include anterior chamber hemorrhage, endophthalmitis, and damage to iris or lens.

Pars Plana Vitrectomy

The techniques of pars plana vitrectomy are covered in BCSC Section 12, *Retina and Vitreous*. A standard 3-port pars plana vitrectomy may be performed for diagnostic and therapeutic purposes. The most common indications for diagnostic vitrectomy include cases in which endophthalmitis, primary intraocular lymphoma or other intraocular malignancy, or infectious etiologies of posterior uveitis or panuveitis are suspected. In addition, chronic uveitis, which has an atypical presentation, an inconclusive systemic workup, and an inadequate response to conventional therapy, may warrant a diagnostic vitrectomy. If the vitreous biopsy could potentially alter the management of uveitis, diagnostic vitrectomy may also be considered. Endophthalmitis is discussed in detail in Chapter 9. Intraocular lymphoma is discussed in Chapter 10. In all these scenarios, undiluted vitreous specimens are typically required for testing. It is possible to obtain 0.5–1.0 cc of undiluted vitreous for evaluation using standard vitrectomy techniques. PCR studies may also be performed on undiluted vitreous if an infectious posterior uveitis or panuveitis is suspected, but the differential must be narrowed to a few causes because "global" PCR testing, even if it were available, would be of little value. However, many different infectious causes may be detected by PCR (Table 6-18).

Therapeutic vitrectomy is performed in selected cases of uveitis to clear the visual axis of opacities or hemorrhage, remove epiretinal membranes, remove subfoveal choroidal neovascular membranes in selected cases, repair complex retinal detachments, reduce intravitreal cytokines and chemokines to help better control inflammation, and reduce CME. Meticulous attention is given to posterior hyaloid separation, thorough vitreous dissection, and removal to the edge of the vitreous base in eyes with uveitis.

Table 6-18 **Infectious Causes of Uveitis Detectable by PCR**

Viral
　Herpes simplex virus types 1, 2
　Varicella-zoster virus
　Cytomegalovirus
　Epstein-Barr virus

Parasitic
　Toxoplasma gondii
　Onchocerca volvulus

Bacterial
　Staphylococcus, Streptococcus, Pseudomonas, Bacillus, Neisseria spp
　Propionibacterium acnes
　Mycobacterium spp
　Borrelia burgdorferi
　Bartonella henselae
　Treponema pallidum
　Tropheryma whipelli

Fungal
　Candida albicans
　Aspergillus spp

Complications of vitrectomy in uveitic eyes can include retinal detachment, suprachoroidal hemorrhage, vitreous hemorrhage, worsening of cataract, worsening of inflammation, and retinal tears or detachment.

Chorioretinal Biopsy

Relentlessly progressive or rapidly progressive posterior uveitic or panuveitic entities, such as necrotizing retinitis, in which the etiology of the disease and thus therapeutic regimen is unknown, may require a chorioretinal biopsy. Suspected intraocular lymphoma confined to the subretinal space is also an indication for a chorioretinal biopsy. This procedure is performed only after all other, less invasive measures, such as serologic, radiologic, and aqueous and vitreous sample testing, have failed to make the diagnosis. It is associated with a high rate of complications and must be performed only by vitreoretinal surgeons with extensive experience with these techniques.

The biopsy may be performed in 3 different ways, depending on the clinical situation, location of the lesion, and the tissue required for diagnosis:

1. Ab interno subretinal aspiration

    a. Perform a pars plana vitrectomy.
    b. Make an incision of the retina over the subretinal deposit with a microvitreoretinal blade parallel to the nerve fiber layer.
    c. Manually aspirate the subretinal material through a silicone-tipped extrusion needle into a 3-cc syringe. Dilute the specimen to 0.5–1.0 cc with fluid from

the central vitreous cavity. Extrude the diluted specimen into a 1-cc collection vial.

    d. Perform an air–fluid exchange and laser photocoagulation around the biopsy site.

2. Ab interno retinal biopsy (posterior lesions)

    a. Perform a pars plana vitrectomy.

    b. Use diathermy to occlude the large vessels leading to the biopsy site.

    c. Make a retinal incision with vertical scissors to excise a 4 × 5-mm patch, leaving the patch attached by 1 corner. Manually aspirate through an 18-gauge needle into a 10-cc syringe and dilute to about 3 cc. Visually confirm specimen in the syringe.

    d. Remove the plunger from the syringe and empty the contents into a sterile Petri dish. Visually confirm the presence of the specimen in the dish.

    e. "Beach" the specimen on the dish by tilting the excess fluid away from it. Carefully aspirate the excess fluid, leaving the specimen isolated in the empty dish. Partition the specimen if necessary for culture. The excess fluid can also be cultured.

    f. Drop a small amount of fixative (usually formalin) onto the tissue and let it "fix" for a few minutes before transferring it to a fixative-filled container.

3. Ab externo chorioretinal biopsy (anterior lesions)

    a. Perform a 360° limbal peritomy. Isolate all 4 rectus muscles on sling sutures.

    b. Sew a Flieringa ring on the sclera, straddling the chosen biopsy site.

    c. Make a circular 90% depth scleral flap reflected anteriorly; the flap is usually at least 5 mm in diameter. Diathermize with a flat needle at the edge of the biopsy site and apply histoacryl glue to strengthen the tissue.

    d. Make an incision with an angled blade at the edge of the biopsy site. Elevate with forceps, holding on to the scleral remnant and glue layer, and transfer to a Petri dish.

    e. Partition the specimen as needed for various studies.

    f. Close the flap with 9-0 nylon. If the closure is not watertight, glue it.

    g. Examine the fundus.

    h. Perform a pars plana vitrectomy, inspect the site, and repair the retinal detachment, or perform the other indicated procedures.

Management of the biopsy specimen from any of these 3 methods is the same. The specimen should be from the margin of normal and inflamed tissue. It should be divided into 3 sections:

1. one frozen for immunopathologic testing if lymphoma is suspected
2. one placed in 4% gluteraldehyde for light and electron microscopic studies
3. one sent for culture, PCR, and microbiologic testing if infection is suspected

Chorioretinal biopsy entails numerous risks, including retinal detachment, cataract, vitreous hemorrhage, and decreased vision or loss of vision due to surgical complications.

The retinal detachment rate may be reduced with meticulous attention to vitreous removal and hyaloidal separation, a careful retinopexy around the biopsy site, and adequate intra-ocular tamponade. Finally, the biopsy may not be useful because of extensive necrosis and chorioretinal separation during fixation that makes pathologic interpretation difficult.

Laser treatment of retinal and choroidal neovascularization is discussed in detail in Chapter 11. Cryoretinopexy in the treatment of pars planitis is discussed in Chapter 7. Other surgical approaches are restorative and address a particular complication, such as cataract extraction or filtering surgery. See Chapter 11, Complications of Uveitis, for further discussion of surgery. See also the volumes of the BCSC that deal with these conditions in detail: Section 10, *Glaucoma;* Section 11, *Lens and Cataract;* and Section 12, *Retina and Vitreous.*

Diagnostic Survey for Uveitis (to be filled in by patient)

FAMILY HISTORY

These questions refer to your grandparents, parents, aunts, uncles, brothers and sisters, children, or grandchildren

Has anyone in your family ever had any of the following?

Cancer	Yes	No
Diabetes	Yes	No
Allergies	Yes	No
Arthritis or rheumatism	Yes	No
Syphilis	Yes	No
Tuberculosis	Yes	No
Sickle cell disease ot trait	Yes	No
Lyme disease	Yes	No
Gout	Yes	No

Has anyone in your family had medical problems in any of the following areas?

Eyes	Yes	No
Skin	Yes	No
Kidneys	Yes	No
Lungs	Yes	No
Stomach or bowel	Yes	No
Nervous system or brain	Yes	No

SOCIAL HISTORY

Age (years):   Current job:

Have you ever lived outside of the United States?	Yes	No
If yes, where?		
Have you ever owned a dog?	Yes	No
Have you ever owned a cat?	Yes	No
Have you ever eaten raw meet or uncooked sausage?	Yes	No
Have you ever had unpasteurized milk or cheese?	Yes	No
Have you ever been exposed to sick animals?	Yes	No
Do you drink untreated stream, well, or lake water?	Yes	No
Do you smoke cigarettes?	Yes	No
Have you ever used intravenous drugs?	Yes	No
Have you ever had bisexual or homosexual relationships?	Yes	No
Have you ever taken birth control pills?	Yes	No

PERSONAL MEDICAL HISTORY

Are you allergic to any medications?	Yes	No
If yes, which medications?		

Please list the medications that you are currently taking, including nonprescription drugs such as aspirin, Advil, antihistamines, etc:

_____

_____

Please list all the eye operations you have had (including laser surgery) and the dates of the surgeries:

_____

_____

_____

_____

Please list all operations you have had and the dates of the surgeries:

_____

_____

_____

_____

Have you ever been told that you have the following conditions?

Anemia (low blood count)	Yes	No
Cancer	Yes	No
Diabetes	Yes	No
Hepatitis	Yes	No
High blood pressure	Yes	No
Pleurisy	Yes	No
Pneumonia	Yes	No
Ulcers	Yes	No
Herpes (cold sores)	Yes	No
Chickenpox	Yes	No
Shingles (zoster)	Yes	No
German measles (rubella)	Yes	No
Measles (rubeola)	Yes	No
Mumps	Yes	No
Chlamydia or trachoma	Yes	No
Syphilis	Yes	No
Gonorrhea	Yes	No
Any other sexually transmitted disease	Yes	No
Tuberculosis (TB)	Yes	No
Leprosy	Yes	No
Leptospirosis	Yes	No
Lyme disease	Yes	No
Histoplasmosis	Yes	No
Candida or moniliasis	Yes	No
Coccidioidomycosis	Yes	No
Sporotrichosis	Yes	No
Toxoplasmosis	Yes	No
Toxocariasis	Yes	No
Cysticercosis	Yes	No
Trichinosis	Yes	No

(Continued)

Whipple disease	Yes	No
AIDS	Yes	No
Hay fever	Yes	No
Allergies	Yes	No
Vasculitis	Yes	No
Arthritis	Yes	No
Rheumatoid arthritis	Yes	No
Lupus (systemic lupus erythematosus)	Yes	No
Scleroderma	Yes	No

Have you ever had any of the following illnesses?

Reiter syndrome	Yes	No
Colitis	Yes	No
Crohn disease	Yes	No
Ulcerative colitis	Yes	No
Adamantiades-Behçet disease	Yes	No
Sarcoidosis	Yes	No
Ankylosing spondylitis	Yes	No
Erythema nodosa	Yes	No
Temporal arteritis	Yes	No
Multiple sclerosis	Yes	No
Serpiginous choroiditis	Yes	No
Fuchs heterochromic iridocyclitis	Yes	No
Vogt-Koyanagi-Harada syndrome	Yes	No

Have you ever had any of the following illnesses?

GENERAL HEALTH

Chills	Yes	No
Fever (persistent or recurrent)	Yes	No
Night sweats	Yes	No
Fatigue (tire easily)	Yes	No
Poor appetite	Yes	No
Unexplained weight loss	Yes	No
Do you feel sick?	Yes	No

HEAD

Frequent or severe headaches	Yes	No
Fainting	Yes	No
Numbness or tingling in your body	Yes	No
Paralysis in parts of your body	Yes	No
Siezures or convulsions	Yes	No

EARS

Hard of hearing or deafness	Yes	No
Ringing or noise in your ears	Yes	No
Frequent or severe ear infections	Yes	No
Painful or swollen ear lobes	Yes	No

NOSE AND THROAT

Sore in your nose or mouth	Yes	No
Severe or recurrent nosebleeds	Yes	No
Frequent sneezing	Yes	No
Sinus trouble	Yes	No
Persistent hoarseness	Yes	No
Tooth or gum infections	Yes	No

SKIN

Rashes	Yes	No
Skin sores	Yes	No
Sunburn easily (photosensitivity)	Yes	No
White patches of skin or hair	Yes	No
Loss of hair	Yes	No
Tick or insect bites	Yes	No
Painfully cold fingers	Yes	No
Severe itching	Yes	No

RESPIRATORY

Severe or frequent colds	Yes	No
Constant coughing	Yes	No
Coughing up blood	Yes	No
Recent flu or viral infection	Yes	No
Wheezing or asthma attacks	Yes	No
Difficulty breathing	Yes	No

Have you ever had any of the following symptoms?

CARDIOVASCULAR

Chest pain	Yes	No
Shortness of breath	Yes	No
Swelling of your legs	Yes	No

BLOOD

Frequent or easy bruising	Yes	No
Frequent or easy bleeding	Yes	No
Have you received blood transfusions?	Yes	No

GASTROINTESTINAL

Trouble swallowing	Yes	No
Diarrhea	Yes	No
Bloody stools	Yes	No
Stomach ulcers	Yes	No
Jaundice or yellow skin	Yes	No

BONES AND JOINTS

Stiff joints	Yes	No
Painful or swollen glands	Yes	No
Stiff lower back	Yes	No
Back pain while sleeping or awakening	Yes	No
Muscle aches	Yes	No

(Continued)

GENITOURINARY

Kidney problems	Yes	No
Bladder trouble	Yes	No
Blood in your urine	Yes	No
Urinary discharge	Yes	No
Genital sores or ulcers	Yes	No
Prostatitis	Yes	No
Testicular pain	Yes	No
Are you pregnant?	Yes	No
Do you plan to be pregnant in the future?	Yes	No

Adapted with permission from Foster CS, Vitale AT. *Diagnosis and Treatment of Uveitis*. Philadelphia: Saunders; 2002.

CHAPTER 7

Noninfectious (Autoimmune) Uveitis

Many different anterior uveitis, intermediate uveitis, posterior uveitis, and panuveitis entities are triggered by environmental, genetic, and innate and adaptive immunologic stimuli. Often the trigger or inciting event or agent that causes the inflammation is unknown or undetectable. No specific infectious pathogen can be clinically isolated in these cases of uveitis. Once the common infectious pathogens have been ruled out and any systemic autoimmune diseases identified by appropriate diagnostic testing, these autoimmune, noninfectious entities can be treated with anti-inflammatory therapy. The noninfectious uveitic entities are discussed in this chapter.

Anterior Uveitis

Anterior uveitis is the most common form of uveitis, accounting for the large majority of uveitis cases, with an annual incidence rate of 8 per 100,000 population. The incidence increases with age to 102.7–341 per 100,000 in patients aged 65 years and older.

> Gritz DC, Wong IG. Incidence and prevalence of uveitis in Northern California. The Northern California Epidemiology of Uveitis Study. *Ophthalmology.* 2004;111:491–500.
>
> Reeves SW, Sloan FA, Lee PP, Jaffe GJ. Uveitis in the elderly; epidemiological data from the National Long-term Care Survey Medicare Cohort. *Ophthalmology.* 2006;113:307–321.

Because uveitis may occur secondarily to inflammation of the cornea and sclera, the physician should evaluate these structures carefully to rule out a primary keratitis or scleritis. Inflammation of the sclera and the cornea is covered in depth in BCSC Section 8, *External Disease and Cornea;* it is not covered in this chapter.

Acute Nongranulomatous Iritis and Iridocyclitis

The classic presentation of acute anterior uveitis is the sudden onset of pain, redness, and photophobia that can be associated with decreased vision. Fine keratic precipitates (KPs) and fibrin dust the corneal endothelium in most cases. Endothelial dysfunction may cause the cornea to become acutely edematous. The anterior chamber shows an intense cellular response and variable flare. Severe cases may show a protein coagulum in the aqueous or, less commonly, a hypopyon (Fig 7-1). Occasionally, a fibrin net forms across the pupillary margin (Fig 7-2),

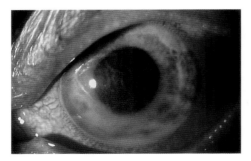

Figure 7-1 Acute HLA-B27–positive anterior uveitis with pain, photophobia, marked injection, fixed pupil, loss of iris detail from corneal edema, and hypopyon. *(Courtesy of David Meisler, MD.)*

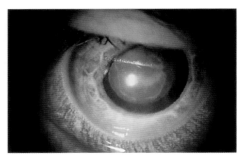

Figure 7-2 Ankylosing spondylitis, acute unilateral iridocyclitis, severe anterior chamber reaction with central fibrinous exudate contracting anterior to the lens capsule, and posterior synechiae from 10 o'clock to 12 o'clock. *(Courtesy of David Meisler, MD.)*

potentially producing a seclusion membrane and iris bombé. Iris vessels may be dilated, and, rarely, a spontaneous hyphema occurs. Cells may also be present in the anterior vitreous, and in rare cases patients develop severe, diffuse vitritis. Fundus lesions are not characteristic, although cystoid macular edema (CME), disc edema, pars plana exudates, or small areas of peripheral localized choroiditis may be noted. Occasionally, IOP may be elevated because of blockage of the trabecular meshwork by debris and cells or by pupillary block.

The attack of inflammation usually lasts several days to weeks up to 3 months. Two patterns may occur. Typically, an attack is acute and unilateral, with a history of episodes alternating between the 2 eyes. Recurrences are common. Either eye may be affected, but recurrence is rarely bilateral. If damage to the vascular endothelium can be minimized, no silent, ongoing damage or low-grade inflammation should occur between attacks. The second pattern is acute and bilateral and occurs simultaneously with tubulointerstitial nephritis.

> Cunningham ET Jr. Diagnosis and management of anterior uveitis. *Focal Points: Clinical Modules for Ophthalmologists.* San Francisco: American Academy of Ophthalmology; 2002, module 1.
>
> D'Alessandro LP, Forster DJ, Rao NA. Anterior uveitis and hypopyon. *Am J Ophthalmol.* 1991;112:317–321.
>
> Rodriguez A, Akova YA, Pedroza-Seres M, Foster CS. Posterior segment ocular manifestations in patients with HLA-B27–associated uveitis. *Ophthalmology.* 1994;101:1267–1274.

Corticosteroids are the mainstay of treatment to reduce inflammation, prevent cicatrization, and minimize damage to the uveal vasculature. Topical corticosteroids are the first line of treatment, and they often need to be given every 1–2 hours. If necessary, periocular or oral corticosteroids may be used for severe episodes. Initial attacks may require all 3 routes of treatment, particularly in the severe cases found mostly in younger patients.

Severely damaged vessels may leak continuously, transforming the typical course from acute and intermittent to chronic and recalcitrant. This chronic course must be avoided at all costs by timely diagnosis, aggressive initial therapy, and patient compliance. Maintenance therapy is not indicated once the active inflammation has been controlled.

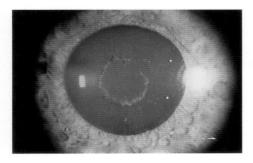

Figure 7-3 Acute iridocyclitis after intensive topical corticosteroids and perilimbal subconjunctival dilating agents, leaving an anterior capsular ring of pigment following posterior synechiolysis. *(Courtesy of John D. Sheppard, Jr, MD.)*

Anti–tumor necrosis factor (TNF) therapy has been effective in decreasing recurrences of anterior uveitis in patients with HLA-B27–associated uveitis.

Cycloplegic/mydriatic agents are used both to relieve pain and to break and prevent synechiae formation. They may be given topically or with conjunctival cotton pledgets soaked in tropicamide (Mydriacyl), cyclopentolate, and phenylephrine hydrochloride (Fig 7-3).

Braun J, Baraliakos X, Listing J, Sieper J. Decreased incidence of anterior uveitis in patients with ankylosing spondylitis treated with the anti-tumor necrosis factor agents infliximab and etanercept. *Arthritis Rheum.* 2005;53:2447–2451.

HLA-B27–related diseases

HLA-B27 denotes a genotype located on the short arm of chromosome 6. Although it is present in only 1.4%–8.0% of the general population, 50%–60% of patients with acute iritis may be HLA-B27–positive. Both racial background and national origin affect the prevalence of HLA-B27 positivity. The precise trigger for acute iritis in genetically susceptible persons is not clear. The HLA-B27 test should be performed on patients with recurrent anterior nongranulomatous uveitis, but the test does not provide an absolute diagnosis.

Power WJ, Rodriguez A, Pedroza-Seres M, Foster CS. Outcomes in anterior uveitis associated with the HLA-B27 haplotype. *Ophthalmology.* 1998;105:1646–1651.

Several autoimmune diseases known as the *seronegative spondyloarthropathies* are strongly associated with both acute anterior uveitis and HLA-B27 positivity. Patients with these diseases, by definition, do not have a positive rheumatoid factor. The seronegative spondyloarthropathies include

- ankylosing spondylitis
- Reiter syndrome (reactive arthritis)
- inflammatory bowel disease
- psoriatic arthritis
- postinfectious, or reactive, arthritis

These entities are sometimes clinically indistinguishable, and all may be associated with spondylitis and sacroiliitis. Women tend to experience more atypical spondyloarthropathies than do men.

Wakefield D, Stahlberg TH, Toivanen A, Granfors K, Tennant C. Serologic evidence of *Yersinia* infection in patients with anterior uveitis. *Arch Ophthalmol.* 1990;108:219–221.

Ankylosing spondylitis Ankylosing spondylitis varies from asymptomatic to severe and crippling. Symptoms of this disorder include lower back pain and stiffness after inactivity. Sacroiliac x-ray films may be difficult to interpret but should show sclerosis and eventual narrowing of the joint space. Ligamentous ossification is frequent. These films are best obtained by ordering a sacroiliac view that tunnels down the joint rather than a lumbosacral spine film, which is obtained by direct anteroposterior imaging and is less likely to clearly reveal sacroiliitis (Figs 7-4, 7-5). Similar disease is found in the pubic symphysis, where localized mineral loss and sclerosis erode the subchondral bone.

Nonsteroidal anti-inflammatory drugs (NSAIDS) are the mainstay of treatment for ankylosing spondylitis. Sulfasalazine may be used in patients whose disease is not controlled with NSAIDS. Morning stiffness and the erythrocyte sedimentation rate decrease in patients taking sulfasalazine, but it is not clear whether it improves pain, function, movement of the spine, or overall well-being. Sulfasalazine appears to reduce the frequency of recurrences of iritis. Side effects of sulfasalazine include skin rashes, stomach upset, and mouth ulcers.

Schmidt WA, Wierth S, Milleck D, Droste U, Gromnica-Ihle E. Sulfasalazine in ankylosing spondylitis: a prospective, randomized, double-blind placebo-controlled study and comparison with other controlled studies. *Z Rheumatol.* 2002;61:159–167.

HLA-B27 is found in up to 90% of patients with ankylosing spondylitis. The chance that an HLA-B27–positive patient will develop spondyloarthritis or eye disease is 1 in 4. Family members may also have ankylosing spondylitis or iritis. Often, symptoms of back disease are lacking in persons with iritis who test positive. Certainly, not all HLA-B27–positive patients develop disease; most do not develop any form of autoimmune disease.

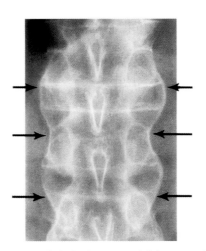

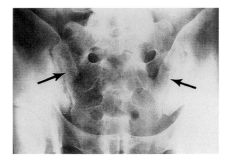

Figure 7-4 Ankylosing spondylitis x-ray film showing total fusion of vertebrae *(arrows)* and marked decalcification. *(Courtesy of John D. Sheppard, Jr, MD.)*

Figure 7-5 Ankylosing spondylitis with moderately severe sacroiliitis shown by tunnel view, with blurring of sacroiliac joint *(arrows)*. *(Courtesy of John D. Sheppard, Jr, MD.)*

The ophthalmologist may be the first physician to suspect ankylosing spondylitis. Symptoms or family history of back problems together with HLA-B27 positivity suggest the diagnosis. Sacroiliac imaging studies (CT, MRI, and/or technicium bone scan) should be obtained when indicated by a suggestive history of morning lower back stiffness that improves with exertion in a patient with ocular disease consistent with HLA-B27 syndrome. Patients with ankylosing spondylitis should be informed of the risk of deformity and must be referred to a rheumatologist. Pulmonary apical fibrosis may develop; aortitis occurs in about 5% of cases and may be associated with aortic valvular insufficiency (Fig 7-6).

Chang JH, McCluskey PJ, Wakefield D. Acute anterior uveitis and HLA-B27. *Surv Ophthalmol.* 2005;50:364–388.

Tay-Kearney M, Schwam BL, Lowder C, et al. Clinical features and associated systemic diseases of HLA-B27 uveitis. *Am J Ophthalmol.* 1996;121:47–56.

Reiter syndrome Reiter syndrome consists of the classic diagnostic triad of nonspecific urethritis, polyarthritis, and conjunctival inflammation often accompanied by iritis. The diagnosis of the syndrome is based on the percentage sensitivity and specificity of various criteria presenting during the initial episode. See Table 7-1.

HLA-B27 is found in 85%–95% of patients, and prostatic fluid culture is negative. The condition occurs most frequently in young adult males, although 10% of patients are female.

Reiter syndrome may be triggered by episodes of diarrhea or dysentery without urethritis. *Chlamydia, Ureaplasma urealyticum, Shigella, Salmonella,* and *Yersinia* have all been implicated as triggering infections. Arthritis begins within 30 days of infection in

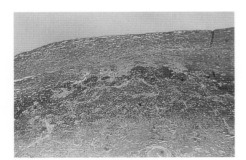

Figure 7-6 Ankylosing spondylitis and aortitis with arterial wall destruction by fibrosis, thickening, and elastic fragmentation. *(Courtesy of John D. Sheppard, Jr, MD.)*

Table 7-1 **Method of Classification of Reiter Syndrome**

	Sensitivity	Specificity
Episode of arthritis of more than 1 month with urethritis and/or cervicitis	84.3%	98.2%
Episode of arthritis of more than 1 month and either urethritis or cervicitis, or bilateral conjunctivitis	85.5%	96.4%
Episode of arthritis of more than 1 month, conjunctivitis, and urethritis	50.6%	98.8%

80% of patients. The knees, ankles, feet, and wrists are affected asymmetrically and in an oligoarticular distribution. Sacroiliitis is present in as many as 70% of patients.

In addition to the classic diagnostic triad, 2 conditions are considered to be major diagnostic criteria:

- *keratoderma blennorrhagicum:* a scaly, erythematous, irritating disorder of the palms and soles of the feet (Figs 7-7, 7-8)
- *circinate balanitis:* a persistent, scaly, erythematous, circumferential rash of the distal penis

The keratoderma blennorrhagicum may resemble pustular psoriasis; this similarity explains the difficulty of distinguishing among the various seronegative spondyloarthropathies.

Numerous minor criteria are also useful in establishing a diagnosis of Reiter syndrome, according to the American Rheumatologic Association guidelines. These include plantar fasciitis (Fig 7-9), Achilles tendonitis (Fig 7-10), sacroiliitis, nailbed pitting, palate ulcers, and tongue ulcers.

Conjunctivitis is the most common eye lesion associated with Reiter syndrome. Conjunctivitis is usually mucopurulent and papillary. Punctate and subepithelial keratitis may also occur, occasionally leaving permanent corneal scars. Acute nongranulomatous iritis occurs in 5%–10% of patients. In some cases, the iritis becomes bilateral and chronic because of a permanent breakdown of the blood–aqueous barrier.

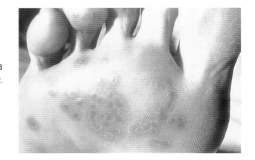

Figure 7-7 Reiter syndrome with keratoderma blennorrhagicum on the sole. *(Courtesy of John D. Sheppard, Jr, MD.)*

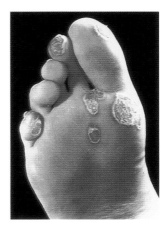

Figure 7-8 Reiter syndrome with pedal discoid keratoderma blennorrhagicum. *(Courtesy of John D. Sheppard, Jr, MD.)*

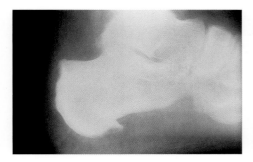 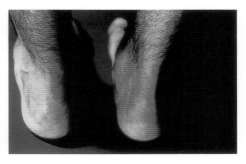

Figure 7-9 Reiter syndrome, x-ray view of calcific plantar fasciitis. *(Courtesy of John D. Sheppard, Jr, MD.)*

Figure 7-10 Reiter syndrome with chronic Achilles tendonitis. *(Courtesy of John D. Sheppard, Jr, MD.)*

Inflammatory bowel disease *Ulcerative colitis* and *Crohn disease (granulomatous ileocolitis)* are both associated with acute iritis. Between 5% and 12% of patients with ulcerative colitis and 2.4% of patients with Crohn disease develop acute anterior uveitis. Occasionally, bowel disease is asymptomatic and follows the onset of iritis. Of patients with inflammatory bowel disease, 20% may have sacroiliitis; of these patients, 60% are HLA-B27–positive. Patients with both acute iritis and inflammatory bowel disease tend to have HLA-B27 as well as sacroiliitis. In contrast, patients with inflammatory bowel disease who develop sclerouveitis tend to be HLA-B27–negative, have symptoms resembling rheumatoid arthritis, and usually do not develop sacroiliitis.

> Salmon JF, Wright JP, Murray AD. Ocular inflammation in Crohn's disease. *Ophthalmology.* 1991;98:480–484.

Psoriatic arthritis From 7% to 25% of patients with psoriatic arthritis develop acute iritis. The iritis in patients with psoriasis without arthritis has distinct clinical features. The mean age of onset is older than in idiopathic or HLA-B27–associated uveitis (30–40 years vs 48). It tends to be bilateral and of longer duration and to require oral treatment with NSAIDs. Retinal vasculitis, CME, and papillitis are frequently seen.

Of patients with psoriatic arthritis, 20% may have sacroiliitis, and inflammatory bowel disease occurs more frequently than would be expected by chance with psoriatic arthritis. Diagnosis is based on the findings of the typical cutaneous changes (Fig 7-11), terminal phalangeal joint inflammation (Fig 7-12), and ungual involvement (Figs 7-13, 7-14).

Treatment consists of mydriatic/cycloplegic agents and corticosteroids, which are usually given topically. In severe cases, periocular or systemic corticosteroids may be required, and chronic cases may require the use of immunomodulatory agents.

> Derhaag PJ, Linssen A, Broekema N, de Waal LP, Feltkamp TE. A familial study of the inheritance of HLA-B27–positive acute anterior uveitis. *Am J Ophthalmol.* 1988;105:603–606.
>
> Durrani K, Foster CS. Psoriatic uveitis: a distinct clinical entity? *Am J Ophthalmol.* 2005;139:106–111.
>
> Rothova A, van Veenedaal WG, Linssen A, Glasius E, Kijlstra A, de Jong PT. Clinical features of acute anterior uveitis. *Am J Ophthalmol.* 1987;103:137–145.

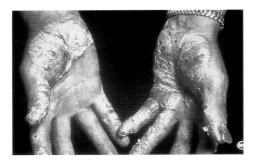

Figure 7-11 Psoriatic arthritis with classic erythematous, hyperkeratotic rash. *(Courtesy of John D. Sheppard, Jr, MD.)*

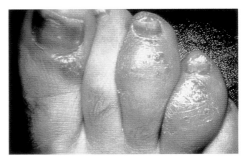

Figure 7-12 Psoriatic arthritis, with sausage digits resulting from tissue swelling and distal interphalangeal joint inflammation. *(Courtesy of John D. Sheppard, Jr, MD.)*

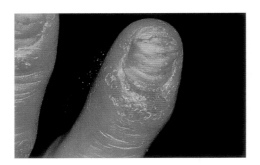

Figure 7-13 Psoriatic arthritis with typical destructive nail changes of subungual hyperkeratosis and onycholysis. *(Courtesy of John D. Sheppard, Jr, MD.)*

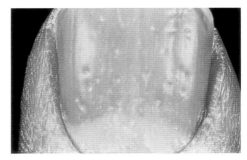

Figure 7-14 Psoriatic arthritis with typical nailbed pitting changes. *(Courtesy of John D. Sheppard, Jr, MD.)*

Tubulointerstitial nephritis uveitis

Tubulointerstitial nephritis uveitis (TINU) occurs predominantly in adolescent girls (11–20 years) and women in their early 30s; the mean age for TINU is 21. Patients present with redness and variable pain, blurred vision, and photophobia. Ocular symptoms and findings are more severe in recurrent disease, with development of fibrin, posterior synechiae, larger KPs, and, rarely, hypopyon. Posterior segment findings may include diffuse vitreous opacities, optic nerve swelling, and retinal exudates.

Patients may present with ophthalmic findings before the development of systemic symptoms such as fever, arthralgias, rashes, and tubulointerstitial nephritis. More commonly, however, patients present with systemic symptoms before the development of iritis. The following criteria are required for a clinical diagnosis of TINU:

- abnormal serum creatinine or decreased creatinine clearance
- abnormal urinalysis with increased β_2-microglobulin, proteinuria, presence of eosinophils, pyuria or hematuria, urinary white cell casts, and normoglycemic glucosuria

- associated systemic illness consisting of fever, weight loss, anorexia, fatigue, arthralgias, and myalgias; patients may also have abnormal liver function, eosinophilia, and an elevated sedimentation rate

The etiology remains unclear. The syndrome has been reported to be associated with HLA-DQ in Caucasians from North America and with HLA-DR14 in Spanish patients. The predominance of activated helper T lymphocytes in the kidney interstitium suggests a role for cellular immunity. Renal biopsies have shown severe interstitial fibrosis. The ophthalmologist plays an important role in the diagnosis of TINU because this disease is very responsive to high-dose oral corticosteroids.

Goda C, Kotake S, Ichiishi A, Namba K, Kitaichi N, Ohno S. Clinical features in tubulointerstitial nephritis and uveitis (TINU) syndrome. *Am J Ophthalmol.* 2005;140:637–641.

Mandeville JT, Levinson RD, Holland GN. The tubulointerstitial nephritis and uveitis syndrome. *Surv Ophthalmol.* 2001;49:195–208.

Glaucomatocyclitic crisis

Glaucomatocyclitic crisis (Posner-Schlossman syndrome) usually manifests as a unilateral mild acute iritis. Symptoms are vague: discomfort, blurred vision, halos. Signs include markedly elevated IOP, corneal edema, fine KPs, low-grade cell and flare, and a slightly dilated pupil. Episodes last from several hours to several days, and recurrences are common over many years. Treatment is with topical corticosteroids and antiglaucoma medication, including, if necessary, carbonic anhydrase inhibitors. Pilocarpine probably should be avoided because it may exacerbate ciliary spasm.

Glaucomatocyclitic crisis, like Vogt-Koyanagi-Harada (VKH) disease, which is discussed later in this chapter, may be associated with the HLA-B54 gene locus. Because Posner-Schlossman syndrome is rare, it should be a diagnosis of exclusion, established only after other, more common syndromes such as herpetic uveitis have been ruled out.

Lens-associated uveitis

Uveitis may result from an immune reaction to lens material. This can occur following disruption of the lens capsule (traumatic or surgical) or from leakage of lens protein through the lens capsule in mature or hypermature cataracts (Figs 7-15 to 7-18).

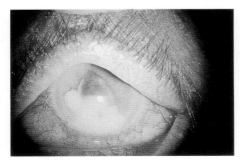

Figure 7-15 Phacoantigenic reaction following phacoemulsification.

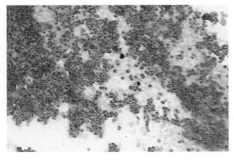

Figure 7-16 Phacoantigenic reaction, histopathology *(aqueous tap)*. Note the neutrophils *(blue)* around the lens *(gray)*.

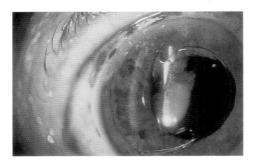

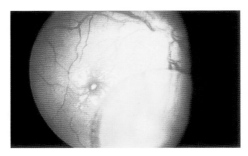

Figure 7-17 Low-grade postoperative uveitis in this patient could be secondary to retained lens cortex or to the anterior chamber IOL. *(Courtesy of John D. Sheppard, Jr, MD.)*

Figure 7-18 Traumatically dislocated nucleus atop the optic nerve produced progressively severe phacoantigenic uveitis and glaucoma, necessitating pars plana lensectomy and vitrectomy. *(Courtesy of John D. Sheppard, Jr, MD.)*

This type of uveitis was once divided into several categories, including phacoanaphylactic endophthalmitis, phacotoxic uveitis, and phacolytic glaucoma. Some of these terms are misleading and do not accurately describe the disease process. For example, the term *phacoanaphylactic* is not appropriate because anaphylaxis involves immunoglobulin E (IgE), mast cells, and basophils, none of which is present in phacogenic uveitis. Also, the term *phacotoxic* is misleading because there is no evidence that lens proteins are directly toxic to ocular tissues.

The exact mechanism of lens-induced uveitis, although unknown, is thought to represent an autoimmune reaction to lens protein. Experimental animal studies suggest that altered tolerance to lens protein leads to the inflammation, which usually has an abrupt onset but may occasionally occur insidiously. Patients previously sensitized to lens protein (eg, after cataract extraction in the fellow eye) can experience inflammation within 24 hours after capsular rupture.

Clinically, patients show an anterior uveitis that may be granulomatous or nongranulomatous. Keratic precipitates are usually present and may be small or large. Anterior chamber reaction varies from mild (eg, postoperative inflammation where there is a small amount of retained cortex) to severe (eg, traumatic lens capsule disruption); hypopyon may be present. Posterior synechiae are common, and IOP is often elevated. Inflammation in the anterior vitreous cavity is common, but fundus lesions do not occur.

Histopathologically, a zonal granulomatous inflammation is centered at the site of lens injury. Neutrophils are present about the lens material with surrounding lymphocytes, plasma cells, epithelioid cells, and occasional giant cells.

Treatment consists of topical and, in severe cases, systemic corticosteroids, as well as mydriatic/cycloplegic agents. Surgical removal of all lens material is usually curative. When small amounts of lens material remain, corticosteroid therapy alone may be sufficient to allow resorption of the inciting material.

Phacolytic glaucoma Phacolytic glaucoma involves an acute increase in IOP caused by clogging of the trabecular meshwork by lens protein and engorged macrophages. This form occurs with hypermature cataracts. The diagnosis is suggested by elevated IOP, lack of KPs, refractile bodies in the aqueous (representing lipid-laden macrophages), and lack of synechiae. Therapy includes pressure reduction, often with osmotic agents and topical medications, and prompt cataract extraction. An aqueous tap may reveal swollen macrophages.

Apple DJ, Mamalis N, Steinmetz RL, Loftfield K, Crandall AS, Olson RJ. Phacoanaphylactic endophthalmitis associated with extracapsular cataract extraction and posterior chamber intraocular lens. *Arch Ophthalmol.* 1984;102:1528–1532.

Meisler DM. Intraocular inflammation and extracapsular cataract surgery. *Focal Points: Clinical Modules for Ophthalmologists.* San Francisco: American Academy of Ophthalmology; 1990, module 7.

Wohl LG, Kline OR Jr, Lucier AC, Galman BD. Pseudophakic phacoanaphylactic endophthalmitis. *Ophthalmic Surg.* 1986;17:234–237.

Postoperative inflammation: infectious

Infectious endophthalmitis must be included in the differential diagnosis of postoperative inflammation and hypopyon. *Propionibacterium acnes* is a cause of delayed or late-onset endophthalmitis following cataract surgery, as are *Staphylococcus epidermidis* and *Candida* species. Infectious endophthalmitis is discussed in more detail in Chapter 9.

Postoperative inflammation: IOL-associated

Intraocular lens–associated uveitis may range from mild inflammation to the *uveitis-glaucoma-hyphema (UGH) syndrome*. Surgical manipulation results in breakdown of the blood–aqueous barrier, leading to vulnerability in the early postoperative period. Intraocular lens implantation can activate complement cascades and promote neutrophil chemotaxis, leading to cellular deposits on the IOL, synechiae formation, capsular opacification, and anterior capsule phimosis. Retained lens material from extracapsular cataract extraction may exacerbate the usual transient postoperative inflammation. Iris chafing caused by the edges or loops of IOLs on either the anterior or the posterior surface of the iris can result in mechanical irritation and inflammation. In particular, metal-loop lenses and poorly polished lenses can cause this reaction. The incidence of this type of complication with modern lenses is 1% or less of cases. The motion of an iris-supported or an anterior chamber IOL may cause intermittent corneal touch and lead to corneal endothelial damage or decompensation, low-grade iritis, peripheral anterior synechiae, recalcitrant glaucoma, and CME (Figs 7-19, 7-20). These lenses should be removed and exchanged when penetrating keratoplasty is performed.

The UGH syndrome still occurs today, although it has become much less common. The syndrome was caused in the past by irritation of the iris root by the warped footplates of poorly made rigid anterior chamber IOLs. Flexible anterior chamber IOLs are less likely to cause UGH syndrome. Various polymers used in the manufacture of IOLs may activate complement and cause neutrophil chemotaxis and resultant inflammation.

Auffarth GU, Wesendahl TA, Brown SJ, Apple DJ. Are there acceptable anterior chamber intraocular lenses for clinical use in the 1990s? An analysis of 4104 explanted anterior chamber intraocular lenses. *Ophthalmology.* 1994;101:1913–1922.

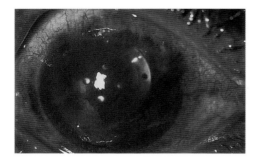 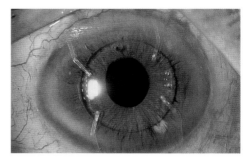

Figure 7-19 Pseudophakic bullous keratopathy and chronic iridocyclitis caused by iris-fixated anterior chamber IOL, with corneal touch, iris stromal erosion, and chronic recalcitrant CME. *(Courtesy of John D. Sheppard, Jr, MD.)*

Figure 7-20 Fixed-haptic anterior chamber IOL (Azar 91Z) associated with peripheral and superior corneal edema, chronic low-grade iridocyclitis, peripheral anterior synechiae, global tenderness, and intermittent microhyphema. *(Courtesy of John D. Sheppard, Jr, MD.)*

As a general rule, the more biocompatible the IOL material, the less likely it is to incite an inflammatory response. Irregular or damaged IOL surfaces as well as polypropylene haptics have been associated with enhanced bacterial and leukocyte binding and probably should be avoided in patients with uveitis. Several attempts have been made to modify the IOL surface to increase its biocompatibility. These modifications include molecular bonding of heparin to the surface of the PMMA lenses *(heparin-surface modification)* and molecular-surface passivation to minimize bacterial and leukocyte adherence.

Foldable implant materials also have been found to be well tolerated in many patients with uveitis. Some studies have shown increased cellular deposition on silicone optics compared with acrylic or hydrogel optics, but others have shown no difference between the lens materials. In general, acrylic IOLs appear to have excellent biocompatibility, with low rates of cellular deposits and capsular opacification.

Randomized, controlled studies still need to be performed to determine the optimal IOL material in these patients. In any event, one of the most important factors in the success of cataract surgery in patients with uveitis is aggressive control of the intraocular inflammation in both the pre- and the postoperative periods. For further discussion and illustrations, see Chapter 11 in this book and BCSC Section 11, *Lens and Cataract.*

Rauz S, Stavrou P, Murray PI. Evaluation of foldable intraocular lenses in patients with uveitis. *Ophthalmology.* 2000;107:909–919.

Ravalico G, Baccara F, Lovisato A, Tognetto D. Postoperative cellular reaction on various intraocular lens materials. *Ophthalmology.* 1997;104:1084–1091.

Drug-induced uveitis

Treatment with certain medications has been associated with the development of intraocular inflammation. Systemic medications reported to cause uveitis include rifabutin (a semisynthetic derivative of rifamycin and rifampin effective in the treatment of *Mycobacterium avium intracellulare*), biphosphanates (inhibitors of bone resorption that are used in the prevention of osteoporosis and in the treatment of hypercalcemia, bone metastasis, and Paget disease), sulfonamides (commonly used in the treatment of urinary tract infections), diethylcarbamazine (an antifilarial agent), and oral contraceptives.

Numerous topical antiglaucoma medications have been associated with uveitis: metipranolol (a nonselective adrenergic blocking agent used in the treatment of glaucoma), anticholinesterase inhibitors, and prostaglandin F2 alpha analogs (travoprost, latanoprost, bimatoprost). Topical glucocorticosteroids have also been reported to be associated with uveitis,

Drugs that are injected directly into the eye have also been associated with uveitis. These include antibiotics, urokinase (a plasminogen activator), and cidofovir (a cytosine analog effective against cytomegalovirus). Treatment is generally with topical corticosteroids and cycloplegic agents, if necessary. Recalcitrant cases may require cessation or tapering of the offending systemic medication.

Certain vaccines, such as bacille Calmette-Guérin (BCG), purified protein derivative (PPD) used in the tuberculin skin test, and influenza, have been implicated as well in the development of uveitis.

Moorthy, Valluri, and Jampol applied 7 criteria proposed by Naranjo and colleagues to determine whether drugs reported to be associated with uveitis were actually the causative agents. Naranjo's criteria were

1. The reaction is a frequently described event that is well documented.
2. Recovery occurs upon withdrawal of the drug.
3. Other possible causes have been excluded.
4. The reaction becomes more severe when the dose of the drug is increased.
5. The adverse event is documented by objective evidence.
6. Similar effects can occur in a given patient with similar drugs.
7. The event should recur on rechallenge with the suspected drug.

They found that only biphosphanates and metipranolol met all 7 criteria, and systemic sulfonamides, rifabutin, and topical corticosteroids met 5 of the criteria for causality.

Faulkner WJ, Burk SE. Acute anterior uveitis and corneal edema associated with travoprost. *Arch Ophthalmol.* 2003;121:1054–1055.

Moorthy RS, Valluri S, Jampol LM. Drug-induced uveitis. *Surv Ophthalmol.* 1998;42:557–570.

Naranjo CA, Busto U, Sellers EM, et al. A method for estimating the probability of adverse drug reactions. *Clin Pharmacol Ther.* 1981;30:239–245.

Chronic Anterior Uveitis (Iridocyclitis)

Inflammation of the anterior segment that is persistent and relapses in less than 3 months after discontinuation of therapy is termed *chronic iridocyclitis;* it may persist for years. This type of inflammation usually starts insidiously, with variable amounts of redness, discomfort, and photophobia. Some patients have no symptoms. The disease can be unilateral or bilateral, and the amount of inflammatory activity is variable. Cystoid macular edema is common.

Juvenile rheumatoid arthritis/juvenile idiopathic arthritis

The classification of juvenile arthritis has been complicated by the differences between the European classification developed by the European League Against Rheumatism (EULAR) and the classification used by the American College of Rheumatology (ACR) and the American Rheumatism Association (ARA). In 1997, the International League of Associations of Rheumatologists (ILAR) adopted the term *juvenile idiopathic arthritis (JIA)* to replace the previously used terms, *juvenile chronic arthritis* and *juvenile rheumatoid arthritis*. However, the ARA has not accepted the term *juvenile idiopathic arthritis*. Table 7-2 offers a comparison of the various systems.

To reflect this situation, we use the term *juvenile rheumatoid arthritis/juvenile idiopathic arthritis (JRA/JIA)* throughout the text.

Cassidy JT, Levinson JE, Bass JC, et al. A study of classification criteria for a diagnosis of juvenile rheumatoid arthritis. *Arthritis Rheum.* 1986;29:274–287.

JRA/JIA is the most common systemic disorder associated with iridocyclitis in the pediatric age group. JRA/JIA is characterized by arthritis beginning before age 16 and lasting for at least 6 weeks.

Ocular involvement in JRA/JIA JRA/JIA is subdivided into 3 types:

1. *systemic onset (Still disease).* This type, usually seen in children under age 5, is characterized by fever, rash, lymphadenopathy, and hepatosplenomegaly. Joint involvement may be minimal or absent initially. This type accounts for approximately 20% of all cases of JRA/JIA, but ocular involvement is rare; fewer than 6% of patients with JRA/JIA have uveitis.
2. *polyarticular onset.* This group shows involvement of 5 or more joints in the first 6 weeks of the disease. It constitutes 40% of JRA/JIA cases overall but only 7%–14% of cases of JRA/JIA-associated iridocyclitis. Patients with a positive rheumatoid factor do not develop uveitis.

Table 7-2 Comparison of the ARA, EULAR, and ILAR Classifications for Childhood Arthritis

ARA/ACR (1972)	EULAR (1977)	ILAR (1997)
Based only on clinical manifestations	Based on clinical and serologic manifestations	Based on clinical and serologic manifestations
Both the onset and the course are important.	Only the onset is important.	Both the onset and the course are important.
Limited to North America	Mostly used by European countries	Mostly used by European countries
Juvenile rheumatoid arthritis (JRA)	Juvenile chronic arthritis (JCA)	Juvenile idiopathic arthritis (JIA)
Systemic onset	Systemic onset	Systemic onset
Polyarticular JRA (RF+/–)	Polyarticular JCA	Polyarthritis (RF-positive) Polyarthritis (RF-negative)
Pauciarticular JRA	Pauciarticular JCA	Oligoarthritis (persistent or extended)
	Juvenile psoriatic arthritis	
	Juvenile ankylosing spondylitis	Psoriatic arthritis
		Enthesitis-related arthritis
	Inflammatory bowel disease–related arthritis	Other arthritis

3. *pauciarticular onset.* This group includes the vast majority (80%–90%) of patients with JRA/JIA who have uveitis. Four or fewer joints may be involved during the first 6 weeks of disease, and patients may have no joint symptoms. This type is subdivided into 2 sets. Type 1 disease is seen in girls under age 5 who typically test positive for antinuclear antibody (ANA); chronic iridocyclitis occurs in up to 25% of these patients. Type 2 disease is seen in older boys, many of whom go on to develop evidence of seronegative spondyloarthropathy (75% are HLA-B27–positive). The uveitis in these patients tends to be acute and recurrent rather than chronic, as in type 1.

The average age of onset of uveitis in patients with JRA/JIA is 6 years. Uveitis generally develops within 5–7 years of the onset of joint disease but may occur as long as 28 years after the development of arthritis. There is usually little or no correlation between ocular and joint inflammation. Risk factors for the development of chronic iridocyclitis in patients with JRA/JIA include female gender, pauciarticular onset, and the presence of circulating ANA. Most patients test negative for rheumatoid factor.

The eye is often white and uninflamed. Symptoms include mild to moderate pain, photophobia, and blurring, although some patients do not have pain. Often, the eye disease is found incidentally during a routine school physical examination. The signs of inflammation include fine KPs, band keratopathy, flare and cells, posterior synechiae, and cataract (Figs 7-21, 7-22). Patients in whom JRA/JIA is suspected should undergo ANA testing and should be evaluated by a pediatric rheumatologist, because the joint disease may be minimal or absent at the time the uveitis is diagnosed. The differential diagnosis in these patients includes Fuchs heterochromic iridocyclitis, sarcoidosis, Adamantiades-Behçet disease, the seronegative spondyloarthropathies, herpetic uveitis, and Lyme disease.

Prognosis Because of the frequently asymptomatic nature of the uveitis in these patients, profound silent ocular damage can occur, and the long-term prognosis often depends on the extent of damage at the time of first diagnosis. Complications are frequent and often severe and include band keratopathy, cataract, glaucoma, vitreous debris, macular edema, chronic hypotony, and phthisis. Children with JRA/JIA, especially those who are ANA-positive or have pauciarticular disease, should undergo regular slit-lamp examinations. Table 7-3 outlines the recommended schedule for screening patients with JRA/JIA for uveitis, as developed by the American Academy of Pediatrics.

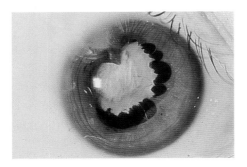

Figure 7-21 JRA/JIA, chronic iridocyclitis, cataract.

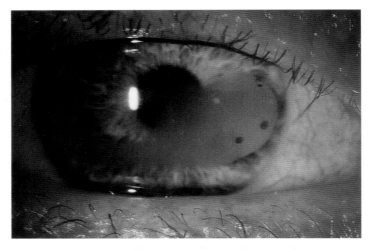

Figure 7-22 Chronic calcific band keratopathy.

Table 7-3 **Recommended Screening Schedule for JRA/JIA Patients Without Known Iridocyclitis**

	Age of Onset	
JRA/JIA Subtype at Onset	**<7 Years[1]**	**≥7 Years[2]**
Pauciarticular		
+ANA	Every 3–4 months[3]	Every 6 months
–ANA	Every 6 months	Every 6 months
Polyarticular		
+ANA	Every 3–4 months[3]	Every 6 months
–ANA	Every 6 months	Every 6 months
Systemic	Every 12 months	Every 12 months

[1] All patients are considered at low risk 7 years after the onset of their arthritis and should have yearly ophthalmic examinations indefinitely.

[2] All patients are considered at low risk 4 years after the onset of their arthritis and should have yearly ophthalmic examinations indefinitely.

[3] If no uveitis 4 years after onset of arthritis, patients should have ophthalmic examinations every 6 months.

Adapted from American Academy of Pediatrics Section on Rheumatology and Section on Ophthalmology. Guidelines for ophthalmologic examinations in children with juvenile rheumatoid arthritis. *Pediatrics.* 1993;92:295–296.

Management The initial treatment for patients with JRA/JIA who have uveitis consists of topical corticosteroids. More severe cases may require systemic or periocular corticosteroids. Corticosteroid therapy is not indicated in patients with chronic aqueous flare in the absence of active cellular reaction. Short-acting mydriatic agents are useful in patients with chronic flare to keep the pupil mobile and to prevent posterior synechiae formation. Use of systemic NSAIDs may permit a lower dose of corticosteroids.

Because of the chronic nature of the inflammation, corticosteroid-induced complications are common. The chronic use of systemic corticosteroids in children presents numerous problems, including growth retardation from premature closure of the epiphyses. In addition, there is evidence that even low-grade inflammation, if present for a prolonged period, can result in unacceptable ocular morbidity and visual loss. For these reasons, many of these children are now treated with weekly low-dose methotrexate. Numerous studies have shown that this treatment regimen can effectively control the uveitis, is generally well tolerated, and can spare patients the complications of chronic corticosteroid use.

Tumor necrosis factor inhibitors are a potential therapeutic modality for JRA/JIA currently under investigation and not FDA approved for JRA/JIA-associated uveitis. Several studies have reported the effectiveness of infliximab, a chimeric monoclonal antibody against TNF-α, in the the treatment of JRA/JIA, with a reduction in ocular inflammation, a decrease in topical and systemic corticosteroid use, and a decrease in the number of recurrences.

Lowder CY, Galor A, Perez VL. Differential effectiveness of etanercept and infliximab in the treatment of ocular inflammation. *Ophthalmology.* Accepted for publication.

Rajaraman RT, Kimura Y, Li S, Haines K, Chu DS. Retrospective case review of pediatric patients with uveitis treated with infliximab. *Ophthalmology.* 2006;113:308–314.

Management of cataracts in patients with JRA/JIA remains a challenge, and the use of IOLs remains controversial. Children who are left aphakic may develop amblyopia. Cataract surgery in patients with JRA/JIA-associated iridocyclitis has been associated with a high rate of complications due to the difficulty in controlling the more aggressive inflammatory response seen in children and especially in patients with JRA/JIA. Lensectomy and vitrectomy via the pars plana have been advocated.

However, more recently, there have been reports of cataract surgery with IOL implants in patients with JRA/JIA. BenEzra reported on 5 children with JRA/JIA who received IOL implants. Although the vision initially improved in 4 of 5 eyes, it later decreased due to the development of retrolental membranes. Lam and colleagues reported good results following cataract extraction and IOL implants in 5 children with JRA/JIA. The major difference between BenEzra's and Lam's studies was the more aggressive, long-term preoperative and postoperative immunomodulatory therapy in Lam's patients.

The following guidelines must be followed when selecting patients with JRA/JIA for cataract surgery with IOL implant:

- The patient's intraocular inflammation must be well controlled for at least 3 months prior to surgery with systemic immunomodulatory therapy and must not require frequent instillation of topical corticosteroids for control of inflammation.
- Only acrylic lenses should be implanted.
- Patients must be followed very frequently following cataract surgery to detect any inflammation, and the inflammation that occurs must be aggressively treated.
- Long-term immunomodulatory therapy must be used pre- and postoperatively, not just perioperatively.

- Due to the lack of long-term results, patients must be strongly advised about the need for careful long-term (lifelong) follow-up in order to detect late complications that may lead to loss of the eye.
- The ophthalmologist must have a low threshold for explantation of the IOL in patients who have persistent postoperative inflammation and recurrent cyclitic membranes,

Patients with band keratopathy should be treated (eg, scraping or chelation with sodium EDTA) and allowed to heal well before cataract surgery is attempted. See also Chapter 11 and BCSC Section 6, *Pediatric Ophthalmology and Strabismus,* Chapter 23.

Glaucoma should be treated with medical therapy initially, although surgical intervention is often necessary in severe cases. Standard filtering procedures are usually unsuccessful, and the use of antifibrotic agents or aqueous drainage devices is usually required for successful control of the glaucoma.

BenEzra D, Cohen E. Cataract surgery in children with chronic uveitis. *Ophthalmology.* 2000;107:1255–1260.

Cunningham ET Jr. Uveitis in children. *Ocul Immunol Inflamm.* 2000;8:251–261.

Dana MR, Merayo-Lloves J, Schaumberg DA, Foster CS. Visual outcomes prognosticators in juvenile rheumatoid arthritis–associated uveitis. *Ophthalmology.* 1997;104:236–244.

Dinning WJ. Uveitis and juvenile chronic arthritis (juvenile rheumatoid arthritis). *Focal Points: Clinical Modules for Ophthalmologists.* San Francisco: American Academy of Ophthalmology; 1990, module 5.

Giannini EH, Brewer EJ, Kuzmina N, et al. Methotrexate in resistant juvenile rheumatoid arthritis. Results of the U.S.A.–U.S.S.R. double-blind, placebo-controlled trial. The Pediatric Rheumatology Collaborative Study Group and The Co-operative Children's Study Group. *N Engl J Med.* 1992;326:1043–1049.

Kanski JJ. Juvenile arthritis and uveitis. *Surv Ophthalmol.* 1990;34:253–267.

Lam L, Lowder CY, Baerveldt G, Smith SD, Traboulsi EI. Surgical management of cataracts in children with juvenile rheumatoid arthritis-associated uveitis. *Am J Ophthalmol.* 2003;135:772–778.

Probst LE, Holland EJ. Intraocular lens implantation in patients with juvenile rheumatoid arthritis. *Am J Ophthalmol.* 1996;122:161–170.

Weiss AH, Wallace CA, Sherry DD. Methotrexate for resistant chronic uveitis in children with juvenile rheumatoid arthritis. *J Pediatr.* 1998;133:266–268.

Fuchs heterochromic iridocyclitis

Fuchs heterochromic iridocyclitis, or *Fuchs uveitis syndrome,* is an entity that is frequently overlooked. Between 2% and 3% of patients referred to various uveitis clinics have Fuchs heterochromic iridocyclitis. This condition is usually unilateral, and its symptoms vary from none to mild blurring and discomfort. Signs include

- diffuse iris stromal atrophy with variable pigment epithelial layer atrophy (Fig 7-23)
- small white stellate KPs scattered *diffusely* over the entire endothelium (Fig 7-24); diffusely distributed KPs also occur with herpetic keratouveitis
- cells presenting in the anterior chamber as well as the anterior vitreous

Synechiae almost never form, but glaucoma and cataracts occur frequently. Generally, fundus lesions are absent, but fundus scars and retinal periphlebitis have been reported on rare occasions. Macular edema seldom occurs.

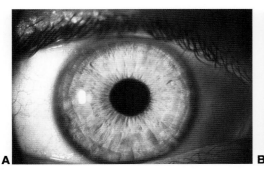
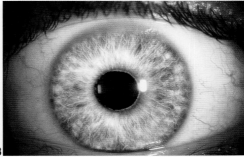

Figure 7-23 Heterochromia in Fuchs heterochromic iridocyclitis. **A,** Right eye. **B,** Left eye. Note the lighter iris color and stromal atrophy *(moth-eaten appearance)* in the left eye, which was the affected eye. *(Courtesy of David Forster, MD.)*

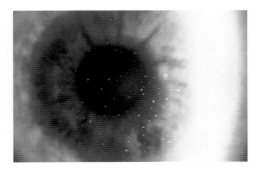

Figure 7-24 Diffusely distributed keratic precipitates in Fuchs heterochromic iridocyclitis. *(Courtesy of David Forster, MD.)*

The diagnosis is based on the distribution of KPs, lack of synechiae, lack of symptoms, and heterochromia. Heterochromia may be subtle in a brown-eyed patient and one must look carefully for signs of iris stromal atrophy. Often, the inflammation is discovered on a routine examination, such as when a unilateral cataract develops. Usually, but not invariably, a lighter-colored iris indicates the involved eye (Fig 7-25). In blue-eyed persons, however, the affected eye may become darker as the stromal atrophy progresses and the darker iris pigment epithelium shows through.

The etiology of Fuchs heterochromic iridocyclitis remains unclear. An association with ocular toxoplasmosis and herpes simplex virus has been suggested. De Groot-Mijnes and colleagues recently reported the association of rubella virus in patients with Fuchs heterochromic iridocyclitis. Thirteen of their 14 patients with the disease demonstrated intraocular immunoglobulin G (IgG) production against rubella virus, whereas none of the patients had antibodies against herpes simplex, herpes zoster, or *Toxoplasma gondii.*

Patients generally do well with cataract surgery, and IOLs can usually be implanted successfully. However, some patients may suffer significant visual disability as a result of extensive vitreous opacification, even after uncomplicated cataract surgery with IOL implantation in the capsular bag. Pars plana vitrectomy should be carefully considered in such patients. Glaucoma control can be difficult. Abnormal vessels may bridge the angle on gonioscopy. These vessels may bleed during surgery, resulting in postoperative hyphema.

Few cases of Fuchs heterochromic iridocyclitis require therapy. The prognosis is good in most cases even though the inflammation persists for decades. Because topical

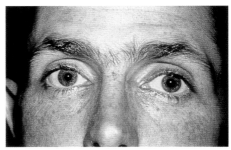

Figure 7-25 Heterochromia in Fuchs heterochromic iridocyclitis in a brown-eyed patient.

corticosteroids can lessen the inflammation but typically do not resolve it, aggressive treatment to eradicate the cellular reaction is not indicated. Cycloplegia is seldom necessary. Histopathology shows plasma cells in the ciliary body, indicating that true inflammation occurs.

de Groot-Mijnes JD, de Visser L, Rothova A, Schuller M, van Loon AM, Weersink AJ. Rubella virus is associated with Fuchs heterochromic iridocyclitis. *Am J Ophthalmol.* 2006;141:212–214.

Jones NP. Fuchs' heterochromic uveitis: a reappraisal of the clinical spectrum. *Eye.* 1991;5: 649–661.

Liesegang TJ. Clinical features and prognosis in Fuchs' heterochromic uveitis syndrome. *Arch Ophthalmol.* 1982;100:1622–1626.

Idiopathic iridocyclitis

In many patients with chronic iridocyclitis, the cause is unknown. Therapy, including cycloplegia, may be necessary before a specific diagnosis is possible. In some cases initially labeled as idiopathic, repeat diagnostic testing at a later date may reveal an underlying systemic condition.

Intermediate Uveitis

The Standardization of Uveitis Nomenclature (SUN) Working Group defines *intermediate uveitis* as the subset of uveitis where the major site of inflammation is in the vitreous. Intermediate uveitis accounts for up to 15% of all cases of uveitis. It is characterized by ocular inflammation concentrated in the anterior vitreous and the vitreous base overlying the ciliary body and peripheral retina–pars plana complex. Anterior vitreous cellular reaction is apparent. Inflammatory cells may aggregate in the vitreous *(snowballs),* where some coalesce. In some patients, inflammatory exudative accumulation on the inferior pars plana *(snowbanking)* seems to correlate with a more severe disease process. There may be associated retinal phlebitis. Anterior chamber reaction may occur, but in adults it is usually mild and attributed to spillover from the vitreous.

Intermediate uveitis is associated with various conditions, including sarcoidosis, multiple sclerosis (MS), Lyme disease, peripheral toxocariasis, syphilis, tuberculosis, primary Sjögren syndrome, and infection with human T-cell lymphotropic virus type 1.

The term *pars planitis* refers to the subset of intermediate uveitis where there is snowbank or snowball formation in the absence of an associated infection or systemic disease. It is the most common form of intermediate uveitis, constituting approximately 85%–90% of cases; the cause is unknown.

Pars Planitis

Pars planitis, previously also known as *chronic cyclitis* and *peripheral uveitis,* most commonly affects persons 5–40 years of age. It has a bimodal distribution, affecting a younger group (5–15 years) and an older group (20–40 years). No overall gender predilection is apparent. The pathogenesis of pars planitis is not well understood but is thought to involve autoimmune reactions against the vitreous, peripheral retina, and ciliary body. An association with the HLA-DR15 and HLA-DR51 alleles and pars planitis has been found. HLA-DR15 is also associated with MS, suggesting a common immunogenetic predisposition to both diseases.

Clinical characteristics

Approximately 80% of cases of pars planitis are bilateral but can often be asymmetric in severity. In children, the initial presentation may consist of significant anterior chamber inflammation accompanied by redness, photophobia, and discomfort. The onset in teenagers and young adults may be more insidious, with the presenting complaint generally being floaters. Ocular manifestations include variable numbers of spillover anterior chamber cells, vitreous cells, snowballs (Fig 7-26), and pars plana exudates. Inferior peripheral retinal phlebitis with retinal venous sheathing is common. With chronic inflammation, CME often develops. Chronic, refractory CME develops in approximately 10% of patients. This is the major cause of visual loss in pars planitis. Ischemia from retinal phlebitis, combined with angiogenic stimuli from intraocular inflammation, can lead to neovascularization along the inferior snowbank in 5%–10% of cases. These neovascular complexes can bleed and result in vitreous hemorrhages, contract, and lead to peripheral tractional and rhegmatogenous retinal detachments; rarely, the complexes evolve into peripheral retinal angiomas. Retinal detachments occur in 10% of patients with pars planitis. With chronicity, posterior synechiae and band keratopathy may also develop. Other possible causes of visual loss associated with chronic inflammation include posterior subcapsular cataracts in 15% of cases, epiretinal membrane in 5%–10% of cases, and vitreous cellular opacification.

Differential diagnosis

The differential diagnosis of pars planitis includes syphilis, Lyme uveitis, sarcoidosis, intermediate uveitis associated with MS, and toxocariasis. Lyme and syphilitic uveitis may simulate any anatomical subtype of uveitis. Lyme antibody titers may be particularly useful in endemic areas, especially in the presence of cutaneous and articular disease. Iridocyclitis and intermediate uveitis may occur in 5%–20% of patients with MS. Sarcoid uveitis presents as an intermediate uveitis in 7% of cases. Periphlebitis and retinal neovascularization frequently occur in sarcoidosis; however, anterior uveitis is much more common. Elevated levels of serum angiotensin-converting enzyme (ACE) and chest CT findings

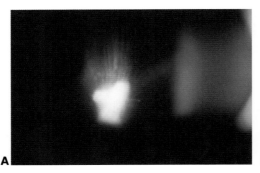 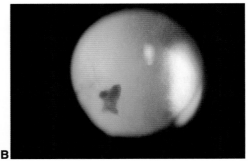

Figure 7-26 **A,** Vitreous snowball opacity in the anterior, inferior retrolental vitreous of a patient with pars planitis. **B,** Same vitreous snowball opacity in retroillumination, showing its location with respect to the lens. Note also the vitreous cellularity as evidenced by retroillumination. *(Courtesy of Ramana S. Moorthy, MD.)*

can help differentiate sarcoidosis from idiopathic pars planitis. A peripheral *Toxocara* granuloma can mimic the unilateral pars plana snowbank in a child and should be ruled out. Serologic testing can be helpful in these cases.

Vitritis without other ocular findings can be suggestive of primary central nervous system lymphoma. These patients are generally much older at presentation than patients with pars planitis, usually in their sixth or higher decades of life. Fuchs heterochromic iridocyclitis can produce mild to dense vitritis but has characteristic KPs and iris heterochromia.

Ancillary tests and histopathology

Diagnosis of pars planitis is based on classic clinical findings. Laboratory workup to exclude other causes of intermediate uveitis, including sarcoidosis, Lyme disease, and syphilis, is essential. Serum ACE, chest CT scanning, Lyme antibody titers, and syphilis serologic investigations should be considered. Fluorescein angiography may show diffuse peripheral venular leakage, disc leakage, and CME. Ultrasound biomicroscopy may be used in cases of a small pupil or dense cataract to demonstrate peripheral exudates or membranes over the pars plana.

Histopathologic examination of eyes with pars planitis shows vitreous condensation and cellular infiltration in the vitreous base. The inflammatory cells consist mostly of macrophages, lymphocytes, and a few plasma cells. Pars planitis is also characterized by peripheral lymphocytic cuffing of venules and a loose fibrovascular membrane over the pars plana.

Prognosis

The clinical course of pars planitis may be divided into 3 categories. Approximately 10% of cases have a self-limiting, benign course; 30% have a smoldering course with remissions and exacerbations; and 60% have a prolonged course without exacerbations. Pars planitis may remain active for many years and has occasionally been documented at more than 30 years. In most cases, the disease "burns out" after 5–15 years. If CME is treated until

neovascularization, although not infrequent structural complications of certain uveitic entities, are not considered essential to the anatomical classification of posterior uveitis. Noninfectious syndromes with primarily posterior segment involvement are included in this section; diagnoses routinely producing both anterior and posterior segment involvement are addressed in the section on panuveitis later in the chapter.

Collagen Vascular Diseases

Systemic lupus erythematosus

Systemic lupus erythematosus (SLE) is a connective tissue disorder with multisystemic involvement that primarily affects women of childbearing age, with higher incidence rates among African Americans and Hispanics in the United States. Although the pathogenesis of SLE is unknown, it is thought to be an autoimmune disorder characterized by B-lymphocyte hyperactivity, polyclonal B-lymphocyte activation, hypergammaglobulinemia, autoantibody formation, and T-lymphocyte autoreactivity with immune complex deposition, leading to end-organ damage. Autoantibodies arising in SLE include ANA, antibodies to both single- and double-stranded DNA (anti-ssDNA and anti-dsDNA), antibodies to cytoplasmic components (anti-Sm, anti-Ro, and anti-La), and antiphospholipid antibodies. The systemic manifestations of SLE are protean and include acute cutaneous diseases in approximately 85% of patients (malar rash, discoid lupus, photosensitivity, mucosal lesions); arthritis in 80%–85% of patients; renal disease in approximately 50%; Raynaud phenomenon in 20%; neurologic involvement in 35%; cardiac, pulmonary, and hepatic disease; and hematologic abnormalities. The diagnosis is essentially clinical, based on the identification of 4 of 11 criteria enumerated by the American College of Rheumatology (Table 7-4).

Ocular manifestations occur in 50% of SLE cases and include cutaneous manifestations on the eyelids (discoid lupus erythematosus), secondary Sjögren syndrome occurring

---

Table 7-4 Revised Criteria for the Diagnosis of Systemic Lupus Erythematosus*

1. Macular rash
2. Discoid rash
3. Photosensitivity
4. Mucosal ulcers
5. Arthritis
6. Serositis (pleuritis, pericarditis)
7. Renal disorder (proteinuria, nephritis)
8. Neurologic disorder (seizures, psychosis)
9. Hematologic disorder (hemolytic anemia, or leukopenia, lymphopenia, or thrombocytopenia)
10. Immunologic disorder (antibody to anti-dsDNA, anti-Sm nuclear antigen, positive antiphospholipid, anticardiolipin antibody or lupus anticoagulant, false-positive test for syphilis)
11. Antinuclear antibody

---

* Diagnosis of systemic lupus erythematosus if 4 or more of the 11 criteria are met.

Adapted from Tan EM, Cohen AS, Fries JF, et al. The 1982 revised criteria for the classification of systemic lupus erythematosus. *Arthritis Rheum.* 1982;25:1271–1277; and Hochberg MC. Updating the American College of Rheumatology revised criteria for the classification of systemic lupus erythematosus [letter]. *Arthritis Rheum.* 1997;40:1725.

in approximately 20% of patients, all subtypes of scleral inflammatory disease, neuro-ophthalmic lesions (cranial nerve palsies, optic neuropathy, and retrochiasmal and cerebral visual disorders), retinal vasculopathy, and, rarely, uveitis.

Lupus retinopathy, the most well recognized posterior segment manifestation, is considered an important marker of systemic disease activity, with a prevalence ranging from 3% among outpatients with mild disease to 29% among those with more active disease. Its clinical spectrum varies from mild to severe and is characterized by the following:

1. Cotton-wool spots with or without intraretinal hemorrhages, occurring independently of hypertension, are thought to be due to the underlying microangiopathy of the disease (Fig 7-27).

2. Severe retinal vascular occlusive disease (arterial and venous thrombosis) resulting in retinal nonperfusion and ischemia, secondary retinal neovascularization, and vitreous hemorrhage (Fig 7-28). More severe retinal vascular occlusive disease in SLE appears to be associated with central nervous system lupus and the presence of antiphospholipid antibodies, including lupus anticoagulant and anticardiolipin antibodies, found in 34% and 44% of these patients, respectively. Antiphospholipid

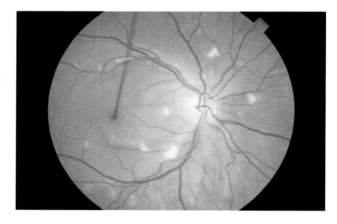

Figure 7-27 Systemic lupus erythematosus, multiple cotton-wool spots. *(Courtesy of E. Mitchel Opremcak, MD.)*

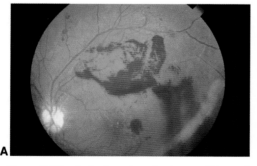 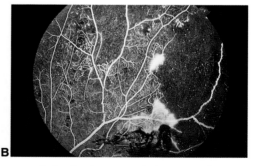

A   B

Figure 7-28 **A,** Ischemic retinal vasculitis and neovascularization in systemic lupus erythematosus. **B,** Fluorescein angiogram of the same patient as in **A** showing capillary nonperfusion. *(Courtesy of E. Mitchel Opremcak, MD.)*

antibodies may also arise primarily, unassociated with other autoimmune diseases, and produce a similar clinical picture; these are frequently associated with spontaneous abortion. Retinal vascular thrombosis is thought to be related to these autoantibodies and to the induction of a hypercoagulable state rather than to an inflammatory retinal vasculitis.

3. Lupus choroidopathy, characterized by serous elevations of the retina, RPE, or both; choroidal infarction; and choroidal neovascularization may be observed with severe systemic vascular disease, due to either hypertension from lupus nephritis or systemic vasculitis (Fig 7-29). SLE-induced hypertension and nephritis may also result in arteriolar narrowing, retinal hemorrhage, and disc edema.

Treatment is directed toward control of the underlying disease, using NSAIDs, corticosteroids, immunomodulatory agents, and systemic antihypertensive medications. Ischemic complications, including proliferative retinopathy, are managed with panretinal photocoagulation.

Dunn JP, Norily SW, Petri M, Finkelstein D, Rosenbaum JT, Jabs DA. Antiphospholipid antibodies and retinal vascular disease. *Lupus.* 1996;5:313–322.

Edworthy SM. Clinical manifestations of systemic lupus erythematosus. In: Harris ED, Budd RC, Firestein GS, et al, eds. *Kelley's Textbook of Rheumatology,* 7th ed. Philadelphia: Saunders; 2005. Vol 1:1201–1224.

Jabs DA, Fine SL, Hochberg MC, Newman SA, Heiner GG, Stevens MB. Severe retinal vaso-occlusive disease in systemic lupus erythematosus. *Arch Ophthalmol.* 1986;104:558–563.

Nguyen QD, Uy HS, Akpek EK, Harper SL, Zacks DN, Foster CS. Choroidopathy of systemic lupus erythematosus. *Lupus.* 2000;9:288–298.

Polyarteritis nodosa

Polyarteritis nodosa (PAN) is an uncommon systemic vasculitis characterized by subacute or chronic focal and episodic necrotizing inflammation of medium-sized and small muscular arteries. The disease presents between the ages of 40 and 60 years and affects men 3 times more frequently than women, with an annual incidence of approximately 0.7 per 100,000 individuals. Although there are no racial or geographic predisposing factors, 10%

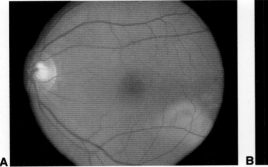
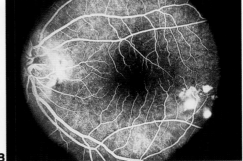

Figure 7-29 **A,** Multifocal choroiditis in systemic lupus erythematosus. **B,** Fluorescein angiogram showing multifocal areas of hyperfluorescence. *(Courtesy of E. Mitchel Opremcak, MD.)*

of the patients are hepatitis B-surface antigen–positive, implicating hepatitis B as an etiologic agent in the development of this disease. Indeed, the demonstration of circulating immune complexes composed of hepatitis B antigen and antibodies to hepatitis B in vessel walls during the early stages of the disease strongly implicate immune-complex–mediated mechanisms in its pathogenesis.

Constitutional symptoms, including fatigue, fever, weight loss, and arthralgia are seen in up to 75% of patients, with mononeuritis multiplex being the most common symptom, if not the initial presenting sign. Renal involvement, related to vasculitis, is common, as is secondary hypertension affecting approximately one third of patients. Gastrointestinal disease with small bowel ischemia and infarction occurs less frequently but may lead to serious complications. Other systemic manifestations include cutaneous involvement (eg, subcutaneous nodules), purpura or Raynaud phenomenon, coronary arteritis, pericarditis, and hematologic abnormalities. Central nervous system disease associated with PAN is rare.

Ocular involvement is present in 10%–20% of patients with PAN, arising as a consequence of the underlying vascular disease. In the posterior pole, this may manifest as hypertensive retinopathy replete with macular star formation, cotton-wool spots, and intraretinal hemorrhage in patients with renal disease; retinal arteriolar occlusive disease; or choroidal infarcts with exudative retinal detachment secondary to vasculitis involving the posterior ciliary arteries and choroidal vessels (Fig 7-30). Elschnig spots may be observed in the posterior pole as a result of choroidal ischemia. Neuro-ophthalmic manifestations include cranial nerve palsies, amaurosis fugax, homonymous hemianopia, Horner syndrome, and optic atrophy. Scleral inflammatory disease of all types, including posterior scleritis, has been reported. Peripheral ulcerative keratitis (PUK), typically accompanied by scleritis, may be the presenting manifestation of PAN.

The diagnosis of PAN is made by fulfilling 3 of the 10 classification criteria:

1. weight loss of more than 4 kg
2. livedo reticularis

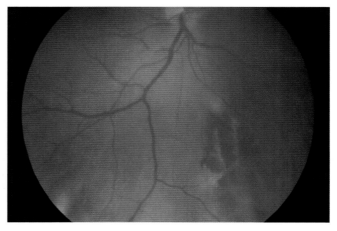

Figure 7-30 Polyarteritis nodosa, retinal vasculitis. *(Courtesy of E. Mitchel Opremcak, MD.)*

3. testicular pain or tenderness
4. myalgia-weakness-polyneuropathy
5. mononeuropathy-polyneuropathy
6. elevated diastolic blood pressure (≥90 mm Hg)
7. elevated blood urea nitrogen
8. positive hepatitis B serology
9. arteriographic abnormalities
10. demonstration of neutrophils on biopsy specimens of small or medium-sized arteries

The presence of antineutrophilic cytoplasmic antibody (ANCA) further suggests the diagnosis (see the discussion on Wegener granulomatosis in the following section). The 5-year mortality rate of untreated PAN is 90%. Although systemic corticosteroids may reduce this rate to 50%, appropriate treatment mandates combination therapy with immunomodulatory medication such as cyclophosphamide, which effects a 5-year survival rate of 80% and may induce long-term remission of the disease. It is therefore important to consider PAN in the differential diagnosis of retinal vasculitis presenting in patients with multiple systemic complaints in which an underlying necrotizing vasculitis is suspected; appropriate diagnosis and management can be life-saving. Tissue biopsy confirms the diagnosis.

Akova YA, Jabbur NS, Foster CS. Ocular presentation of polyarteritis nodosa. Clinical course and management with steroid and cytotoxic therapy. *Ophthalmology.* 1993;100:1775–1781.

Gayraud M, Guillevin L, Cohen P, et al. Treatment of good-prognosis polyarteritis nodosa and Churg-Strauss syndrome: comparison of steroids and oral or pulse cyclophosphamide in 25 patients. French Cooperative Study Group for Vasculitides. *Br J Rheumatol.* 1997;36:1290–1297.

Kielar RA. Exudative retinal detachment and scleritis in polyarteritis. *Am J Ophthalmol.* 1976;82:694–698.

Perez VL, Chavala SH, Ahmed M, et al. Ocular manifestations and concepts of systemic vasculitides. *Surv Ophthalmol.* 2004;49:399–418.

Wegener granulomatosis

Wegener granulomatosis is a multisystemic autoimmune disorder characterized by the classic triad of necrotizing granulomatous vasculitis of the upper and lower respiratory tract, focal segmental glomerulonephritis, and necrotizing vasculitis of small arteries and veins. A limited form of Wegener has also been described, consisting of granulomatous inflammation involving the respiratory tract without overt involvement of the kidneys; however, subclinical renal disease may be present on tissue biopsy. Involvement of the paranasal sinuses is the most characteristic clinical feature of this disorder, followed by pulmonary and renal disease. Renal involvement may or may not be evident at presentation, but its early detection is important, as up to 85% of patients develop glomerulonephritis during the course of the disease, which, if left untreated, carries significant disease-associated mortality.

Patients may present with constitutional symptoms, sinusitis associated with bloody nasal discharge, pulmonary symptomatology, and arthritis. Dermatologic involvement is seen in approximately half of patients, with purpura involving the lower extremities being seen most frequently; less commonly seen are ulcers and subcutaneous nodules. Nervous system involvement may be seen in approximately one third of patients with peripheral neuropathies, the most common being mononeuritis multiplex; less frequently observed are cranial neuropathies, seizures, stroke syndromes, and cerebral vasculitis.

Ocular or orbital involvement is seen in 15% of patients at presentation and in 29%–52% of patients during the course of Wegener granulomatosis. Orbital involvement, one of the most frequently reported ocular findings, is usually secondary to contiguous extension of the granulomatous inflammatory process from the nasal sinus into the orbit. Orbital pseudotumor, distinct from the sinus inflammation; orbital cellulitis; and dacriocystitis may occur from the involved and secondarily infected nasal mucosa. Scleritis of any type, particularly diffuse anterior or necrotizing disease, with or without PUK, affects 16%–38% of patients. Posterior scleritis has also been reported.

Approximately 10% of patients with Wegener granulomatosis and ocular involvement have been reported to have an associated nonspecific unilateral or bilateral anterior, intermediate, or posterior uveitis, with varying degrees of vitritis. Retinal involvement is relatively uncommon, occurring in approximately 5%–12% of patients. Retinal vascular manifestations range from relatively benign cotton-wool spots, with or without associated intraretinal hemorrhages, to more severe vaso-occlusive disease, including branch or central retinal artery or vein occlusion. Retinitis has been reported in 10%–20% of patients; those with accompanying retinal vasculitis may develop retinal neovascularization, vitreous hemorrhage, and neovascular glaucoma (Fig 7-31). Optic nerve involvement, especially ischemic optic neuropathy, is not uncommon. Vision loss in Wegener

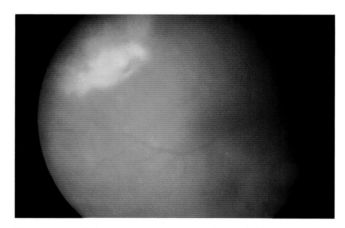

Figure 7-31 Wegener granulomatosis, retinitis. *(Courtesy of E. Mitchel Opremcak, MD.)*

granulomatosis may be seen in 8%–37% of patients, especially among those with long-standing or inadequately treated disease.

Tissue biopsy establishes the histologic diagnosis, whereas laboratory evaluation and imaging studies may disclose nodular, diffuse, or cavitary lesions on chest x-ray; protein-uria or hematuria; elevated sedimentation rate; C-reactive protein; and the presence of ANCAs. These are specific markers for a group of related systemic vasculitides, including Wegener granulomatosis, PAN, microscopic polyarteritis nodosa, Churg-Strauss syndrome, and pauci-immunoglomerulonephritis. Specifically, ANCAs are antibodies directed against cytoplasmic azurophilic granules of neutrophils and monocytes, of which 2 classes have been described based on the pattern seen on immunofluorescence. The cytoplasmic pattern, or c-ANCA, is both sensitive and specific for Wegener granulomatosis in particular, whereas the perinuclear pattern, or p-ANCA, is associated with PAN, microscopic polyarteritis nodosa, relapsing polychondritis, and renal vasculitis. Between 85% and 95% of all ANCA found in Wegener granulomatosis is c-ANCA, with antigen specificity for proteinase 3 (PR3), which is highly specific for the disease; the remainder is p-ANCA, directed against myeloperoxidase (MPO). In contrast, the diagnostic sensitivity of c-ANCA and p-ANCA for PAN is only 5% and 15%, respectively; in patients with microscopic polyarteritis nodosa, p-ANCA (MPO) positivity is more common (50%–80%), with a smaller percentage (40%) having the c-ANCA (anti-PR3) marker.

As with PAN, appropriate treatment mandates combination therapy with oral corticosteroids and immunomodulatory agents, specifically with cyclophosphamide. Without therapy, the 1-year mortality rate is 80%. However, 93% of patients treated with cyclophosphamide and corticosteroids successfully achieve remission with resolution of ocular manifestations. Also as with PAN, ophthalmologists must be intimately familiar with Wegener granulomatosis, as ocular inflammatory manifestations are frequently present, and timely diagnosis and treatment is essential in reducing not only ocular morbidity but overall patient mortality.

Bullen CL, Liesegang TJ, McDonald TJ, DeRemee RA. Ocular complications of Wegener's granulomatosis. *Ophthalmology.* 1983;90:279–290.

Hoffman GS, Kerr GS, Leavitt RY, et al. Wegener's granulomatosis: an analysis of 158 patients. *Ann Intern Med.* 1992;116:488–498.

Inflammatory Chorioretinopathies of Unknown Etiology

The inflammatory chorioretinopathies, or white dot syndromes, as they are commonly called, are a heterogeneous group of inflammatory disorders with overlapping clinical features that share the common presence of discrete, multiple, well-circumscribed yellow-white lesions at the level of the retina, outer retina, RPE, choriocapillaris, and choroid during some phase of their disease course. The white dot syndromes consist of the predominantly noninfectious ocular syndromes listed in Table 7-5. Their differential diagnosis includes systemic and ocular infectious entities such as syphilis, diffuse unilateral subacute neuroretinitis (DUSN), and ocular histoplasmosis syndrome (OHS), as well as noninfectious entities such as sarcoidosis, sympathetic ophthalmia, VKH syndrome, and intraocular lymphoma (Table 7-6). Common presenting symptoms include photopsias,

Table 7-5 Inflammatory Choroidopathies

	Birdshot	APMPPE	Serpiginous Choroiditis	MCP	PIC	SFU	MEWDS	ARPE	AZOOR
Age	Older (30–70)	Young (20–50)	Young, middle-age (20–60)	Young (9–69)	Young (18–40)	Young (14–34)	Young (10–47)	Young (16–40)	Young (13–63)
Sex	F>M	M=F	M=F	F (3:1)	F (90%)	F (100%)	F (3:1)	M=F	F (3:1)
Laterality	Bilateral	Bilateral	Bilateral, asymmetric	Bilateral	Bilateral	Asymmetric	Unilateral	Unilateral (75%)	Unilateral (24%), bilateral (76%)
Systemic associations	80%–98% HLA-A29+, lymphocyte proliferation to retinal S-antigen	Viral prodrome, cerebrovasculitis, CSF abnormalities	HLA-B7	None	None	None	Viral prodrome (50%)	None	Systemic autoimmune disease (28%)
Pathogenesis	Autoimmune ?	Viral ?	Autoimmune? Infectious (herpes)?	Viral ?	Variant of MCP? Limited myopic degeneration?	Autoimmune	Viral? Common non–disease-specific genetics?	Viral?	Viral vs autoimmune
Onset	Insidious	Acute	Variable	Insidious	Acute	Insidious	Acute	Acute	Insidious
Course	Chronic, recurrent	Self-limited	Chronic, recurrent	Chronic, recurrent	Self-limited	Chronic, recurrent	Self-limited	Self-limited	Chronic, recurrent (31%)
Symptoms	Blurred vision, floaters, photopsias, disturbed night and color vision	Blurred vision, scotomata, photopsias	Blurred vision, scotomata	Blurred vision, floaters, photopsias, metamorphopsia, scotomata	Paracentral scotomata, photopsias, metamorphopsia	Blurred vision, decreased vision	Blurred or decreased vision, scotomata, photopsias	Central metamorphopsia, scotomata	Photopsias

	Birdshot	APMPPE	Serpiginous Choroiditis	MCP	PIC	SFU	MEWDS	ARPE	AZOOR
Exam	Vitritis; ovoid, creamy, white-yellow, postequatorial lesions (50–1500 μm), do not pigment	Multifocal, flat, gray-white lesions, 1–2 disc areas, outer retina/RPE with evolving pigmentation	Geographic, yellow-gray, peripapillary, macular chorioretinal lesions with centripedal extension; activity at leading, peripheral edge with RPE/choriocapillaris atrophy in its wake	Myopia, iridocyclitis (50%), vitritis (100%), active white-yellow chorioretinal lesions (50–200 μm) evolving to punched-out scars	Myopia, vitritis absent, white-yellow chorioretinal lesions	Moderate vitritis, 50–500 μm yellow-white lesions posterior pole to midperiphery, RPE, hypertrophy, atrophy, large stellate zones of subretinal fibrosis	Myopia; mild iridocyclitis; vitritis; small white-orange, evanescent, perifoveal dots (100–200 μm) outer retina/RPE; macular granularity	Small, hyperpigmented lesions with yellow halo (100–200 μm), unassociated vitritis	Initially normal to subtle RPE changes, late pigment migration, focal perivenous sheathing
Structural complications	Retinal vasculitis, disc edema, CME, CNVM (6%)	Disc edema	CNVM (25%), RPE mottling, scarring, loss of choriocapillaris	Optic disc edema, peripapillary pigment changes, CME (14%–44%), CNVM (33%)	CNVM (17%–40%), serous detachment over confluent lesions	Neurosensory retinal detachment, CME, CNVM	Disc edema, venous sheathing	None	RPE mottling, occasional CME
Fluorescein angiography (FA)	Early hypofluorescence vs silence, subtle late stain; leakage from disc, vessels, CME; delayed retinal circulation time	Acute lesions: early block-age, late staining; late window defects	Early hypofluorescence, late staining/leak of active border, leakage in presence of CNVM	Early block-age, late staining of lesions, leakage from CME, CNVM	Early hyperfluorescence, variable late leakage/staining acute lesions, leakage in presence of CME, CNVM	Multiple areas of alternating hypo- and hyperfluorescence; early, late staining	Early punctate hyperfluorescence, wreathlike configuration, late staining of lesions, optic nerve	Early hyperfluorescence with surrounding halo of hyperfluorescence and late staining	In acute stage, normal with increased retinal circulation time; in late stage, diffuse hyperfluorescence, RPE atrophy

(Continued)

Table 7-5 (continued)

	Birdshot	APMPPE	Serpiginous Choroiditis	MCP	PIC	SFU	MEWDS	ARPE	AZOOR
Indocyanine green angiography (ICG)	Corresponding hypofluorescent lesions more numerous than on exam, FA	Hypofluorescent spots corresponding to those seen on exam, FA	Early hypofluorescence, late staining, more widespread extent than seen on exam, FA	Multiple hypofluorescent lesions, confluence around optic nerve, more numerous than on exam, FA	Multiple hypofluorescent, peripapillary, posterior pole lesions, corresponding to those seen on exam, FA		Multiple hypofluorescent spots, more numerous than on exam, FA		
Electrophysiology, visual fields (VF)	ERG: abnormal rod and cone responses	EOG: variably abnormal	ERG: normal	ERG: abnormal, extinguished responses	ERG: normal VF: enlargement of blind spot (41%)	VF, ERG, and EOG markedly attenuated	ERG: diminished a wave, early receptor potentials (reversible); VF: enlarged blind spot, paracentral scotomata	ERG: normal EOG: abnormal	ERG, MF ERG: abnormal; VF: temporal, superior defects, enlarged blind spot
Visual prognosis	Guarded without treatment	Good	Guarded	Guarded	Good in absence of CNVM	Guarded	Excellent	Excellent	Guarded
Treatment	Systemic corticosteroids, immunomodulation	Observation, systemic corticosteroids with CNS involvement	Systemic corticosteroids, immunosuppression, laser for CNVM	Systemic corticosteroids, immunomodulation, laser for CNVM	Observation, systemic/periocular corticosteroids, laser for CNVM	Corticosteroids for CME, immunomodulatory therapy of equivocal efficacy long term	Observation	None	Corticosteroids, immunosuppressives, antivirals of equivocal efficacy

APMPPE = acute posterior multifocal placoid pigment epitheliopathy, ARPE = actue retinal pigment epitheliitis, AZOOR = acute zonal occult outer retinopathy, CNVM = choroidal neovascular membrane, MCP = multifocal choroiditis and panuveitis syndrome, MEWDS = multiple evanescent white dot syndrome, PIC = punctate inner choroiditis, SFU = subretinal fibrosis and uveitis syndrome

Table 7-6 Differential Diagnoisis for Retinochoroidopathies

Syphilis
Diffuse unilateral subacute neuroretinitis (DUSN)
Ocular histoplasmosis syndrome (OHS)
Tuberculosis
Toxoplasmosis
Pneumocystis choroidopathy
Candidiasis
Acute retinal necrosis (ARN)
Ophthalmomyasis
Sarcoidosis
Sympathetic ophthalmia
Vogt-Koyanagi-Harada (VKH) syndrome
Intraocular lymphoma

blurred vision, nyctalopia, floaters, and field loss contiguous with a blind spot. In many cases, a prodromal viral syndrome can be identified. Bilateral involvement, albeit asymmetrically (with the exception of multiple evanescent white dot syndrome [MEWDS]), is the rule. Other than patients with birdshot retinochoroidopathy and serpiginous choroidopathy, the majority of individuals are younger than 50 years of age. A female predominance is more commonly observed in patients with MEWDS, birdshot retinochoroidopathy, multifocal choroiditis and panuveitis (MCP), punctate inner choroiditis (PIC), and acute zonal occult outer retinopathy (AZOOR).

The etiology of the white dot syndromes is unknown. Some investigators have postulated an infectious cause; others have suggested an autoimmune/inflammatory pathogenesis arising among individuals with common non–disease-specific genetics, triggered by some exogenous agent. Whether the white dot syndromes represent a clinical spectrum of a single disease entity or are discrete diseases themselves awaits identification of the underlying mechanisms. Although they have similarities, the white dot syndromes can be differentiated clinically based on their variable lesion morphology and evolution, distinct natural histories, and angiographic behavior. This has important implications with respect to disease-specific indications for treatment and predictions of the ultimate visual prognosis.

Gass JD. Are acute zonal occult outer retinopathy and the white dot syndromes (AZOOR complex) specific autoimmune diseases? *Am J Ophthalmol.* 2003;135:380–381.

Jampol LM, Becker KG. White spot syndromes of the retina: a hypothesis based on the common genetic hypothesis of autoimmune/inflammatory disease. *Am J Ophthalmol.* 2003;135:376–379.

Quillen DA, Davis JB, Gottlieb JL, et al. The white dot syndromes. *Am J Ophthalmol.* 2004;137:538–550.

Birdshot retinochoroidopathy

Birdshot retinochoroidopathy (vitiliginous chorioretinitis) is an uncommon disease presenting in predominantly Caucasian females of northern European descent past the fourth decade of life. Although there is no consistent systemic disease association, birdshot retinochoroidopathy is highly correlated with the presence of the HLA-A29 haplotype (80%–98%), which confers considerably increased risk for the development of this disease. HLA-A29 is confirmatory rather than diagnostic, as 7% of the general population carries this haplotype, and in the absence of characteristic clinical features, an alternative diagnosis should be considered. Retinal autoimmunity is thought to play an important role in the pathogenesis of birdshot, as is suggested by the similarities between it and experimental autoimmune uveitis (EAU) and by the demonstration of lymphocyte proliferation to retinal S-antigen. Alternatively, it has been hypothesized that an infectious agent may enhance the expression, by the HLA-A29 molecule, of self-peptides to T lymphocytes. Both T and B lymphocytes, but no organisms, have been seen on histopathologic examination of the chorioretinal lesions from autopsy eyes with birdshot.

Presenting symptoms include blurred vision, floaters, nyctalopia, and disturbance of color vision. Anterior segment inflammation may be minimal or lacking; however, varying degrees of vitritis are commonly noted. Funduscopy reveals characteristic multifocal, hypopigmented, ovoid, cream-colored lesions (50–1500 μm) at the level of the choroid and RPE in the postequatorial fundus; typically these show a nasal and radial distribution, emanating from the optic nerve, and frequently they follow the underlying choroidal vessels (Fig 7-32). They do not pigment over time and are best appreciated by indirect ophthalmoscopy. Retinal vasculitis, CME, and optic nerve head inflammation are important components of active disease. Late complications include optic atrophy, epiretinal membrane (ERM) formation, and, rarely, choroidal neovascularization.

Fluorescein angiography (FA) does not typically highlight the birdshot lesions themselves but rather is useful in identifying active retinal vasculitis, CME, and optic nerve head leakage (Figs 7-33, 7-34). Indocyanine green (ICG) angiography discloses multiple hypofluorescent spots, which are typically more numerous than those seen on clinical examination or on FA (Fig 7-35). Progressive visual field loss and electroretinogram (ERG) abnormalities are commonly seen with extended follow-up, suggesting that a more diffuse retinal dysfunction not fully explained by the presence of CME or other structural abnormalities contributes to visual loss. These tests also may be useful in following the disease course and response to therapy.

Although it has been reported that 20% of patients may have self-limiting disease, the course is generally marked by multiple exacerbations and remissions, with few

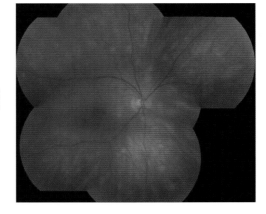

Figure 7-32 Birdshot chorioretinitis with multiple postequatorial, cream-colored ovoid lesions. *(Courtesy of Ramana S. Moorthy, MD.)*

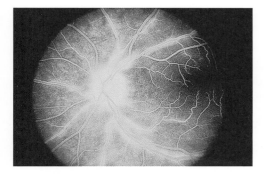

Figure 7-33 Fluorescein angiogram showing diffuse retinal phlebitis. *(Courtesy of E. Mitchel Opremcak, MD.)*

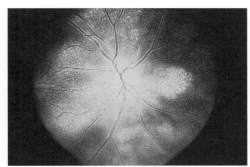

Figure 7-34 Fluorescein angiogram showing cystoid retinal edema in birdshot chorioretinitis. *(Courtesy of E. Mitchel Opremcak, MD.)*

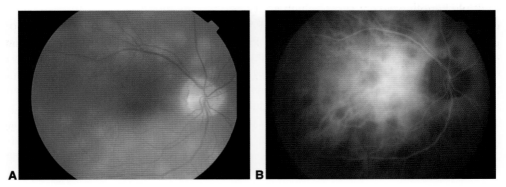

Figure 7-35 Birdshot retinochoroidopathy. Fundus photograph **(A)** and ICG angiogram **(B)** showing numerous, midphase, hypofluorescent spots corresponding to fundus lesions. *(Courtesy of Albert T. Vitale, MD.)*

patients maintaining good vision without treatment. It has been recently reported that among patients with disease duration of greater than 30 months, more than two thirds had a visual acuity of worse than 20/50 and a third had visual acuity of worse than 20/200. The overall 5-year cumulative incidence of acuity of 20/200 or worse was 20%.

Treatment consists of the initial administration of systemic corticosteroids, with an early introduction of corticosteroid-sparing immunomodulatory agents, because birdshot is typically incompletely responsive to corticosteroids as monotherapy, and extended treatment is anticipated in most patients. Corticosteroid-sparing immunomodulators include low-dose cyclosporine (2–5 mg/kg/day), mycophenolate mofetil, azathioprine, methotrexate, daclizumab, and intravenous polyclonal immunoglobulin (IV-Ig). Periocular corticosteroid injections are useful as adjunctive therapy in managing CME and inflammatory recurrences. This approach is effective in reducing intraocular inflammation, inflammatory recurrences, and the risk of developing CME, and in preserving visual acuity.

Gaudio PA, Kaye DB, Crawford JB. Histopathology of birdshot retinochoroidopathy. *Br J Ophthalmol.* 2002;86:1439–1441.

Kiss S, Ahmed M, Letko E, Foster CS. Long-term follow-up of patients with birdshot retinochoroidopathy treated with corticosteroid-sparing systemic immunomodulatory therapy. *Ophthalmology.* 2005;112:1066–1071.

Levinson RD, Gonzales CR. Birdshot retinochoroidopathy: immunopathogenesis, evaluation, and treatment. *Ophthalmol Clin North Am.* 2002;15:343–350.

Nussenblatt RB, Mittal KK, Ryan S, Green WR, Maumenee AE. Birdshot retinochoroidopathy associated with HLA-A29 antigen and immune responsiveness to retinal S-antigen. *Am J Ophthalmol.* 1982;94:147–158.

Sobrin L, Lam BL, Liu M, Feuer WJ, Davis JL. Electroretinographic monitoring in birdshot chorioretinopathy. *Am J Ophthalmol.* 2005;140:52–64.

Thorne JE, Jabs DA, Peters GB, Hair D, Dunn JP, Kempen JH. Birdshot retinochoroidopathy: ocular complications and visual impairment. *Am J Ophthalmol.* 2005;140:45–51.

Vitale AT, Rodriguez A, Foster CS. Low-dose cyclosporine therapy in the treatment of birdshot retinochoroidopathy. *Ophthalmology.* 1994;101:822–831.

Acute posterior multifocal placoid pigment epitheliopathy

Acute posterior multifocal placoid pigment epitheliopathy (APMPPE) is an uncommon condition presenting in otherwise healthy young adults, typically surrounding an influenza-like illness (50%), with men and women being affected equally. A genetic predisposition for the development of this disease may be present given the association of HLA-B7 and HLA-DR2 with this entity. A number of noninfectious systemic conditions have been reported in association with APMPPE, including erythema nodosum, Wegener granulomatosis, polyarteritis nodosa, cerebral vasculitis, scleritis and episcleritis, sarcoidosis, and ulcerative colitis. Infectious conditions have also been associated with APMPPE, including group A Streptococcal infection, tuberculosis, Lyme disease, mumps, and following vaccination with hepatitis B. These diverse disease associations reinforce the concept that APMPPE is an immune-driven vascular alteration.

Patients typically present with a sudden onset of bilateral, asymmetric visual loss associated with central and paracentral scotomata, with the fellow eye becoming involved within days to weeks. Photopsias may precede visual loss. There is minimal anterior segment inflammation, but vitritis of a mild to moderate degree is present in 50% of patients. Funduscopic findings include multiple, large, flat, yellow-white placoid lesions at the level of the RPE, varying in size from 1 to 2 disc areas, located throughout the posterior pole to the equator (Fig 7-36). New peripheral lesions may appear in a linear or radial array over the next 3 weeks. Papillitis may be observed, but CME is uncommon. Atypical findings include retinal vasculitis, retinal vascular occlusive disease, retinal neovascularization, and exudative retinal detachment. The lesions resolve over a period of 2 to 6 weeks, leaving a permanent geographic-shaped alteration in the RPE consisting of alternating depigmentation and pigment clumping.

The diagnosis of APMPPE is based on the characteristic clinical presentation and characteristic FA findings during the acute phase of the disease: early hypofluorescence (blockage) corresponding to the lesion areas and late hyperfluorescent staining (Fig 7-37). ICG angiography reveals choroidal hypofluorescence in both the acute and inactive stages of the disease, with these lesions becoming smaller in the inactive stages (Fig 7-38). Whether the lesions themselves are due primarily to involvement of the RPE or represent choroidal hypoperfusion at the level of the precapillary arteriole with secondary involvement of the RPE and photoreceptors, or some combination of the 2, remains controversial. An important consideration in the differential diagnosis is serpiginous choroidopathy. APMPPE is an acute, usually nonrecurrent disease, whereas serpiginous choroidopathy is insidious and relentlessly progressive. A variant of APMPPE (ampiginous choroidopathy) has been reported that has features of both diseases, being chronic or recurrent, with progressive destruction of the retina and loss of central acuity (Fig 7-39).

Although visual acuity returns to 20/40 or better in the majority of patients within 6 months, 20% are left with residual visual dysfunction. The risks of visual loss include foveal involvement at presentation, older age at presentation, unilateral disease, longer interval between initial and fellow eye involvement, and recurrence. There are no convincing data to

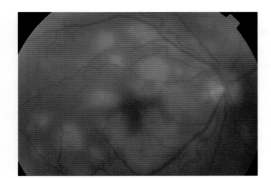

Figure 7-36 APMPPE. Multifocal, placoid lesions in the macula. *(Courtesy of Albert T. Vitale, MD.)*

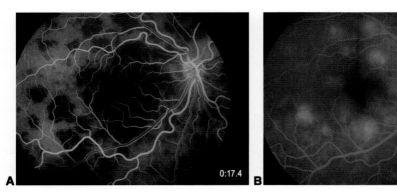

Figure 7-37 APMPPE, fluorescein angiogram. **A,** Early blockage of choroidal circulation. **B,** Late-phase staining. *(Courtesy of Albert T. Vitale, MD.)*

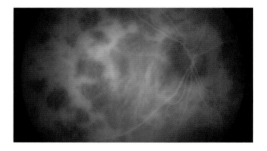

Figure 7-38 APMPPE. ICG angiogram showing multiple midphase hypofluorescent spots. *(Courtesy of Albert T. Vitale, MD.)*

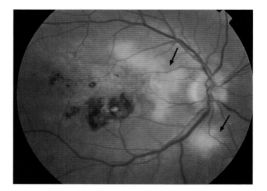

Figure 7-39 Ampiginous choroidopathy. RPE hyperpigmentation and atrophy in the central macula in areas of previous inflammation, with new, yellow-white foci of active disease nasal and inferior to the optic nerve *(arrows)*. *(Courtesy of Albert T. Vitale, MD.)*

suggest that treatment with systemic corticosteroids is beneficial in altering the visual outcome. Some authorities, however, advocate their use in patients presenting with extensive macular involvement in an effort to limit subsequent retinal pigment epithelial derangement of the foveal center and in patients with an associated central nervous system vasculitis.

Jones BE, Jampol LM, Yannuzzi LA, et al. Relentless placoid chorioretinitis: a new entity or an unusual variant of serpiginous chorioretinitis? *Arch Ophthalmol.* 2000;118:931–938.

Pagliarini S, Piguet B, Ffytche TJ, Bird AC. Foveal involvement and lack of visual recovery in APMPPE associated with uncommon features. *Eye.* 1995;9:42–47.

Stanga PE, Lim JI, Hamilton P. Indocyanine green angiography in chorioretinal diseases: indications and interpretation: an evidence-based update. *Ophthalmology.* 2003;110:15–21.

Williams DF, Mieler WF. Long-term follow-up of acute multifocal posterior placoid pigment epitheliopathy. *Br J Ophthalmol.* 1989;73:985–990.

Wolf MD, Folk JC, Panknen CA, Goeken NE. HLA-B7 and HLA-DR2 antigens and acute posterior multifocal placoid pigment epitheliopathy. *Arch Ophthalmol.* 1990;108:698–700.

Serpiginous choroidopathy

Serpiginous choroidopathy, also known as *geographic* or *helicoid choroidopathy,* is an uncommon, chronic, progressive inflammatory condition affecting adult men and women equally in the second to sixth decades of life. Its etiology is unknown, but it is thought to represent an immune-mediated occlusive vasculitis, as suggested by the finding of lymphocytes in the choroidal infiltrates of patients with this disease as well as by the increased frequency of HLA-B7 and retinal S-antigen associations. An infectious etiology has been suggested by the demonstration of elevated antibacterial antibodies, such as antistreptolysin O antibodies, and the association of viral meningitis in patients with this disease. A possible association with herpesviruses has also been postulated but not conclusively demonstrated.

Patients present with unilateral decreased vision with minimal vitreous involvement and a quiet anterior chamber. Funduscopy reveals asymmetric bilateral disease with characteristic gray-white lesions at the level of the RPE projecting in a pseudopodial or geographic manner from the optic nerve in the posterior fundus (Fig 7-40). Less commonly, macular or peripheral lesions may be present. Disease activity is typically confined to the leading edge of the advancing lesion and may be associated with shallow subretinal fluid. Occasionally, vascular sheathing has been reported along with RPE detachment and neovascularization of the disc. Late findings include atrophy of the choriocapillaris, RPE, and retina, with extensive RPE hyperpigmentation and subretinal fibrosis, and choroidal neovascularization occurring at the border of the old scar in up to 25% of patients.

The disease course is marked by progressive centrifugal extension, with marked asymmetry between the 2 eyes. New lesions and recurrent attacks are typical, with 12%–38% of patients reaching a final visual acuity of between 20/200 and counting fingers in the affected eye. Fluorescein angiography shows blockage of the choroidal flush in the early phase of the study and staining of the active edge of the lesion in the later stage of the angiogram (Fig 7-41). In contrast, early hyperfluorescence with late leakage is indicative of the presence of choroidal neovascularization. ICG angiography reveals early hypofluorescence of the acute lesions with late staining. ICG may detect more extensive disease than is seen on FA or on clinical examination and so may be useful in detecting occult disease and in monitoring disease progression and response to treatment.

Given the small number of patients with this disorder, there is no consensus with respect to the optimal treatment regimen or its efficacy. Systemic immunomodulation has been suggested as first-line therapy for patients with serpiginous choroidopathy because corticosteroids alone are ineffective. Cyclosporine has been effectively used as monotherapy in small numbers of patients, as has triple therapy with prednisone, cyclosporine,

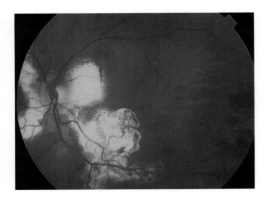

Figure 7-40 Serpiginous choroidopathy. *(Courtesy of Albert T. Vitale, MD.)*

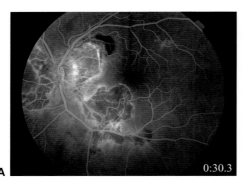 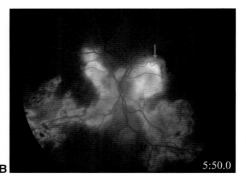

Figure 7-41 Serpiginous choroidopathy, fluorescein angiogram. **A,** Early blocked fluorescence *(arrow).* **B,** Late staining and leakage at the active margin of the lesion *(arrow). (Courtesy of Albert T. Vitale, MD.)*

and azathioprine. Although this approach may induce rapid remission of acute disease, prolonged therapy is required because disease recurrence is typical as agents are tapered. Recently, cytotoxic therapy with cyclophosphamide or chlorambucil has been shown to induce long drug-free remissions. Laser photocoagulation is an important adjunct in the treatment of associated choroidal neovascularization.

Akpek EK, Jabs DA, Tessler HH, Joondeph BC, Foster CS. Successful treatment of serpiginous choroiditis with alkylating agents. *Ophthalmology.* 2002;109:1506–1513.

Christmas NJ, Oh KT, Oh DM, Folk JC. Long-term follow-up of patients with serpiginous choroiditis. *Retina.* 2002;22:550–556.

Hooper PL, Kaplan HJ. Triple agent immunosuppression in serpiginous choroiditis. *Ophthalmology.* 1991;98:944–951.

Lim WK, Buggage RR, Nussenblatt RB. Serpiginous choroiditis. *Surv Ophthalmol.* 2005;50: 231–244.

Priya K, Madhavan HN, Reiser BJ, et al. Association of herpesviruses in the aqueous humor of patients with serpiginous choroiditis: a polymerase chain reaction-based study. *Ocul Immunol Inflamm.* 2002;10:253–261.

Multifocal choroiditis and panuveitis syndrome

Multifocal choroiditis and panuveitis syndrome (MCP), PIC, and subretinal fibrosis and uveitis syndrome (SFU) represent a subset of the white dot syndromes in that some authorities regard them as discrete entities and others view them as a single disease with a variable severity continuum. MCP, although classified as a panuveitis, is presented here among the white dot syndromes given its characteristic funduscopic appearance and for the sake of consistency.

MCP is an idiopathic inflammatory disorder of unknown etiology affecting the choroid, retina, and vitreous that presents asymmetrically, most often in young myopic females. The ophthalmoscopic hallmarks include the presence of punched-out white-

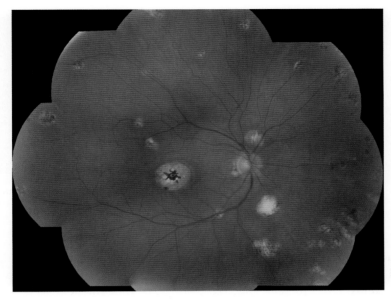

Figure 7-42 Multifocal choroiditis and panuveitis syndrome (MCP). *(Courtesy of E. Mitchel Oprem-cak, MD.)*

yellow dots (50–200 µm) in a peripapillary, midperipheral, and anterior equatorial distribution (Fig 7-42). An associated vitritis is uniformly present, effectively excluding a diagnosis of OHS and PIC. The lesions are smaller than those seen in birdshot retinochoroidopathy and evolve into atrophic scars with varying degrees of hyperpigmentation. They are larger and more pigmented than those seen in PIC. New lesions may appear, and peripheral chorioretinal streaks and peripapillary pigment changes similar to those seen in OHS have been observed. Macular edema (14%–41%) and choroidal neovascularization (33%) are frequent complications leading to poor vision.

Fluorescein angiography shows early blockage and late staining of the lesions, as well as leakage in the presence of macular edema and choroidal neovascularization (Fig 7-43). As it does with birdshot retinochoroidopathy, ICG angiography shows multiple midphase hypofluorescent lesions that are more numerous than those seen on examination or on FA. These spots may fade with treatment and resolution of the intraocular inflammation.

A viral etiology has been postulated involving herpes simplex and Epstein-Barr virus; however, neither has been conclusively demonstrated. Pathologic specimens obtained from eyes with MCP have shown variable findings, ranging from large numbers of B lymphocytes in the choroid to a predominance of T lymphocytes. This suggests that different immune mechanisms may produce a similar clinical picture and that an initial viral infection may trigger an autoimmune process.

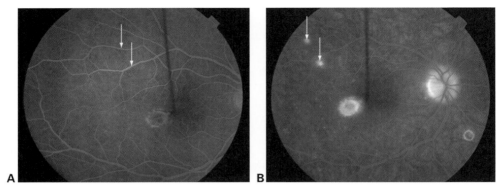

Figure 7-43 Multifocal choroiditis and panuveitis, fluorescein angiogram. **A,** Early blocked fluorescence *(arrows)*. **B,** Late staining of lesions *(arrows)*. *(Courtesy of Ramana S. Moorthy, MD.)*

The diagnosis is one of exclusion, as many other conditions, such as sarcoidosis, syphilis, and tuberculosis, may cause MCP. The visual prognosis is guarded, with permanent visual loss occurring in up to 70% of patients in at least 1 eye as a result of the complications associated with chronic, recurrent inflammation. In one study, an overall final visual acuity of 20/54 was observed among 47 eyes, with 60% of these having a final visual acuity of 20/40 or better and 32% reaching a visual acuity of 20/200 or worse.

Systemic and periocular corticosteroids may be effective for the treatment of macular edema and have been shown to induce the regression of choroidal neovascularization in some patients. Corticosteroid-sparing strategies with immunomodulatory therapy are frequently required due to the chronic, recurrent nature of the inflammation; these have been successful in achieving inflammatory quiescence and preserving visual acuity. Laser photocoagulation using thermal and photodynamic therapy (PDT) modalities, as well as the emerging application of anti-VEGF treatment as described for OHS, are important adjuncts to the treatment of choroidal neovascularization.

Dryer RF, Gass JD. Multifocal choroiditis and panuveitis: a syndrome that mimics ocular histoplasmosis. *Arch Ophthalmol.* 1984;102:1776–1784.

Michel SS, Ekong A, Baltatzis S, Foster CS. Multifocal choroiditis and panuveitis: immunomodulatory therapy. *Ophthalmology.* 2002;109:378–383.

Parnell JR, Jampol LM, Yannuzzi LA, Gass JD, Tittl MK. Differentiation between presumed ocular histoplasmosis syndrome and multifocal choroiditis with panuveitis based on morphology of photographed fundus lesions and fluorescein angiography. *Arch Ophthalmol.* 2001;119:208–212.

Slakter JS, Giovannini A, Yannuzzi LA, et al. Indocyanine green angiography of multifocal choroiditis. *Ophthalmology.* 1997;104:1813–1819.

Spaide RF, Sugin S, Yannuzzi LA, DeRosa JT. Epstein-Barr virus antibodies in multifocal choroiditis and panuveitis. *Am J Ophthalmol.* 1991;112:410–413.

Punctate inner choroiditis

Punctate inner choroiditis (PIC) is an idiopathic inflammatory disorder that, like MCP, occurs in otherwise healthy, Caucasian, myopic females between the ages of 18 and 40. Patients with PIC present with metamorphopsia, paracentral scotomata, photopsias, and asymmetric loss of central acuity. In contrast to the lesions of MCP, those of PIC (100–200 μm) rarely extend to the midperiphery and are never associated with vitritis (Fig 7-44). They progress to atrophic scars, typically leaving a halo of pigmentation, and are deeper and more punched out than those of MCP. New lesions and CME are rarely seen, whereas serous retinal detachment may be seen over confluent PIC lesions. As with MCP, choroidal neovascularization is commonly observed (17%–40%) and recurrences are common (Fig 7-45).

Fluorescein angiography shows early hyperfluorescence with late staining of the lesions, in contrast to what is seen in MCP (Figs 7-46, 7-47). ICG angiography displays midphase hypofluorescence throughout the posterior pole in a peripapillary distribution that corresponds to the lesions seen on FA and on clinical examination, which may be useful in delineating the disease extent and monitoring its activity (Fig 7-48).

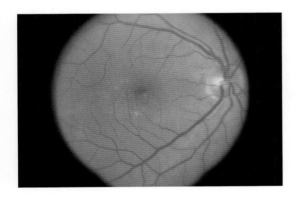

Figure 7-44 Punctate inner choroiditis (PIC). *(Courtesy of E. Mitchel Opremcak, MD.)*

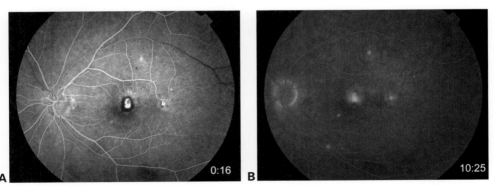

Figure 7-45 PIC with associated CNV. **A,** Fluorescein angiogram showing early hyperfluorescence of the PIC lesions, with lacey hyperfluorescence of CNV. **B,** Late hyperfluorescence and staining of PIC lesions and leakage due to CNV. *(Courtesy of Albert T. Vitale, MD.)*

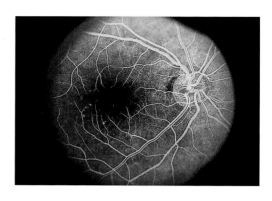

Figure 7-46 PIC. Fluorescein angiogram showing blocked fluorescence early in the study. *(Courtesy of E. Mitchel Opremcak, MD.)*

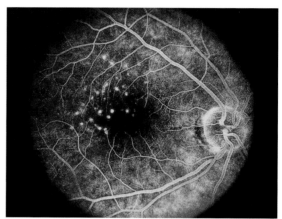

Figure 7-47 PIC. Fluorescein angiogram showing late hyperfluorescence. *(Courtesy of E. Mitchel Opremcak, MD.)*

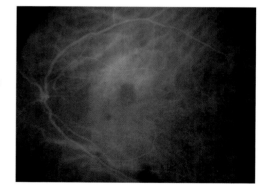

Figure 7-48 PIC. ICG angiogram showing multiple midphase hypofluorescent spots. *(Courtesy of Albert T. Vitale, MD.)*

The visual prognosis is favorable in eyes not complicated by choroidal neovascularization involving the foveal center. Treatment options include observation or periocular and/or systemic corticosteroids for eyes presenting with poor initial visual acuity or multiple acute PIC lesions proximate to the fovea. Laser photocoagulation, with or without intravitreal corticosteroids or antiangiogenic agents, and submacular surgery may be considered in eyes with choroidal neovascularization, as previously described.

Brown J Jr, Folk JC, Reddy CV, Kimura AE. Visual prognosis of multifocal choroiditis, punctate inner choroidopathy, and the diffuse subretinal fibrosis syndrome. *Ophthalmology.* 1996;103:1100–1105.

Spaide RF, Freund KB, Slakter J, Sorenson J, Yanuzzi LA, Fisher Y. Treatment of subfoveal choroidal neovascularization associated with multifocal choroiditis and panuveitis with photodynamic therapy. *Retina.* 2002;22:545–549.

Subretinal fibrosis and uveitis syndrome

Subretinal fibrosis and uveitis syndrome (SFU) is a panuveitis of unknown etiology affecting otherwise healthy, young, myopic females between the ages of 14 and 34 years of age. A mild to moderate vitritis is typically present bilaterally, with 50–500-μm white-yellow lesions located in the posterior pole to midperiphery at the level of the RPE. These lesions may fade without RPE alterations, become atrophic, or enlarge and coalesce into large stellate zones of subretinal fibrosis (Figs 7-49, 7-50). Serous neurosensory retinal detachment, CME, and choroidal neovascularization may also be observed.

Immune mechanisms have been implicated in the pathogenesis of SFU, as suggested by the presence of local antibodies directed against the RPE, granulomatous infiltration of the choroid, enhanced expression of the Fas-Fas ligand in the retina, choroidal scars, and choroidal granulomas. The disease course is marked by chronic recurrent inflammation and the visual prognosis is guarded. Treatment with systemic corticosteroids and immunomodulatory agents is of equivocal efficacy.

Fluorescein angiography shows multiple areas of blocked choroidal fluorescence and hyperfluorescence in the early stages of the study; in the late phase, staining of the lesions without leakage is observed. Again, the differential diagnosis includes ocular inflammatory conditions producing panuveitis and those in the differential diagnosis of the white

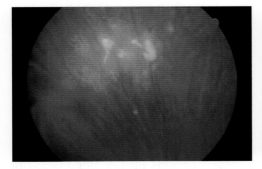
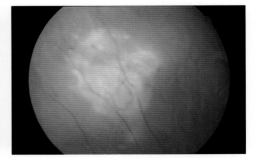

Figure 7-49 Subretinal fibrosis and uveitis syndrome *(SFU).* Fundus photograph showing multifocal white subretinal lesions. *(Courtesy of E. Mitchel Opremcak, MD.)*

Figure 7-50 SFU. Fundus photograph from the same patient as in Figure 7-49, showing progressive subretinal fibrosis. *(Courtesy of E. Mitchel Opremcak, MD.)*

dot syndromes, including sarcoidosis, OHS, APMPPE, syphilis, tuberculosis, birdshot retinochoroidopathy, pathologic myopia, sympathetic ophthalmia, and toxoplasmosis.

Brown J Jr, Folk JC. Current controversies in the white dot syndromes. Multifocal choroiditis, punctate inner choroidopathy, and the diffuse subretinal fibrosis syndrome. *Ocul Immunol Inflamm.* 1998;6:125–127.

Chan CC, Matteson DM, Li Q, Whitcup SM, Nussenblatt RB. Apoptosis in patients with posterior uveitis. *Arch Ophthalmol.* 1997;115:1559–1567.

Palestine AG, Nussenblatt RB, Parver LM, Knox DL. Progressive subretinal fibrosis and uveitis. *Br J Ophthalmol.* 1985;68:667–673.

Multiple evanescent white dot syndrome

Multiple evanescent white dot syndrome (MEWDS) is an idiopathic inflammatory condition of the retina that typically presents with acute, unilateral (80%) blurred or decreased vision with central or peripheral scotomata in otherwise healthy young (10–47 years), moderately myopic females (90%), frequently surrounding a flulike prodrome. Funduscopy during the acute phase of the disease reveals multiple, discrete white orangish spots

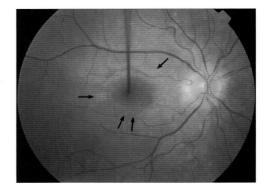

Figure 7-51 Multiple evanescent white dot syndrome *(MEWDS)*. Multiple, discrete, punctate yellowish perifoveal dots *(arrows)*. *(Courtesy of Albert T. Vitale, MD.)*

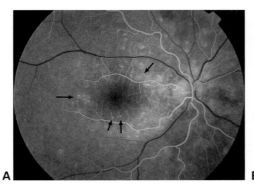
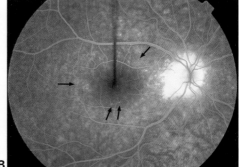

Figure 7-52 MEWDS, fluorescein angiogram. **A,** Early phase with multiple punctate hyperfluorescent lesions surrounding the fovea *(arrows)*. **B,** The lesions stain late in a wreathlike configuration *(arrows)*. *(Courtesy of Albert T. Vitale, MD.)*

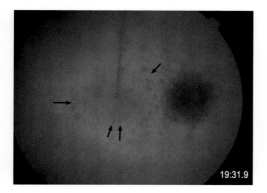

Figure 7-53 MEWDS. ICG angiogram of the same patient as in Figure 7-52, showing multiple, midphase, hypofluorescent spots, more numerous than appreciated on a fluorescein angiogram or clinical examination *(arrows)*. *(Courtesy of Albert T. Vitale, MD.)*

(100–200 μm) at the level of the RPE or deep retina, typically in a perifoveal location (Fig 7-51). These spots are transitory and are frequently missed; they leave instead a granular macular pigmentary change, a pathognomonic finding. There may be few associated vitreous cells, mild blurring of the optic disc, and, in rare instances, isolated vascular sheathing.

Fluorescein angiography is characteristic, revealing punctate hyperfluorescent lesions in a wreathlike configuration surrounding the fovea that stain late (Fig 7-52). ICG angiography shows multiple hypofluorescent lesions that are more numerous than those seen on examination or on FA and that typically fade with resolution of the disease (Fig 7-53). Visual field abnormalities are variable and include generalized depression, paracentral or peripheral scotomata, and enlargement of a blind spot. Electroretinographic abnormalities include diminished a-wave and early receptor potential (ERP) amplitudes, both of which are reversible. The multifocal ERG and electro-oculogram (EOG) localize the disease process to the RPE/photoreceptor complex.

The prognosis is excellent, and vision is completely recovered in 2–10 weeks without treatment. Recurrences are uncommon, occurring in 10%–15% of patients, and bilateral disease is rare. MEWDS has been reported in association with MCP and with acute macular neuroretinopathy (AMN). The latter is a rare condition, occurring among otherwise healthy young females, and is characterized by the acute onset of visual impairment and multifocal scotomata that correspond precisely to reddish, flat, wedge-shaped lesions in the macula. Although most patients experience a minimal decrease in visual acuity, symptoms frequently persist despite resolution of the fundus lesions. No treatment is required, given the condition's favorable natural history.

Bryan RG, Freund KB, Yannuzi LA, Spaide RF, Huang SJ, Costa DL. Multiple evanescent white dot syndrome in patients with multifocal choroiditis. *Retina.* 2002;22:317–322.

Jampol LM, Sieving PA, Pugh D, Fishman GA, Gilbert H. Multiple evanescent white dot syndrome. I. Clinical findings. *Arch Ophthalmol.* 1984;102:671–674.

Olitsky SE. Multiple evanescent white-dot syndrome in a 10-year-old child. *J Pediatr Ophthalmol Strabismus.* 1998;35:288–289.

Sieving PA, Fishman GA, Jampol LM, Pugh D. Multiple evanescent white dot syndrome. II. Electrophysiology of the photoreceptors during retinal pigment epithelial disease. *Arch Ophthalmol.* 1984;102:675–679.

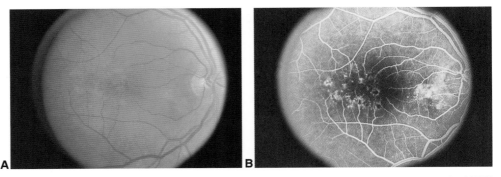

Figure 7-54 **A,** Acute retinal pigment epitheliitis (ARPE). **B,** Fluorescein angiogram in ARPE showing honeycomb lesions at the level of the RPE. *(Courtesy of E. Mitchel Opremcak, MD.)*

Acute retinal pigment epitheliitis

Acute retinal pigment epitheliitis (ARPE), or Krill disease, is a benign, acute, self-limiting inflammatory disorder of the RPE of unknown etiology. It typically presents in otherwise healthy young adults between the ages of 16 and 40 years with acute unilateral visual loss, central metamorphopsia, and scotomata. Ophthalmoscopic findings include clusters of small, discrete, hyperpigmented lesions, typically with a yellow halo in the posterior pole unassociated with vitritis or other funduscopic abnormalities (Fig 7-54). Fluorescein angiography shows early hyperfluorescence of the pinpoint dots with a surrounding halo of hyperfluorescence and late staining. Visual field testing shows central scotomata. A normal ERG and an abnormal EOG localize the disease process to the RPE. No treatment is required, as the lesions resolve without sequelae with excellent visual acuity over 6–12 weeks.

Deutman AF. Acute retinal pigment epitheliitis. *Am J Ophthalmol.* 1974;78:571–578.

Luttrull J, Chittum EM. Acute retinal pigment epitheliitis. *Am J Ophthalmol.* 1995;120:389–391.

Acute zonal occult outer retinopathy (AZOOR)

Acute zonal occult outer retinopathy (AZOOR) is typified by acute loss of 1 or more zones of outer retinal function associated with photopsia, minimal funduscopic changes, and ERG abnormalities affecting 1 or both eyes. Patients are typically young, myopic females who present with acute unilateral visual disturbances and apparently normal funduscopic examination, not infrequently associated with a mild vitritis (50%) and visual acuity in the 20/40 range. Electrophysiology may demonstrate a consistent pattern of dysfunction, not only at the photoreceptor/RPE complex but also at the inner retinal level. Essentially these consist of a delayed 30-Hz–flicker ERG and a reduction in the EOG light rise, which, when present with classic symptomatology, may be helpful diagnostically.

With extended follow-up, the majority of patients develop bilateral disease, with recurrences in approximately one third of patients. Similarly, the funduscopic appearance varies with the stage of the disease, ranging from initial subtle RPE changes with depigmentation in areas of visual loss to vessel attenuation, late pigment migration, and focal perivenous sheathing. Visual field abnormalities typically stabilize in approximately three quarters of patients and partially improve in about 25%. Visual acuity remains in the

20/40 range in 68% of patients; however, legal blindness has been reported in as many as 18% with long-term follow-up.

The considerable similarities between AZOOR and other white dot syndromes—namely, MEWDS, MCP, PIC, AMN, OHS, and acute idiopathic blind spot enlargement syndrome (AIBSE) has led some investigators to group these entities together in the so-called AZOOR complex of diseases. Although an infectious etiology has been postulated, systemic autoimmune disease has been observed in 28% of patients, supporting the notion that these diseases are of an inflammatory etiology arising among patients with a common non–disease-specific genetic background.

Cancer-associated retinopathy and retinitis pigmentosa should be considered in the differential diagnosis. It is unclear whether treatment with systemic corticosteroids or immunomodulatory therapy alters the disease course or visual outcome.

Francis PJ, Marinescu A, Fitzke FW, Bird AC, Holder GE. Acute zonal occult outer retinopathy: towards a set of diagnostic criteria. *Br J Ophthalmol.* 2005;89:70–73.

Gass JD, Agarwal A, Scott IU. Acute zonal occult outer retinopathy: a long-term follow-up study. *Am J Ophthalmol.* 2002;134:329–339.

Panuveitis

Although intraocular inflammation can originate as an iritis, retinitis, or choroiditis, the designation "panuveitis," or *diffuse uveitis,* by definition, requires involvement of all anatomical compartments of the eye—namely, the anterior chamber, vitreous, retina and/or choroid—with no single predominant site of inflammation. As with posterior uveitis, structural complications such as macular edema, retinal or choroidal neovascularization, or vasculitis, although not infrequent accompaniments, are not considered essential in the anatomical classification of panuveitis. Generally, panuveitis is bilateral, although 1 eye may be first and the severity is not necessarily symmetric. The discussion of panuveitis in this chapter is limited to the noninfectious entities.

Sarcoidosis

Sarcoidosis is a multisystem granulomatous disorder of unknown etiology with protean, systemic, and ocular manifestations. Although intrathoracic manifestations are most common (90%), other organs frequently involved by sarcoidosis include the lymph nodes, skin, eyes, central nervous system, bones, and joints. Between 15% and 50% of patients with systemic sarcoidosis may exhibit ocular involvement, with uveitis being the most frequent manifestation. In most large series, sarcoidosis accounts for between 3% and 10% of all cases of uveitis.

Sarcoidosis has a worldwide distribution, with all races being affected. In the United States, however, the disease is 10–20 times more prevalent among African Americans than among Caucasians. Both sexes are affected, albeit with a slight female predominance, usually between the ages of 20 and 50 years. Pediatric involvement is uncommon, and the clinical course is atypical. Children with early-onset sarcoidosis (younger than 5 years of age) are less likely than adults to manifest pulmonary disease and far more likely to have cutaneous and articular involvement; the disease course in older children (ages 8–15 years) approximates that in adults.

A variety of infectious agents and environmental allergens have been implicated in the pathogenesis of sarcoidosis, but none has been conclusively demonstrated. A possible genetic predisposition for the development of the disease is suggested by the increased frequency of HLA-DRB1 in patients with biopsy-confirmed sarcoidosis. Patients with the disease characteristically exhibit peripheral anergy on skin testing due to depression in delayed-type hypersensitivity, but at the target organ site, an active helper T-lymphocyte (CD4+) and macrophage-driven immunologic response is present, leading to granuloma formation.

The basic pathologic lesion of sarcoidosis is a noncaseating epithelioid cell granuloma, or tubercle (Fig 7-55). The epithelioid cell is a polyhedral mononuclear histiocyte that is derived from monocytes of the peripheral blood or macrophages of the tissue. The tubercle of sarcoidosis is composed of the following:

- epithelioid cells
- multinucleate giant cells of the Langhans type, with nuclei at the periphery of the cell arranged in an arc or incomplete circle
- a thin rim of lymphocytes

Central areas of the tubercle seldom undergo fibrinoid degeneration or, in skin lesions (lupus pernio), micronecrosis. Various types of inclusion bodies may occur in the cytoplasm of giant cells, including

- *Schaumann,* or *lamellar bodies:* ovoid, basophilic, calcific bodies measuring up to 100 μm in diameter and also containing iron
- *asteroid bodies:* star-shaped acidophilic bodies measuring up to 25 μm in diameter

Systemic sarcoidosis may present acutely, frequently with associated iridocyclitis in young patients, and spontaneously remit within 2 years of onset. *Löfgren syndrome* consists of erythema nodosum, febrile arthropathy, bilateral hilar adenopathy, and acute iritis and is quite responsive to systemic corticosteroids; it has a good long-term prognosis. *Heerfordt syndrome* (uveoparotid fever) is characterized by uveitis, parotitis, fever, and facial nerve palsy. Chronic sarcoidosis presents insidiously and is characterized by persistent disease of more than 2 years' duration, frequently with interpulmonary involvement

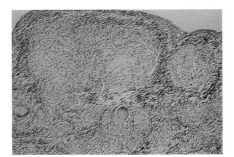

Figure 7-55 Sarcoidosis, histopathologic view of conjunctival biopsy. Note the giant cells and granulomatous inflammation.

and chronic uveitis. Extended corticosteroid therapy may be required. Pulmonary disease is the major cause of morbidity; overall mortality from sarcoidosis approaches 5% but may be as high as 10% with neurosarcoidosis.

Sarcoidosis may affect any ocular tissue, including the orbit and adnexa. Cutaneous involvement is frequent, and orbital and eyelid granulomas are common (Fig 7-56). Palpebral and bulbar conjunctival nodules may also be observed and provide a readily accessible site for tissue biopsy (Fig 7-57). Lacrimal gland infiltration may cause keratoconjunctivitis sicca.

Anterior uveitis, presenting either acutely or as a chronic granulomatous iridocyclitis, is the most common ocular lesion, occurring in approximately two thirds of patients with ocular sarcoidosis. Symptoms of uveal involvement are variable and frequently include mild to moderate blurring of vision and aching around the eyes. Typical findings include

- mutton-fat KPs (Fig 7-58)
- Koeppe and Busacca iris nodules (Fig 7-59)
- white clumps of cells (snowballs) in the inferior anterior vitreous

Although the cornea is infrequently involved, nummular corneal infiltrates and inferior corneal endothelial opacification may be seen; band keratopathy may develop due to either chronic uveitis or hypercalcemia. Large iris granulomas, together with extensive posterior synechiae, may lead to iris bombé and angle-closure glaucoma. Peripheral

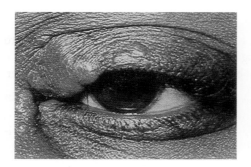

Figure 7-56 Sarcoidosis, skin lesions.

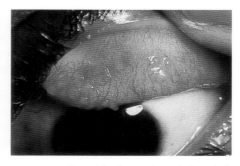

Figure 7-57 Sarcoidosis, conjunctival nodules.

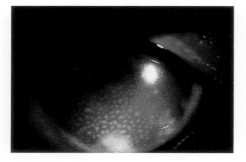

Figure 7-58 Sarcoidosis, keratic precipitates and iridocyclitis.

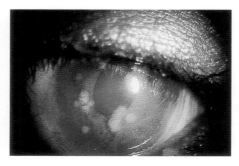

Figure 7-59 Sarcoidosis, iris nodules.

anterior synechiae (PAS) may also be extensive, encompassing the entire angle for 360° in advanced cases. Secondary glaucoma, together with sarcoid uveitis, may be severe and portends a poor prognosis with associated severe visual loss.

Posterior segment lesions occur in approximately 14%–20% of patients with ocular sarcoidosis. Vitreous infiltration is common and may be diffuse or appear more classically as yellowish white aggregates, so-called snowballs, or linearly, as a "string of pearls." Nodular granulomas measuring ¼ to 1 disc diameter may be observed on the optic nerve, in both the retina and the choroid, either posteriorly or peripherally (Fig 7-60). Perivascular sheathing is also common, appearing most often as either a linear or segmental periphlebitis (Fig 7-61). Irregular nodular granulomas along venules have been termed *candlewax drippings,* or *taches de bougie.* Occlusive retinal vascular disease, especially branch retinal vein occlusion and, less commonly, central retinal vein occlusion, together with peripheral retinal capillary nonperfusion, may lead to retinal neovascularization and vitreous hemorrhage. Cystoid macular edema is frequently present, and optic disc

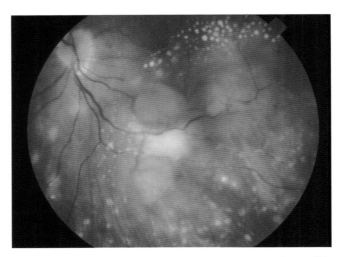

Figure 7-60 Multiple retinal and choroidal nodular granulomas, perivasculitis, and vitritis in a patient with sarcoid-associated posterior segment involvement. *(Courtesy of Albert T. Vitale, MD.)*

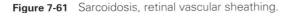

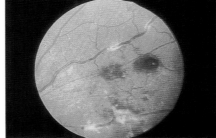

Figure 7-61 Sarcoidosis, retinal vascular sheathing.

edema without granulomatous invasion of the optic nerve may be observed in patients with papilledema and neurosarcoidosis.

Diagnosis and management

Given its heterogeneous presentation, sarcoidosis should be considered in the differential diagnosis of any patient presenting with intraocular inflammation. Early-onset sarcoidosis in children (5 years of age or younger) must be differentiated from JRA/JIA-associated iridocyclitis and from familial juvenile systemic granulomatosis, given the overlap of ocular and articular involvement.

A chest radiograph is the single best screening test for the diagnosis of sarcoidosis, because it is abnormal in approximately 90% of patients with this disease. Thin-cut, spiral computed tomographic (CT) imaging is a more sensitive imaging modality and may be particularly valuable in the setting of a normal chest radiograph in which there remains a high clinical index of suspicion for disease. In such cases, parenchymal, mediastinal, and hilar structures with distinctive CT patterns that are virtually pathognomonic for sarcoidosis may lead to the diagnosis. Although the serum ACE and lysozyme levels may be abnormally elevated, neither are diagnostic or specific; rather, they are reflective of the total-body granuloma content and, as such, may be useful in following patients with active disease. Similarly, gallium scanning in combination with an elevated ACE level appears to be highly specific for sarcoidosis in patients with active disease in whom the clinical suspicion of sarcoidosis is high. However, routine screening of patients with uveitis with both ACE levels and gallium scanning may be inappropriate given the low positive predictive value in this clinical setting. Ultimately, the diagnosis of sarcoidosis is made histopathologically, from tissue obtained from the lungs, mediastinal lymph nodes, skin, peripheral lymph nodes, liver, conjunctiva, or minor salivary glands (lacrimal gland). Biopsy sites exhibiting readily accessible and clinically evident lesions (such as those on the skin, palpable lymph nodes, and nodules on the conjunctiva) should be sought because such lesions are associated with a high yield and low morbidity and may obviate the need for more invasive transbronchial biopsy.

Topical, periocular, and systemic corticosteroids are the mainstays of therapy. Cycloplegia is useful for comfort and for prevention of synechiae. Vision-threatening posterior segment lesions generally require, and are responsive to, systemic corticosteroids (prednisone, 40–80 mg/day). Systemic immunomodulatory therapy with methotrexate, azathioprine, mycophenolate mofetil, or cyclosporine may be required in patients who either are intolerant of or fail to respond to systemic corticosteroids. Recently, the TNF-α inhibitor infliximab has been shown to be effective in the treatment of sarcoid-associated uveitis. Prognostic factors associated with visual loss in patients with ocular sarcoidosis include the presence of chronic posterior uveitis, glaucoma, a delay in presentation to a uveitis specialist of more than 1 year, and the presence of intermediate or posterior uveitis. The likelihood of significant visual improvement is substantially increased with systemic therapy.

Bonfioli AA, Orefice F. Sarcoidosis. *Semin Ophthalmol.* 2005;20:177–182.

Dana MR, Merayo-Lloves J, Schaumberg DA, Foster CS. Prognosticators for visual outcome in sarcoid uveitis. *Ophthalmology.* 1996;103:1846–1853.

Dev S, McCallum RM, Jaffe GJ. Methotrexate treatment for sarcoid-associated panuveitis. *Ophthalmology.* 1999;106:111–118.

Duker JS, Brown GC, McNamara JA. Proliferative sarcoid retinopathy. *Ophthalmology.* 1988;95:1680–1686.

Jabs DA, Johns CJ. Ocular involvement in chronic sarcoidosis. *Am J Ophthalmol.* 1986;102:297–301.

Kaiser PK, Lowder CY, Sullivan P, et al. Chest computerized tomography in the evaluation of uveitis in elderly women. *Am J Ophthalmol.* 2002;133:499–505.

Power WJ, Neves RA, Rodriguez A, Pedroza-Seres M, Foster CS. The value of combined serum angiotensin-converting enzyme and gallium scan in diagnosing ocular sarcoidosis. *Ophthalmology.* 1995;102:2007–2011.

Sympathetic Ophthalmia

Sympathetic ophthalmia (SO) is a rare, bilateral, diffuse granulomatous, nonnecrotizing panuveitis that may develop after either surgical or accidental trauma to 1 eye (the exciting eye), followed by a latent period and the appearance of uveitis in the uninjured fellow eye (the sympathizing eye). Although the precise incidence of SO is difficult to ascertain due to its rarity, significant improvements in the management of ocular trauma, together with the more widespread use of immunomodulaatory therapy, has led to an overall decrease in its incidence. Earlier estimates of the incidence of SO ranged from 0.2% to 0.5% in eyes with nonsurgical trauma and 10 cases in 100,000 following intraocular surgery. Although the most recent minimum incidence estimate is low (at 0.03/100,000), SO remains a disease with a persistent and potentially devastating presence.

Accidental penetrating ocular trauma had been identified as the classic, most common precipitating event for SO until recently. Ocular surgery—particularly vitreoretinal surgery—has now emerged as the main risk for the development of SO. In the early 1980s, the prevalence of SO following pars plana vitrectomy was reported to be 0.01%, increasing to 0.06% when performed in the context of other penetrating ocular injuries. More recent studies suggest that the risk of developing SO following pars plana vitrectomy is more than twice this figure and may be significantly greater than that of infectious endophthalmitis following vitrectomy. Improved access to emergency surgical care following penetrating ocular trauma and improved microsurgical technique have undoubtedly influenced this etiologic shift from penetrating ocular injury to surgical trauma. Similarly, the demographic of SO has changed from earlier reports, in which there was higher prevalence among males, children, and the elderly (due to their presumed increased risk of accidental trauma), to more recent studies, which show no sex predominance and a lower risk in children (due in part to a reduced incidence of pediatric ocular injuries) and an increased risk in the elderly (likely due to an increased frequency of ocular surgery and retinal detachment in this population). Finally, although SO has been traditionally reported to develop in 80% of patients within 3 months of injury and in 90% within 1 year, this time interval may be longer than previously assumed; in recent series, only one third of patients developed SO within 3 months and less than half did so within 1 year of injury.

Patients with SO typically present with asymmetric bilateral panuveitis, with more severe inflammation in the exciting eye than in the sympathizing eye, at least initially.

Signs and symptoms in the sympathizing eye vary in their severity and onset, ranging from minimal problems in near vision, mild photophobia, and slight redness to severe granulomatous anterior uveitis. Both eyes may show mutton-fat KPs, thickening of the iris from lymphocytic infiltration, posterior synechiae formation, and elevated IOP due either to trabeculitis or to hypotony as a result of ciliary body shutdown (Fig 7-62).

Posterior segment findings include moderate to severe vitritis with characteristic yellowish white, midequatorial choroidal lesions, so-called Dalen-Fuchs nodules, that may become confluent. Peripapillary choroidal lesions and exudative retinal detachment may also develop (Fig 7-63). Structural complications of SO include cataract, chronic CME, choroidal neovascularization, and optic atrophy. Extraocular findings similar to those observed with VKH, including cerebral spinal fluid pleocytosis, sensory neural hearing disturbance, alopecia, poliosis, and vitiligo may be observed, although they are uncommon.

During the acute stage of the disease, FA reveals multiple hyperfluorescent sites of leakage at the level of the RPE during the venous phase, which persists into the late stage of the study (Fig 7-64). Pooling of dye is observed beneath areas of exudative neurosensory retinal detachment. Less common fluorescein angiographic patterns are determined by the status of the overlying RPE, with Dalen-Fuchs nodules appearing hypofluorescent early, simulating the pattern seen in APMPPE, or hyperfluorescent with late staining. ICG angiography reveals numerous hypofluorescent foci, which are best visualized during the

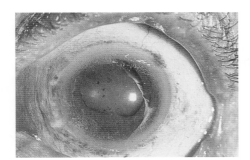

Figure 7-62 Sympathetic ophthalmia, sympathizing eye with synechiae.

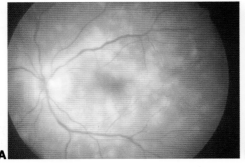
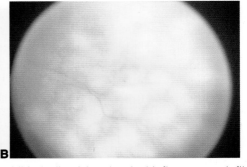

Figure 7-63 A, Peripapillary and multifocal choroiditis (yellowish subretinal inflammatory infiltrates) with exudative retinal detachment in the macula. **B,** Peripheral multifocal choroiditis and hazy view due to vitritis. *(Courtesy of Ramana S. Moorthy, MD.)*

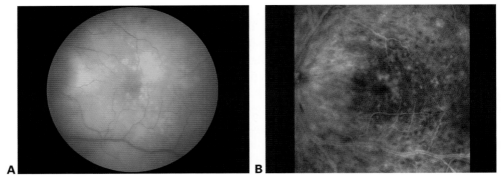

Figure 7-64 Sympathetic ophthalmia. **A,** Fundus photograph showing a multifocal choroiditis. **B,** Corresponding fluorescein angiogram disclosing multiple areas of alternating hyperfluorescence and blocked fluorescence at the level of the RPE. *(Courtesy of Albert T. Vitale, MD.)*

Figure 7-65 Sympathetic ophthalmia, ICG angiogram of the same patient as in Figure 7-64. Multiple, midphase hypofluorescent foci corresponding to, and more numerous than, the choroidal lesions seen on clinical examination or FA.

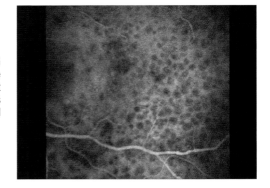

intermediate phase of the angiogram; some of these foci may become isofluorescent in the late stage of the study (Fig 7-65). B-scan ultrasonography frequently reveals choroidal thickening.

The histopathologic features of SO are similar for both the exciting and sympathizing eyes and include the following (Figs 7-66, 7-67):

- diffuse, granulomatous, nonnecrotizing infiltration of the choroid with a predominance of lymphocytes; some epithelioid cells; few giant cells, and plasma cells; and eosinophils in the inner choroid, particularly in heavily pigmented persons
- nodular clusters of epithelioid cells containing pigment, located between the RPE and Bruch's membrane, corresponding to the Dalen-Fuchs nodules; although present in one third of patients with SO, Dalen-Fuchs nodules are not pathognomonic, as they may also be seen in patients with VKH and sarcoidosis.
- absence of inflammatory involvement of the choriocapillaris and retina
- phagocytosis of uveal pigment by epithelioid cells
- extension of the granulomatous process into the scleral canals, the optic disc, vessels, macula, and periphery

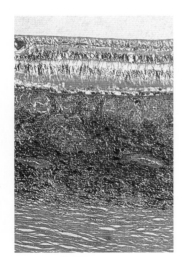

Figure 7-66 Diffuse granulomatous inflammation in sympathetic ophthalmia.

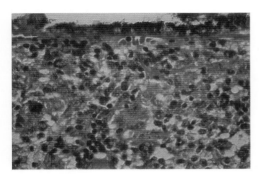

Figure 7-67 Sympathetic ophthalmia (histopathologic view). Note the giant cells in the choroid.

The precise etiology of SO is unknown; however, in the overwhelming majority of patients, there is a history of penetrating ocular injury complicated by incarceration of uveal tissue. Although it has been speculated that an infectious agent or a bacterial antigen may, through molecular mimicry of an endogenous ocular antigen, precipitate an immune response resulting in the development of SO, no organism has been consistently isolated from eyes with this disease, and it has not been reproduced in animal models following injection of a putative infectious agent. However, animal studies do support the notion that SO may result from altered T-lymphocyte responses to ocular self-antigens such as retinal S-antigen or to other retinal or choroidal melanocyte antigens. Furthermore, there may be a genetic predisposition to the development of the disease, as patients with SO are more likely to express HLA-DR4, -DRw53, and -DQw3 haplotypes. Recent studies from both the United Kingdom and Japan report the highest relative risk for haplotypes HLA-DRB1*04 and -DQB1*04. It should be noted that the immunogenetics of SO and VKH are virtually identical, as the same associations have been found in both diseases.

The diagnosis of SO is clinical and should be suspected in the presence of bilateral uveitis following any ocular trauma or surgery. Table 7-7 lists surgical procedures and injuries known to be associated with SO. Differential diagnostic considerations include other causes of panuveitis, including tuberculosis, sarcoidosis, syphilis, and fungi, as well

Table 7-7 Surgical Procedures and Injuries That May Lead to Sympathetic Ophthalmia

Surgical procedures associated with sympathetic ophthalmia
Vitrectomy
Secondary IOL placement
Trabeculectomy
Iridencleisis
Contact and noncontact YAG laser cyclodestruction
Cyclocryotherapy
Proton beam and helium ion irradiation for choroidal melanoma
Cataract extraction, particularly when the iris is entrapped within the wound

Injuries associated with sympathetic ophthalmia
Perforating ulcers
Severe contusion
Subconjunctival scleral rupture
Any perforating injury, with or without direct uveal involvement or uveal prolapse

as traumatic or postoperative endophthalmitis. Phacoanaphylaxis has been reported in association with SO in up to 25% of cases and may present with a similar clinical picture. The clinical presentations of SO and VKH may be strikingly similar; however, systemic signs and symptoms are generally present, whereas a history of prior ocular injury is typically absent in patients with VKH.

The course of SO is chronic, with frequent exacerbations, and if left untreated, leads to loss of vision and phthisis bulbi. Every attempt should be made to salvage eyes with a reasonable prognosis for useful vision with meticulous and prompt closure of penetrating injuries; however, enucleation within 2 weeks of injury to prevent the development of SO should be considered in grossly disorganized globes with no discernible visual function. Although controversial, enucleation may still be preferred to evisceration as the operation of choice for the removal of ocular contents in severely injured eyes because it eliminates the possibility of residual uveal tissue, which may predispose to the development of sympathetic disease. BCSC Section 7, *Orbit, Eyelids, and Lacrimal System,* discusses the advantages and disadvantages of enucleation and evisceration in greater detail. Enucleation of the exciting eye once SO has become established has not been shown to be beneficial in altering the disease course of the sympathizing eye.

The mainstay of therapy for SO is immunomodulatory therapy, initially with systemic corticosteroids, with the frequent addition of corticosteroid-sparing agents such as azathioprine, methotrexate, mycophenolate mofetil, cyclosporine, chlorambucil, and cyclophosphamide, as extended therapy is anticipated in most patients. Topical corticosteroids, together with cycloplegic/mydriatic agents, are essential in the treatment of acute anterior uveitis associated with SO, as are periocular corticosteroids in the management of inflammatory recurrences and CME. With prompt and aggressive systemic immunomodulation, the visual prognosis of SO is good, with 50% of patients achieving a final visual acuity of 20/40 or better in at least 1 eye.

Bilyk JR. Enucleation, evisceration, and sympathetic ophthalmia. *Curr Opin Ophthalmol.* 2000;11:372–386.

Chan CC, Roberg RG, Whitcup SM, Nussenblatt RB. 32 cases of sympathetic ophthalmia: a retrospective study at the National Eye Institute, Bethesda, MD, from 1982 to 1992. *Arch Ophthalmol.* 1995;113:597–600.

Davis JL, Mittal KK, Freidlin V, et al. HLA associations and ancestry in Vogt-Koyanagi-Harada disease and sympathetic ophthalmia. *Ophthalmology.* 1990;97:1137–1142.

Gass JD. Sympathetic ophthalmia following vitrectomy. *Am J Ophthalmol.* 1982;93:552–558.

Kilmartin DJ, Dick AD, Forrester JV. Prospective surveillance of sympathetic ophthalmia in the UK and Republic of Ireland. *Br J Ophthalmol.* 2000;84:259–263.

Kilmartin DJ, Dick AD, Forrester JV. Sympathetic ophthalmia following vitrectomy: should we counsel patients? *Br J Ophthalmol.* 2000;84:448–449.

Kilmartin DJ, Wilson D, Liversidge J, et al. Immunogenetics and clinical phenotype of sympathetic ophthalmia in British and Irish patients. *Br J Ophthalmol.* 2001;85:281–286.

Liddy BS, Stuart J. Sympathetic ophthalmia and Vogt-Koyanagi-Harada syndrome. *Int Ophthalmol Clin.* 1990;30:279–285.

Lubin JR, Albert DM, Weinstein M. Sixty-five years of sympathetic ophthalmia. A clinico-pathologic review of 105 cases (1913–1978). *Ophthalmology.* 1980;87:109–121.

Marak GE Jr . Recent advances in sympathetic ophthalmia. *Surv Ophthalmol.* 1979;24:141–156.

Rao NA, Robin J, Hartmann D, Sweeney JA, Marak GE Jr. The role of the penetrating wound in the development of sympathetic ophthalmia: experimental observations. *Arch Ophthalmol.* 1983;101:102–104.

Shindo Y, Ohno S, Usui M, et al. Immunogenetic study of sympathetic ophthalmia. *Tissue Antigens.* 1997;49:111–115.

Winter FC. Sympathetic uveitis, a clinical and pathological study of the visual result. *Am J Ophthalmol.* 1955;39:340–347.

Vogt-Koyanagi-Harada Disease

Vogt-Koyanagi-Harada (VKH) disease is an uncommon multisystemic disease of presumed autoimmune etiology that is characterized by chronic, bilateral, diffuse, granulomatous panuveitis with accompanying integumentary, neurologic, and auditory involvement. Although the disease most commonly affects darkly pigmented ethnic groups (Asians, Asian Indians, Hispanics, Native Americans, and Middle Easterners) and is uncommon among Caucasians, VKH is also rare among Africans, suggesting that other factors, in addition to skin pigmentation, are important in its pathogenesis. The incidence of VKH varies geographically, accounting for 1%–4% of all uveitis referrals in the United States and 8% in Japan. In Brazil and Saudi Arabia, it is the most commonly encountered cause of noninfectious uveitis. Women appear to be affected more often than men except in the Japanese population.

The precise etiology and pathogenesis of VKH are unknown, but current clinical and experimental evidence suggests a cell-mediated autoimmune process driven by T lymphocytes directed against self-antigens associated with melanocytes in genetically susceptible individuals. Sensitization to melanocytic antigenic peptides by cutaneous injury or viral infection has been proposed as a possible trigger of this autoimmune process. Tyrosinase or tyrosinase-related proteins and unidentified 75-kDa protein and S-100 protein have been implicated as target antigens on the melanocytes. A genetic predisposition for the development of the disease and an immune dysregulatory pathogenesis is further supported by the strong association with HLA-DR4 among Japanese patients with VKH; the strongest associated risk is observed with the HLA-DRB1*0405 and HLA-DRB1*0410 haplotypes. Among Hispanic patients from southern California with VKH disease, 84% were found to have HLA-DR1 or HLA-DR4, with the HLA-DR1 conferring a higher relative risk than the HLA-DR4 haplotype.

Histopathologic findings in VKH vary depending on the stage of the disease. There are 4 stages: prodromal, acute uveitic, convalescent, and chronic recurrent. During the acute uveitic stage, diffuse, nonnecrotizing, granulomatous inflammation consisting of lymphocytes and macrophages admixed with epithelioid and multinucleate giant cells is found throughout the uvea. Proteinaceous fluid exudates are observed in the subretinal space between the detached neurosensory retina and the RPE. Although the peripapillary choroid is the predominant site for the granulomatous inflammatory infiltration, the ciliary body and iris may also be affected. Focal aggregates of epithelioid histiocytes admixed with RPE, or Dalen-Fuchs nodules, appear between Bruch's membrane and the RPE. In the convalescent stage, choroidal inflammation subsides and the number of choroidal melanocytes decreases; the clinical appearance of numerous focal yellowish, round lesions in the inferior peripheral fundus corresponds to the focal loss of RPE cells histologically. Although Dalen-Fuchs nodules are present in both VKH and SO, plasma cells are readily observed in VKH and involvement of the choriocapillaris is more common than in SO. These differences notwithstanding, the numerous similarities between SO and VKH clinically and pathologically suggest that they share a similar immunopathogenesis, albeit vis-à-vis different triggering events and modes of sensitization.

The clinical features of VKH vary depending on the stage of the disease. The prodromal stage is marked by flulike symptoms. Patients present with headache, nausea, meningismus, dysacusia, tinnitus, fever, orbital pain, photophobia, and hypersensitivity of the skin and hair to touch several days preceding the onset of ocular symptoms. Focal neurologic signs, although rare, may develop and include cranial neuropathies, hemiparesis, aphasia, transverse myelitis, and ganglionitis. Cerebrospinal fluid analysis reveals lymphocytic pleocytosis with normal glucose in more than 80% of patients, which may persist for up to 8 weeks. Auditory problems are observed in 75% of patients, frequently coincident with the onset of ocular disease. Central dysacusia, usually involving higher frequencies, or tinnitus occurs in approximately 30% of patients early in the disease course, typically improving within 2 to 3 months; however, persistent deficits may remain.

The acute uveitic stage is heralded by the onset of sequential blurring of vision in both eyes, 1 to 2 days after the onset of central nervous system signs, and is marked by bilateral granulomatous anterior uveitis, a variable degree of vitritis, thickening of the posterior choroid with elevation of the peripapillary retinal choroidal layer, hyperemia and edema of the optic nerve, and multiple serous retinal detachments (Fig 7-68). The focal serous retinal detachments are often shallow, with a cloverleaf pattern around the posterior pole, but may coalesce and evolve into large bullous exudative detachments (Fig 7-69). Profound visual loss may be seen during this phase. Less commonly, mutton-fat KPs and iris nodules at the pupillary margin may be observed. Intraocular pressure may be elevated; the anterior chamber may be shallow due to forward displacement of the lens iris diaphragm from ciliary body edema or annular choroidal detachment, or it may be low, secondary to ciliary body shutdown.

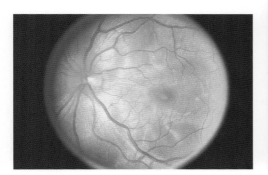

Figure 7-68 Disc hyperemia and multiple serous retinal detachments in the posterior pole of the left eye of an Hispanic patient in the acute phase of VKH disease. *(Reprinted with permission from Moorthy RS, Inomata H, Rao NA. Vogt-Koyanagi-Harada syndrome. Surv Ophthalmol. 1995;39:271, 272.)*

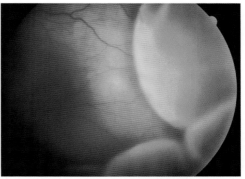

Figure 7-69 Bullous exudative retinal detachment in the acute phase of VKH disease. *(Courtesy of Albert T. Vitale, MD.)*

The convalescent stage occurs several weeks later and is marked by resolution of the exudative retinal detachments and gradual depigmentation of the choroid, resulting in the classic orange-red discoloration known as the *sunset-glow fundus appearance* (Fig 7-70). In addition, small, round, discrete depigmented lesions develop in the inferior peripheral fundus, representing resolved Dalen-Fuchs nodules (Fig 7-71). Juxtapapillary depigmentation may also be seen (see Fig 7-70). In Hispanics, the sunset-glow fundus may show focal areas of retinal hyperpigmentation or hypopigmentation. Perilimbal vitiligo (Sugiura sign) may be found in up to 85% of Japanese patients but is rarely observed among Caucasians (Fig 7-72). Integumentary changes, including vitiligo, alopecia, and poliosis, typically appear during the convalescent stage in about 30% of patients and correspond with the development of fundus depigmentation (Figs 7-73, 7-74). In general, skin and hair changes occur weeks to months following the onset of ocular inflammation, but in some cases they may appear simultaneously. Between 10% and 63% of patients develop vitiligo, depending on ethnic background, with the incidence of cutaneous and other extraocular manifestations being relatively low among Hispanics.

Patients inadequately treated during the uveitic and convalescent stages may enter the chronic recurrent stage. This is marked by recurrent bouts of granulomatous anterior uveitis, with the development of KPs, posterior synechiae, iris nodules, iris depigmentation, and stromal atrophy. Recurrent posterior uveitis with exudative retinal detachment is uncommon during this stage. Visually debilitating sequelae of chronic inflammation develop during this stage and include posterior subcapsular cataract, glaucoma, CNV, and subretinal fibrosis.

Based on these clinical features and their distinctive appearance within the overall disease course, comprehensive diagnostic criteria for the complete, incomplete, or probable forms of VKH have been recently revised (Table 7-8). Regardless of the form of the disease, essential features for the diagnosis of VKH include bilateral involvement, the absence of a history of penetrating ocular trauma, and no evidence of other ocular or systemic disease.

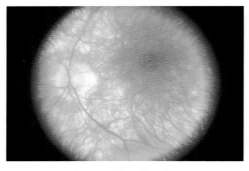

Figure 7-70 Sunset-glow fundus appearance in the chronic phase of VKH disease in an Hispanic patient. *(Reprinted with permission from Moorthy RS, Inomata H, Rao NA. Vogt-Koyanagi-Harada syndrome. Surv Ophthalmol. 1995;39:271, 272.)*

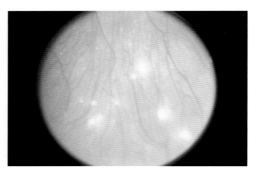

Figure 7-71 Multiple inferior peripheral punched-out chorioretinal lesions representing resolved Dalen-Fuchs nodules in the chronic phase of VKH disease. *(Courtesy of Ramana S. Moorthy, MD.)*

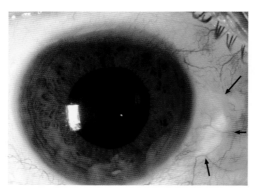

Figure 7-72 Perilimbal vitiligo of a Sugiura sign *(arrows). (Courtesy of Albert T. Vitale, MD.)*

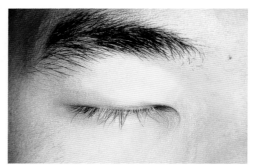

Figure 7-73 Vitiligo of the upper eyelid and marked poliosis in the chronic phase of VKH disease. *(Courtesy of Ramana S. Moorthy, MD.)*

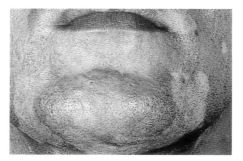

Figure 7-74 VKH disease, skin lesion.

The diagnosis of VKH is essentially a clinical one, but in patients presenting without extraocular changes, FA, ICG angiography, optical coherence tomography (OCT), lumbar puncture, and ultrasonography may be useful confirmatory tests. During the acute uveitic stage, FA typically reveals numerous punctate hyperfluorescent foci at the level of the RPE

Table 7-8 Revised Diagnostic Criteria for Vogt-Koyanagi-Harada Disease

Complete Vogt-Koyanagi-Harada disease
1. No history of penetrating ocular trauma or surgery
2. No clinical or laboratory evidence of other ocular or systemic disease
3. Bilateral ocular disease (either a or b below must be met):
    a. Early manifestations
        i. Diffuse choroiditis as manifested by either:
            (1) Focal areas of subretinal fluid, or
            (2) Bullous serous subretinal detachments
        ii. With equivocal fundus findings, then both:
            (1) Fluorescein angiography showing focal delayed choroidal perfusion, pinpoint leakage, large placoid areas of hyperfluorescence, pooling of dye within subretinal fluid, and optic nerve staining
            (2) Ultrasonography showing diffuse choroidal thickening without evidence of posterior scleritis
    b. Late manifestations
        i. History suggestive of findings from 3a, and either both ii and iii below, or multiple signs from iii
        ii. Ocular depigmentation
            (1) Sunset-glow fundus, or
            (2) Sugiura's sign
        iii. Other ocular signs
            (1) Nummular chorioretinal depigmentation scars, or
            (2) RPE clumping and/or migration, or
            (3) Recurrent or chronic anterior uveitis
4. Neurologic/auditory findings (may have resolved by time of exam):
    a. Meningismus
    b. Tinnitus
    c. Cerebrospinal fluid pleocytosis
5. Integumentary findings (not preceding CNS/ocular disease)
    a. Alopecia
    b. Poliosis
    c. Vitiligo

Incomplete Vogt-Koyanagi-Harada disease
Criteria 1 to 3 and either 4 or 5 from above

Probable Vogt-Koyanagi-Harada disease
Criteria 1 to 3 from above must be present
Isolated ocular disease

Adapted from Read RW, Holland GN, Rao NA, et al. Revised diagnostic criteria for Vogt-Koyanagi-Harada disease: report of an international committee on nomenclature. *Am J Ophthalmol.* 2001;131:647–652.

in the early stage of the study followed by pooling of dye in the subretinal space in areas of neurosensory detachment (Fig 7-75). The vast majority of patients show disc leakage, but CME and retinal vascular leakage are uncommon. In the convalescent and chronic recurrent stages of the disease, focal RPE loss and atrophy produces multiple hyperfluorescent window defects without progressive staining.

ICG angiography highlights the choroidal pathology, disclosing a delay in choriocapillaris and choroidal vessel perfusion, together with multiple hypofluorescent spots throughout the fundus, thought to correspond to foci of lymphocytic infiltration, and hyperfluorescent pinpoint changes within areas of exudative retinal detachment. These

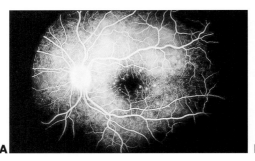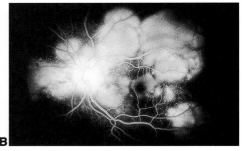

A **B**

Figure 7-75 **A,** Early arteriovenous phase fluorescein angiogram showing multiple pinpoint foci of hyperfluorescence in the posterior pole of the left eye of a patient in the acute phase of VKH disease. **B,** Late arteriovenous phase fluorescein angiogram showing fluorescein pooling in multiple serous retinal detachments in the posterior pole in the same eye. *(Courtesy of Ramana S. Moorthy, MD.)*

hypofluorescent spots may be present even when the funduscopic examination and FA are unremarkable.

Ultrasonography may be helpful in establishing the diagnosis, especially in the presence of media opacity. Findings include diffuse, low-to-medium reflective thickening of the posterior choroid, most prominent in the peripapillary area, with extension to the equatorial region, exudative retinal detachment, vitreous opacification, and posterior thickening of the sclera.

OCT may be useful in the diagnosis and monitoring of serous macular detachments, CME, and choroidal neovascular membranes.

In highly atypical cases—particularly patients presenting early in the course of the disease with prominent neurologic signs and a paucity of ocular findings—a lumbar puncture, revealing lymphocytic pleocytosis, may be useful diagnostically. However, in the vast majority of cases, the history and clinical examination, together with FA and/or ultrasonography, are sufficient to establish the diagnosis of VKH disease.

The differential diagnosis of VKH includes SO, uveal effusion syndrome, posterior scleritis, primary intraocular lymphoma, uveal lymphoid infiltration, APMPPE, and sarcoidosis. These entities may be differentiated from VKH by a thorough history, review of systems, and physical examination, together with a directed laboratory evaluation.

The acute stage of VKH is exquisitely responsive to early and aggressive treatment with topical, periocular, and systemic corticosteroids and cycloplegic/mydriatic agents. Initial doses typically range from 1.0 to 1.5 mg/kg/day of oral prednisone or 200 mg of intravenous methylprednisolone for 3 days, followed by high-dose oral corticosteroids. Systemic corticosteroids are tapered slowly according to the clinical response, usually over a 6-month period, in an effort to prevent progression of the disease to the chronic recurrent stage and to minimize the incidence and severity of extraocular manifestations. Recurrent episodes of inflammation become increasingly corticosteroid-resistant and require treatment with immunomodulatory therapy, including cyclosporine, azathioprine, mycophenolate mofetil, chlorambucil, or cyclophosphamide. The overall visual prognosis for patients managed in this fashion is fair, with nearly 60%–70% of patients retaining vision of 20/40 or better. Structural complications associated with ocular morbidity include cataract formation (50%); glaucoma (33%); CNV (10%–15%); and subretinal fibrosis, the development of which is associated with increased duration of the disease, more frequent recurrences, and an older age of disease onset. Recently, the use of either oral corticosteroids or immunomodulatory drug therapy with extended follow-up has been shown to reduce the risk of vision loss and the development of some structural complications. Specifically, with systemic corticosteroids, the risk of CNV and of subretinal fibrosis was reduced by 82%, and the risk of visual acuity loss to 20/200 or worse in better-seeing eyes was reduced by 67%. The use of immunomodulatory drug therapy was associated with a risk reduction of 67% for vision loss to 20/50 or worse in better-seeing eyes and of 92% for vision loss to 20/200 or worse in better-seeing eyes.

Bouchenaki N, Herbort CP. The contribution of indocyanine green angiography to the appraisal and management of Vogt-Koyanagi-Harada disease. *Ophthalmology.* 2001;108:54–64.

Bykhovskaya I, Thorne JE, Kempen JH, Dunn JP, Jabs DA. Vogt-Koyanagi-Harada disease: clinical outcomes. *Am J Ophthalmol.* 2005;140:674–678.

Gocho K, Kondo I, Yamaki K. Identification of autoreactive cells in Vogt-Koyanagi-Harada disease. *Jpn J Ophthalmol.* 2001;42:2004–2009.

Hayakawa K, Ishikawa M, Yamaki K. Ultrastructural changes in rat eyes with experimental Vogt-Koyanagi-Harada disease. *Jpn J Ophthalmol.* 2004;48:222–227.

Inomata H, Rao NA. Depigmented atrophic lesions in sunset-glow fundi of Vogt-Koyanagi-Harada disease. *Am J Ophthalmol.* 2001;131:607–614.

Moorthy RS, Inomata H, Rao NA. Vogt-Koyanagi-Harada syndrome. *Surv Ophthalmol.* 1995;39:265–292.

Ohno S, Char DH, Kimura SJ, O'Connor GR. Vogt-Koyanagi-Harada syndrome. *Am J Ophthalmol.* 1977;83:735–740.

Read RW, Holland GN, Rao NA, et al. Revised diagnostic criteria for Vogt-Koyanagi-Harada disease: report of an international committee on nomenclature. *Am J Ophthalmol.* 2001;131:647–652.

Read RW, Rechodouni A, Butani N, et al. Complications and prognostic factors in Vogt-Koyanagi-Harada disease. *Am J Ophthalmol.* 2001;131:599–606.

Rubsamen PE, Gass JD. Vogt-Koyanagi-Harada syndrome. Clinical course, therapy, and long-term visual outcome. *Arch Ophthalmol.* 1991;109:682–687.

Shindo Y, Ohno S, Yamamoto T, Nakamura S, Inoko H. Complete association of the HLA-DRB1*04 and DQB1*04 alleles with Vogt-Koyanagi-Harada disease. *Hum Immunol.* 1994;39:169–176.

Weisz JM, Holland GN, Roer LN, et al. Association between Vogt-Koyanagi-Harada syndrome and HLA-DR1 and -DR4 in Hispanic patients living in southern California. *Ophthalmology.* 1995;102:1012–1015.

Adamantiades-Behçet Disease

Adamantiades-Behçet disease (ABD) is a chronic, relapsing occlusive vasculitis (Fig 7-76) of unknown etiology that is characterized, in part, by a uveitis that can affect both the anterior and the posterior segments of the eye, often simultaneously. The symptoms of this disease were described as early as 2500 years ago, but it was only in the early 20th century that its clinical features were more completely described by Adamantiades and Behçet. ABD occurs in many ethnic populations all over the world. It is most common in the eastern Mediterranean countries and in countries in the eastern rim of Asia, in the

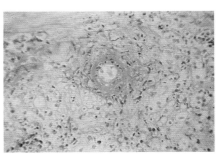

Figure 7-76 Adamantiades-Behçet disease, histopathologic view of perivascular inflammation.

Northern Hemisphere, particularly along the Old Silk Route, made famous by traders such as Marco Polo. The prevalence of ABD varies from as high as 80–300 cases per 100,000 inhabitants in Turkey, to 8–10 per 100,000 in Japan, to 0.4 per 100,000 in the United States. The complete type of ABD is more common in men and the incomplete type is equally frequent in men and women. Throughout the world, the main age of onset is between 25 and 35 years. Although there have been some familial cases of ABD, most cases are sporadic.

The diagnosis of ABD is a clinical one and is based on the presence of multiple systemic findings. The diagnostic system for ABD given in Table 7-9 was suggested by researchers in Japan. Another diagnostic system, which was suggested by the International Study Group for ABD, is shown in Table 7-10. According to the Japanese classification system, the 4 major criteria for ABD are recurrent oral aphthae, skin lesions (including erythema nodosum and acneiform eruptions), recurring genital ulcers, and intraocular inflammation. The presence of all 4 major symptoms is considered the *complete form* of Adamantiades-Behçet disease. The *incomplete form* has 3 major criteria, which can occur at different times, or typical ocular inflammatory disease that is recurrent, plus 1 other major criterion. The *suspect type* of ABD is associated with only 2 major symptoms and no ocular symptoms. The *possible type* has only 1 main criterion or symptom. Although ABD is a multisystem disease, it can predominantly affect 1 of these systems; thus, special clinical types of ABD occur—namely, neuro-ABD, ocular-ABD, intestinal-ABD, and vascular-ABD. Laboratory tests that can help confirm the diagnosis include a pathergy test (skin prick), HLA-B51, and nonspecific immunologic factors such as ESR and C-reactive protein. These diagnostic tests may be beneficial in confirming the suspected clinical diagnosis. They are not, in and of themselves, diagnostic of ABD.

Nonocular systemic manifestations

Oral aphthae are the most frequent finding in ABD (Fig 7-77). These are mucosal ulcers that produce significant discomfort and pain and are recurrent. They can occur on the lips, gums, palate, tongue, uvula, and posterior pharynx. They are round or oval, discrete white ulcerations that vary in size from 2 to 15 mm with a red rim. They recur every 5 to 10 days or every month. They last from 7 to 10 days and then heal without much scarring unless they are large.

Skin lesions can include painful or recurrent lesions of erythema nodosum, often over extensor surfaces such as the tibia, but also the face, neck, and buttocks. They disappear with minimal, if any, scarring. Acne vulgaris or folliculitis-like skin lesions may frequently

Table 7-9   Diagnostic System for Adamantiades-Behçet Disease (Japan)

Major Criteria
Recurrent oral aphthous ulcers
Skin lesions (erythema nodosum, acneiform pustules, folliculitis)
Recurrent genital ulcers
Ocular inflammatory disease

Minor Criteria
Arthritis
Gastrointestinal ulceration
Epididymitis
Systemic vasculitis or associated complications
Neuropsychiatric symptoms

Types of ABD
Complete (4 major criteria)
Incomplete (3 major criteria or ocular involvement with 1 other major criterion)
Suspect (2 major criteria with no ocular involvement)
Possible (1 major criterion)

Adapted from Foster CS, Vitale AT. *Diagnosis and Treatment of Uveitis*. Philadelphia: W.B. Saunders; 2002.

Table 7-10   Diagnostic System for Adamantiades-Behçet Disease (International Study Group for Behçet Disease)

Recurrent oral aphthous ulcers (at least 3 or more times per year) plus 2 of the following criteria:
1. Recurrent genital ulcers
2. Ocular inflammation
3. Skin lesions
4. Positive cutaneous pathergy test

Adapted from Foster CS, Vitale AT. *Diagnosis and Treatment of Uveitis*. Philadelphia: W.B. Saunders; 2002.

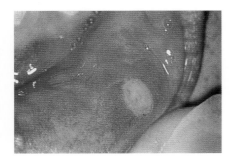

Figure 7-77   Adamantiades-Behçet disease, mucous membrane ulcers.

appear on the upper thorax and face. Nearly 40% of patients with ABD exhibit cutaneous pathergy, which is characterized by the development of a sterile pustule at the site of a venipuncture or an injection but is not pathognomic of ABD.

Genital ulcers appear grossly similar to oral aphthous ulcers. In male patients, they can occur on the scrotum or penis. In female patients, they can appear on the vulva and the vaginal mucosa. These lesions have variable amounts of pain associated with them.

Systemic vasculitis may also occur, and any size artery or vein in the body may be affected. This may occur in up to 25% of patients with ABD. Four different vascular complications can develop from the systemic vasculitis of ABD: arterial occlusion, aneurysm, venous occlusion, and varices.

Cardiac involvement from ABD can include granulomatous endocarditis, myocarditis, endomyocardial fibrosis, coronary arteritis, and pericarditis. These can occur in up to 17% of patients with ABD. Gastrointestinal involvement can include multiple ulcers involving the esophagus, stomach, and intestines. Pulmonary involvement is mainly that of pulmonary arteritis with aneurysmal dilatation of the pulmonary artery. Fifty percent of patients with ABD develop arthritis; in 50% of these patients, the knee is most affected.

Neurologic involvement is probably the most serious of all manifestations of ABD, and it is well recognized. Central nervous system involvement may occur in up to 10% of patients with ABD. Neuro-ABD occurs many years after the initial onset of ABD. Ten percent of patients with neuro-ABD can have ocular involvement, and 30% of patients with ocular-ABD may have neurologic involvement. Central nervous system involvement mainly affects the motor portion of the central nervous system. Widespread vasculitis in the central nervous system can result in headaches. Central nervous system symptoms such as strokes, palsies, and a confusional state may develop in 25% of patients. Mortality has been reported to be as high as 10% in patients with neuro-ABD, but today it may be better, especially with the use of immunomodulatory medications. More men than women appear to develop neuro-ABD. Neuro-ophthalmic involvement can include cranial nerve palsies, central scotomata caused by papillitis, visual field defects, and papilledema resulting from thrombosis of the superior saggital sinus or other venous sinuses.

Ocular manifestations

Ocular manifestations carry serious implications in ABD because they are often recurrent and relapsing, resulting in permanent, often irreversible, ocular damage. Severe vision loss can occur in up to 25% of ABD patients. Ocular disease appears to be more severe in men, and more men are affected; 80% of cases can be bilateral. Ocular involvement as an initial presenting problem is relatively uncommon, occurring in about 10% of patients. The intraocular inflammation is characterized by a nongranulomatous necrotizing obliterative vasculitis that can affect any or all portions of the uveal tract.

Anterior uveitis may be the only ocular manifestation in ABD; it presents with a hypopyon in about 25% of cases (Fig 7-78). This inflammation is nongranulomatous. Redness, pain, photophobia, and blurred vision are common findings. On clinical examination, the hypopyon can shift with the patient's head position and may not be visible unless viewed by gonioscopy. Although anterior uveitis may be very severe, it can spontaneously resolve even without treatment; however, the nature of ocular ABD is one of explosive onset over the course of just a few hours. With relapses, posterior synechiae, iris bombé, and angle-closure glaucoma may all develop. Other, less common, anterior segment findings of ABD can include cataract, episcleritis, scleritis, conjunctival ulcers, and corneal immune ring opacities.

The posterior segment manifestations of ocular-ABD are often profoundly sight-threatening. The essential retinal finding is that of an obliterative, necrotizing retinal vasculitis (Fig 7-79) that affects both the arteries and the veins in the fundus. Posterior

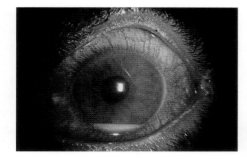

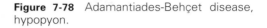

Figure 7-78 Adamantiades-Behçet disease, hypopyon.

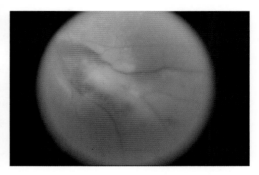

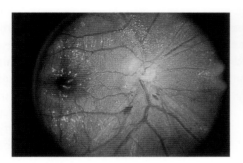

Figure 7-79 Adamantiades-Behçet disease, retinal vasculitis.

Figure 7-80 Retinitis and vasculitis with retinal hemorrhage in a patient with Adamantiades-Behçet disease. The retinitis seen here appears similar to necrotizing herpetic retinitis with retinal whitening and occlusive retinal vasculitis. *(Courtesy of Ramana S. Moorthy, MD.)*

manifestations can include branch retinal vein occlusion, isolated branch artery occlusions, combined branch retinal vein and branch retinal artery occlusions, and vascular sheathing with variable amounts of vitritis, plus associated CME. Retinal ischemia can lead to the development of retinal neovascularization and even of neovascularization of the iris and neovascular glaucoma. After repeated episodes of retinal vasculitis and vascular occlusions, retinal vessels may become white and sclerotic. Active areas of retinal vasculitis may be accompanied by multifocal areas of chalky white retinitis. The ischemic nature of the vasculitis and accompanying retinitis may produce a funduscopic appearance that may be confused with ARN syndrome or other necrotizing herpetic entities (Fig 7-80; also see Chapter 8). The optic nerve is affected in 25% of ABD patients. Optic papillitis can occur, but progressive optic atrophy may occur as a result of the vasculitis affecting the arterioles that supply blood to the optic nerve.

Pathogenesis and immunology of ABD

The underlying etiology of ABD is unknown. Many environmental factors have been suggested as a potential cause, but none of them has been proven. No infectious agent or microorganisms have been reproducibly isolated from lesions of patients with ABD. Although ABD may be considered an autoimmune disease—and autoimmune mechanisms have been intimated in its pathogenesis—there are many differences between classic autoimmune diseases and ABD. These differences include a male preponderance; a lack of association with other autoimmune diseases; a lack of definite T-lymphocyte hypofunction;

the hyperactivity of B lymphocytes; and a lack of association with HLA alleles, often found in other autoimmune disease.

Specific HLA associations have been found in certain systemic forms of ABD. HLA-B12 is associated with B12 mucocutaneous lesions, HLA-B27 may be associated with arthritis, and HLA-B5 may be associated with ocular lesions. These are not reproducible in all populations. Histopathologically, the lesions of ABD will resemble delayed-type hypersensitivity reactions early on; late lesions resemble immune-complex–type reactions.

Diagnosis of ABD is based on clinical findings and the diagnostic criteria given in Tables 7-9 and 7-10. HLA testing, cutaneous pathergy testing, and nonspecific serologic markers of inflammation such as ESR and C-reactive protein may be useful for confirming the diagnosis. Fluorescein angiography demonstrates marked dilatation and occlusion of retinal capillaries with perivascular staining, evidence of retinal ischemia, leakage of fluorescein into the macula with the development of CME, and retinal neovascularization that may leak. Radiologic imaging, including chest radiography, chest CT, and MRI of the brain with contrast enhancement, may be helpful, as indicated by clinical presentation.

Differential diagnosis

The differential diagnosis for ABD includes HLA-B27–associated anterior uveitis; Reiter syndrome; sarcoidosis; and systemic vasculitides, including systemic lupus, erythematosus, polyarteritis nodosa, and Wegner granulomatosis. Viral retinitis caused by herpes simplex virus or varicella-zoster virus should also be included in the differential diagnosis.

Treatment

The goal of treatment is not only to treat the explosive onset of acute disease but also to prevent or decrease the number of relapses of the ocular inflammatory disease. The use of immunomodulatory agents is imperative. The most commonly used agents include corticosteroids, cytotoxic drugs, colchicine, cyclosporine, and tacrolimus.

Corticosteroids Corticosteroids may be used to treat explosive-onset anterior segment and posterior segment inflammation, although most patients will eventually become resistant to corticosteroid therapy. Neverthess, corticosteroids (eg, 1.5 mg/kg/day of prednisone with a gradual taper) are extremely useful in controlling acute inflammation. Often, the immediate anti-inflammatory effect of corticosteroids is beneficial to patients waiting for cytotoxic therapeutic drugs to take full effect.

Immunomodulatory medications Azathioprine has been found to be useful in preserving visual acuity in patients with established ocular-ABD. It can also be effective in controlling oral and genital ulcers and arthritis. Chlorambucil has been found to be effective and safe in the treatment of ABD even at relatively low doses. As a single agent, chlorambucil may be the most effective of the immunomodulatory agents. Cyclophosphamide has been used with some success in Japan to treat ABD patients. It is an attractive alternative to chlorambucil although somewhat less effective. Both chlorambucil and cyclophosphamide have been shown to be more effective than cyclosporine A in the management of posterior segment ocular-ABD. Effective therapeutic reduction of white blood cell counts and proper hematologic monitoring are essential and can be quite complex with these alkylating agents. Cyclosporine A, at 5 mg/kg/day, has been used with some limited success in the management of ocular-ABD, but these lower, nonnephrotoxic doses appear to be not as effective as other cytotoxic agents in the management of posterior segment ocular-ABD. Low doses of cyclosporine may be combined with other cytotoxic immunomodulators for greater efficacy in controlling ocular-ABD. Tacrolimus may also be used as a substitute for cyclosporine A; it has been successfully used in Japan to treat ABD. Colchicine, at 0.6 mg/day, is used as a prophylaxis for current inflammatory episodes rather than as treatment for active disease. It is ineffective as a single agent for treating ocular symptomatology. Mycophenolate mofetil has been used in small case series to treat ABD and has been successful in treating ocular-ABD. The role of etanercept and infliximab in the treatment of ABD is under investigation. Infliximab appears promising for the treatment of ocular-ABD. Recent reports in the European literature emphasize the efficacy and good tolerance of IFN-α2a in patients with Adamantiades-Behçet disease.

Prognosis

Prognosis for vision is guarded in patients with ABD. Complications such as complex cataract, glaucoma, secondary and neovascular glaucoma, retinal and optic disc neovascularization, and vitreous hemorrhage all require complex surgical intervention (see Chapter 11) and have a profound impact on final visual outcomes. The chronic relapsing nature of this disease, with frequent exacerbations after long periods of remission, makes it difficult to predict the visual outcomes. Older clinical studies reported that severe vision loss can occur in up to 25% of ABD patients, but in the past 15 years, earlier initiation of immunomodulatory therapy has resulted in better visual outcomes.

Evereklioglu C. Current concepts in the etiology and treatment of Behçet disease. *Surv Ophthalmol.* 2005;50:297–350.

Feron EJ, Rothova A, van Hagen PM, Baarsma GS, Suttorp-Schulten MS. Interferon-alpha 2b for refractory ocular Behcet's disease. *Lancet.* 1994;343:1428.

Hashimoto T, Takeuchi A. Treatment of Behçet's disease. *Curr Opin Rheumatol.* 1992;4:31–34.

Kotter I, Zierhut M, Eckstein AK, et al. Human recombinant interferon alfa-2a for the treatment of Behçet's disease with sight threatening posterior or panuveitis. *Br J Ophthalmol.* 2003;87:423–431.

Nussenblatt RB, Palestine AG, Chan CC, Mochizuki M, Yancey K. Effectiveness of cyclosporin therapy for Behçet's disease. *Arthritis Rheum.* 1985;28:671–679.

Sfikakis PP, Theodossiadis PG, Katsiari CG, Kaklamanis P, Markomichelakis NN. Effect of infliximab on sight-threatening panuveitis in Behçet disease. *Lancet.* 2001;358:295–296.

Whitcup SM, Salvo EC Jr, Nussenblatt RB. Combined cyclosporine and corticosteroid therapy for sight-threatening uveitis in Behçet's disease. *Am J Ophthalmol.* 1994;118:39–45.

Yazici H, Pazarli H, Barnes CG, et al. A controlled trial of azathioprine in Behçet's syndrome. *N Engl J Med.* 1990;322:281–285.

Zafirakis P, Foster CS. Adamantiades-Behçet disease. In Foster CS, Vitale AT. *Diagnosis and Treatment of Uveitis.* Philadelphia: W.B. Saunders; 2002:632–652.

CHAPTER 8

Infectious Uveitis

Viruses, fungi, protozoa, helminths, and bacteria can all cause infectious uveitis. Because these organisms may produce inflammation in different parts of the uveal tract, this chapter has been organized based on the causative organism and, if appropriate, subcategorized into the anatomical location of the intraocular inflammation. The most common primary site of inflammation has been identified for each entity. Some agents, such as herpes simplex virus, may cause anterior and/or posterior uveitis. Others, such as syphilis, Lyme borreliosis, and onchocerciasis, usually cause panuveitis.

Viral Uveitis

Herpesviridae Family (HSV, VZV, CMV, and EBV)

Herpes simplex virus and varicella-zoster virus

Anterior uveitis   Acute anterior uveitis is often associated with herpetic viral disease. BCSC Section 8, *External Disease and Cornea,* extensively discusses herpes simplex virus (HSV) and varicella-zoster virus (VZV) (Figs 8-1, 8-2, 8-3). Usually, the uveal inflammation associated with these herpesviruses is a keratoiritis secondary to corneal disease. On occasion, the iritis may occur without noticeable keratitis. In many cases, the inflammation becomes chronic. Varicella-zoster virus may be considered in the differential diagnosis of chronic unilateral iridocyclitis, even if the cutaneous component of the condition occurred in the past or was minimal even when present. Some patients may develop iridocyclitis without ever having had a cutaneous component (varicella-zoster sine herpete).

Varicella (chickenpox), which is caused by the same virus responsible for secondary varicella-zoster virus (VZV) reactivation, is frequently associated with an acute, mild, nongranulomatous, self-limiting, bilateral iritis or iridocyclitis. Cutaneous vesicles at the side of the tip of the nose *(Hutchinson sign)* indicate nasociliary nerve involvement and a greater likelihood that the eye will be affected (see Fig 8-1). Most patients are asymptomatic, but as many as 40% of patients with primary varicella-zoster virus infection may develop iritis when examined prospectively.

Patients with intraocular viral infections, particularly the herpes group infections, which also includes cytomegalovirus, may occasionally develop stellate keratic precipitates (KPs). This morphology is also seen in Fuchs heterochromic iridocyclitis and

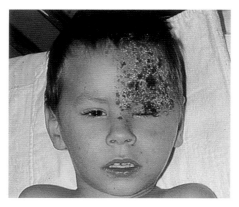

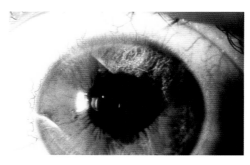

Figure 8-2 Iris stromal atrophy in a patient with varicella-zoster iridocyclitis. *(Courtesy of David Forster, MD.)*

Figure 8-1 Varicella-zoster virus, skin lesions.

Figure 8-3 Varicella-zoster virus, necrosis of long ciliary nerve.

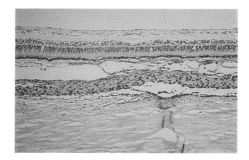

toxoplasmosis. These stellate KPs usually assume a diffuse distribution, as opposed to the usual distribution, which occurs in the inferior third of the cornea known as the Arlt triangle. In addition, the KPs are fine and fibrillar, often with a distinctly stellate pattern on high-magnification biomicroscopy. The identification of diffuse or stellate KPs is useful in the differential diagnosis of anterior segment inflammation but not diagnostic of any particular condition. In patients with herpetic disease and concomitant keratopathy, however mild, anterior segment inflammation may also be associated with diffuse or localized decreased corneal sensation and neurotrophic keratitis.

Glaucoma is a frequent complication of herpetic uveitis and is thus a helpful diagnostic hallmark. Most inflammatory syndromes are associated with decreased IOP as a result of ciliary body hyposecretion. However, just as the herpesvirus can localize to corneal, cutaneous, or conjunctival tissues, herpetic reactivation may directly cause trabeculitis and thus increase IOP, often to as high as 50–60 mm Hg. In addition, inflammatory cells may contribute to trabecular obstruction and congestion. Hyphema may occur in herpetic uveitis.

Iris atrophy is also characteristic of herpetic inflammation and can be seen with either herpes simplex or varicella-zoster. The atrophy may be patchy or sectoral (see Fig 8-2). Such atrophy is best demonstrated with retroillumination at the slit lamp.

Viral retinitis (discussed in the following section) may occur with these entities, particularly in immunocompromised hosts. Vasculitis commonly occurs with varicella-zoster ophthalmicus, and it may lead to anterior segment ischemia, retinal artery occlusion, and scleritis. Vasculitis in the orbit may lead to cranial nerve palsies.

Treatment for viral anterior uveitis usually includes topical corticosteroids and cycloplegic agents. Topical antiviral agents are usually ineffective in the treatment of herpetic uveitis but may be indicated in patients with herpes simplex keratouveitis to prevent dendritic keratitis during topical corticosteroid therapy. Systemic antivirals such as acyclovir, famciclovir, or valacyclovir are often beneficial in cases of severe uveitis. Initiation of oral antiviral therapy within the first few days after the onset of varicella-zoster is now recommended. Patients with herpetic uveitis may require prolonged corticosteroid therapy with very gradual tapering. In fact, some patients with varicella-zoster require chronic, albeit extremely low, doses of topical corticosteroids (as infrequent as 1 drop per week) to remain quiescent. Systemic corticosteroids are necessary at times. Long-term, low-dose antiviral therapy may be beneficial in patients with herpetic uveitis, but controlled studies are lacking. The oral dosages are acyclovir 400 mg twice a day or valacyclovir 500 mg daily for patients with herpes simplex disease and acyclovir 800 mg twice a day or valacyclovir 1g daily for varicella-zoster disease. Consultation with an infectious disease specialist may be appropriate.

Barron BA, Gee L, Hauck WW, et al. Herpetic Eye Disease Study: a controlled trial of oral acyclovir for herpes simplex stromal keratitis. *Ophthalmology*. 1994;101:1871–1882.

Parrish CM. Herpes simplex virus eye disease. *Focal Points: Clinical Modules for Ophthalmologists*. San Francisco: American Academy of Ophthalmology; 1997, module 2.

Sandor EV, Millman A, Croxson TS, Mildvan D. Herpes zoster ophthalmicus in patients at risk for the acquired immune deficiency syndrome (AIDS). *Am J Ophthalmol*. 1986;101:153–155.

Siverio Junior CD, Imai Y, Cunningham ET Jr. Diagnosis and management of herpetic anterior uveitis. *Int Ophthalmol Clin*. 2002;42:43–48.

van der Lelij A, Ooijman FM, Kijlstra A, Rothova A. Anterior uveitis with sectoral iris atrophy in the absence of keratitis: a distinct clinical entity among herpetic eye diseases. *Ophthalmology*. 2000;107:1164–1170.

Wilhelmus KR, Gee L, Hauck WW, et al. Herpetic Eye Disease Study: a controlled trial of topical corticosteroids for herpes simplex stromal keratitis. *Ophthalmology*. 1994;101:1883–1895.

Acute retinal necrosis syndrome, progressive outer retinal necrosis, nonnecrotizing herpetic retinitis   The acute retinal necrosis (ARN) syndrome is part of a spectrum of necrotizing herpetic retinopathies the clinical expression of which appears to be influenced by both host and viral factors. Originally described in 1971 among otherwise healthy adults, ARN has also been reported in children and among immunocompromised patients, including those with AIDS. Acute, fulminant disease may arise without a systemic prodrome years after primary infection or following cutaneous or systemic herpetic infection such as dermatomal zoster, chickenpox, or herpetic encephalitis. The prevalence is nearly equal between the sexes, with the majority of cases clustering between the fifth and seventh decades. A genetic predisposition may increase the relative risk of developing ARN among patients with specific human leukocyte antigen (HLA) haplotypes, including HLA-DQw7 antigen and phenotype -Bw62 and -DR4 in Caucasian patients in the United States and HLA-Aw33, -B44, and -DRw6 in Japanese patients. The American Uveitis Society has established mandatory and supporting criteria for the diagnosis of ARN that are based solely on the clinical findings

Table 8-1 American Uveitis Society Criteria for Diagnosis of Acute Retinal Necrosis Syndrome

One or more foci of retinal necrosis with discrete borders, located in the peripheral retina*
Rapid progression in the absence of antiviral therapy
Circumferential spread
Occlusive vasculopathy with arteriolar involvement
Prominent vitritis, anterior chamber inflammation
Optic neuropathy/atrophy, scleritis, pain supportive but not required

*Macular lesions do not exclude diagnosis in the presence of peripheral retinitis.

Adapted from Holland GN. Standard diagnostic criteria for the acute retinal necrosis syndrome. Executive Committee of the American Uveitis Society. *Am J Ophthalmol.* 1994;117:663–667.

and disease progression, independent of viral etiology or host immune status (Table 8-1). Retinal lesions of presumed herpetic etiology that are not characteristic of well-recognized syndromes such as cytomegalovirus (CMV) retinitis or progressive outer retinal necrosis are grouped under the umbrella designation *necrotizing herpetic retinopathy.*

Patients with ARN usually present with acute unilateral loss of vision, photophobia, floaters, and pain. Fellow eye involvement may occur in approximately 36% of cases, usually within 6 weeks of disease onset, but involvement may be delayed for up to 26 years following initial presentation. Significant anterior segment inflammation replete with corneal edema, KPs, posterior synechiae, and elevated IOP are frequently observed, together with heavy vitreous cellular infiltration. Within 2 weeks, the classic triad of occlusive retinal arteriolitis, vitritis, and a multifocal yellow-white peripheral retinitis has evolved. Early on, the peripheral retinal lesions are discontinuous and have scalloped edges that appear to arise in the outer retina. Within days, however, they coalesce to form a confluent 360° creamy retinitis that progresses posteriorly, leaving full-thickness retinal necrosis, arteriolitis, phlebitis, and occasional retinal hemorrhage in its wake (Figs 8-4, 8-5). Widespread necrosis of the midperipheral retina, multiple posterior retinal breaks, and proliferative vitreoretinopathy predispose to combined traction-rhegmatogenous retinal detachments in 75% of patients (Fig 8-6). The posterior pole tends to be spared, but an exudative retinal detachment may arise with severe inflammation. The optic nerve is frequently involved, as evidenced by disc swelling and a relative afferent defect.

In most instances, the diagnosis is made clinically, with important differential considerations, including CMV retinitis, atypical toxoplasmic retinochoroiditis, syphilis, lymphoma, leukemia, and autoimmune retinal vasculitis such as Adamantiades-Behçet disease. ARN may also be seen in association with concurrent or antecedent herpetic encephalitis (herpes simplex virus type 1[HSV-1], herpes simplex virus type 2 [HSV-2]). When the diagnosis is uncertain, intraocular fluid analysis of aqueous and/or vitreous samples should be performed.

Intraocular antibody production as a measure of the host response to a specific microbial pathogen can be computed using the Goldmann-Witmer (GW) coefficient: the ratio of specific antibody (aqueous or vitreous)/total IgG (aqueous or vitreous) to specific antibody (serum)/total IgG (serum), as measured by enzyme-linked immunosorbent assay (ELISA) or radioimmunoassay. (See also Chapter 6, Clinical Approach to Uveitis.) A ratio of greater

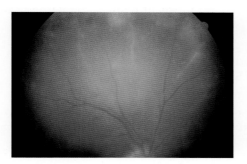

Figure 8-4 Acute retinal necrosis, vitritis, arteriolitis, and multiple peripheral "thumb-print" areas of retinitis. *(Courtesy of E. Mitchel Opremcak, MD.)*

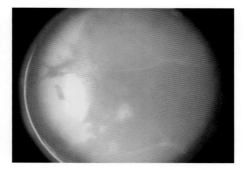

Figure 8-5 Acute retinal necrosis, confluent peripheral retinitis. *(Courtesy of E. Mitchel Opremcak, MD.)*

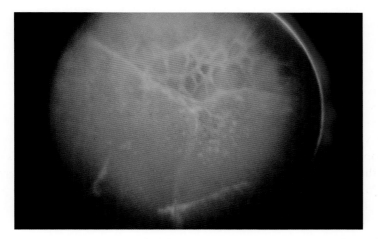

Figure 8-6 Acute retinal necrosis, retinal detachment with multiple, posterior retinal breaks. *(Courtesy of E. Mitchel Opremcak, MD.)*

than 4 is considered diagnostic of local antibody production. Aqueous humor analysis is most frequently performed following simple anterior chamber paracentesis. It has been used more widely in Europe than in the United States as an adjunct to the diagnosis of toxoplasmosis and necrotizing herpetic retinitis due to HSV and VZV, but it is of little value in the diagnosis of CMV retinitis. The combination of the GW coefficient with polymerase chain reaction (PCR) may increase diagnostic yield, especially in viral infections.

Polymerase chain reaction is probably the most sensitive, specific, and rapid diagnostic method for detecting infectious posterior uveitis in general and ARN specifically, largely supplanting viral culture, intraocular antibody titers, and serology. PCR may be performed on either aqueous humor or vitreous biopsy specimens; however, for most cases of ARN, aqueous sampling is usually sufficient. Quantitative PCR may add additional information with respect to viral load, disease activity, and response to therapy. Recent studies using PCR-based assays suggest that the most common cause of ARN is VZV, followed by HSV-1, HSV-2, and, in rare instances, CMV. Patients with ARN due to HSV-1 and VZV tend to be older (mean age 40 years), whereas those with ARN due to HSV-2 tend to be younger (less than 25 years of age). There is a higher risk of encephalitis and meningitis among patients with ARN due to HSV-1 than among those with ARN due to VZV. In rare instances where PCR is negative but the clinical suspicion for herpetic necrotizing retinitis is high, endoretinal biopsy may be diagnostic.

Timely diagnosis and prompt antiviral therapy are essential given the rapidity of disease progression, the frequency of retinal detachment, and the guarded visual prognosis. Intravenous acyclovir, at 10 mg/kg/day in 3 divided doses over 10–14 days, remains the classic regimen; it is effective against HSV and VZV. Reversible elevations in the serum creatinine and liver function tests may occur, and, in the presence of frank renal insufficiency, the dosage will need to be reduced. For infection with VZV, oral acyclovir at 800 mg orally 5 times daily or an equivalent dose of valacyclovir (1 g orally 3 times daily) or famciclovir (500 mg orally 3 times daily) should be continued for 3 months following the intravenous induction. For ARN associated with HSV-1 infection, the dose is one half what it is for VZV. Antiviral therapy may reduce the incidence of contralateral disease or bilateral acute retinal necrosis (BARN) by 80% over 1 year. After 24–48 hours of antiviral therapy, systemic corticosteroids (prednisone, 1 mg/kg/day) are introduced and subsequently tapered over several weeks to treat active inflammation. Aspirin and other anticoagulation agents have been used to treat an associated hypercoagulable state and prevent vascular occlusions, but the results have been uncertain.

More recently, intravitreal ganciclovir (0.2–2.0 mg/0.1 mL) and foscarnet (1.2–2.4 mg/0.1 mL) have been used to achieve a rapid induction in combination with oral valacyclovir as first-line therapy or in patients who fail to respond to systemic acyclovir (see Chapter 12). The superiority of intravitreal plus oral therapy has not been demonstrated over the classic intravenous approach. Given the short intravitreal half-life of these drugs, injections may need to be repeated twice weekly until retinitis is controlled. Effective treatment inhibits the development of new lesions and promotes lesion regression over 4 days.

Retinal detachment occurs within the first weeks to months following the onset of retinitis. Given the location and multiplicity of retinal breaks, prophylactic barrier laser photocoagulation, applied to the areas of healthy retina at the posterior border of the necrotic lesions, may prevent retinal detachment and is recommended as soon as the view permits. Early vitrectomy combined with endolaser photocoagulation has been proposed to help eliminate the contribution of vitreous traction on the necrotic retina. Due to the presence of proliferative vitreoretinopathy and multiple posterior retinal tears, internal repair using vitrectomy techniques, air–fluid exchange, endolaser photocoagulation, long-acting gas, or silicone oil tamponade is more successful in achieving a high rate of anatomical attachment than are standard scleral buckling procedures. Untreated, approximately two thirds of eyes obtain a final visual acuity of 20/200 or worse due to retinal detachment, concurrent optic atrophy, or macular pathology. With early recognition, aggressive antiviral therapy, and laser photocoagulation, this prognosis may be significantly improved, as shown in one study in which 46% of 13 eyes achieved a visual acuity of 20/40 or better and 92% of eyes a visual acuity of better than 20/400.

Progressive outer retinal necrosis (PORN) is essentially a morphologic variant of acute necrotizing herpetic retinitis, occurring most often in patients with advanced stages

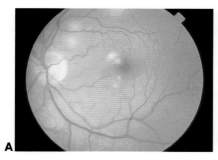 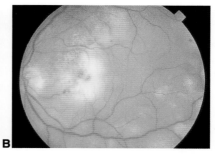

Figure 8-7 **A,** Multifocal areas of white retinitis in a patient with PORN. **B,** Fundus photograph taken 5 days later showing rapid disease progression and confluence of the areas of the viral retinitis. *(Courtesy of E. Mitchel Opremcak, MD.)*

of HIV/AIDS (CD4$^+$ T lymphocytes $\leq$50 cells/μL) or in patients who are otherwise profoundly immunomodulated. The most common cause of PORN is VZV; however, HSV has also been implicated. As with ARN, the retinitis begins as patchy areas of outer retinal whitening that coalesce rapidly; however, in contrast to ARN, the posterior pole may be involved early in the course of the disease, vitreous inflammatory cells are typically absent, and the retinal vasculature is minimally involved, at least initially (Fig 8-7). In addition, a previous history of cutaneous zoster (67%) and eventual bilateral involvement (71%) is frequently observed in patients with PORN and HIV/AIDS, who have a similarly high rate (70%) of retinal detachment. The visual prognosis is poor, with 67% of patients having a final visual acuity of no light perception in the largest series reported to date. Although the disease is often resistant to intravenous acyclovir alone, successful management has been reported with combination systemic and intraocular therapy with foscarnet and ganciclovir. Long-term suppressive antiviral therapy is required in patients with HIV/AIDS who are not able to achieve immune reconstitution on highly active antiretroviral therapy (HAART). See also BCSC Section 12, *Retina and Vitreous.*

Nonnecrotizing posterior uveitis (nonnecrotizing herpetic retinitis, NNHR) may occur in patients with herpetic infections, including acute retinochoroiditis with diffuse hemorrhages in children following acute varicella infection and a chronic choroiditis or retinal vasculitis in adults. In a recent study, using PCR-based assays and local antibody analysis of aqueous fluid samples for herpesviruses, a viral etiology was confirmed in 13% of cases deemed "idiopathic posterior uveitis." Inflammation is typically bilateral, presenting with cystoid macular edema (CME), as a birdshot-like retinochoroidopathy, or as an occlusive bilateral retinitis. Patients are initially resistant to conventional therapy with systemic corticosteroids and/or immunomodulatory therapy but achieve a favorable response when switched to systemic antiviral medication.

Blumenkranz M, Clarkson J, Culbertson WW, Flynn HW, Lewis ML, Young GM. Visual results and complications after retinal reattachment in the acute retinal necrosis syndrome. The influence of operative technique. *Retina.* 1989;9:170–174.

Bodaghi B, Rozenberg F, Cassoux N, Fardeau C, LeHoang P. Nonnecrotizing herpetic retinopathies masquerading as severe posterior uveitis. *Ophthalmology.* 2003;110:1737–1743.

Chau Tran TH, Cassoux N, Bodaghi B, LeHoang P. Successful treatment with combination of systemic antiviral drugs and intravitreal ganciclovir injections in the management of severe necrotizing herpetic retinitis. *Ocul Immunol Inflamm.* 2003;11:141–144.

Crapotta JA, Freeman WR. Visual outcome in acute retinal necrosis. *Retina.* 1994;14:382–383.

Engstrom RE Jr, Holland GN, Margolis TP, et al. The progressive outer retinal necrosis syndrome. A variant of necrotizing herpetic retinopathy in patients with AIDS. *Ophthalmology.* 1994;101:1488–1502.

Ganatra JB, Chandler D, Santos C, Kuppermann B, Margolis TP. Viral causes of the acute retinal necrosis syndrome. *Am J Ophthalmol.* 2000;129:166–172.

Holland GN. Standard diagnostic criteria for the acute retinal necrosis syndrome. Executive Committee of the American Uveitis Society. *Am J Ophthalmol.* 1994;117:663–667.

Holland GN, Cornell PJ, Park MS, et al. An association between acute retinal necrosis syndrome and HLA-DQw7 and phenotype Bw62, DR4. *Am J Ophthalmol.* 1989;108:370–374.

Scott IU, Luu KM, Davis JL. Intravitreal antivirals in the management of patients with acquired immunodeficiency syndrome with progressive outer retinal necrosis. *Arch Ophthalmol.* 2002;120:1219–1222.

Van Gelder RN, Willig JL, Holland GN, Kaplan HJ. Herpes simplex virus type 2 as a cause of acute retinal necrosis syndrome in young patients. *Ophthalmology.* 2001;108:869–876.

Cytomegalovirus

Cytomegalovirus is a double-stranded DNA virus in the Herpesviridae family. It is the most common cause of congenital viral infection, with clinical disease occurring among neonates and immunocompromised patients with leukemia, lymphoma, or conditions requiring systemic immunomodulation; and in patients with HIV/AIDS. CMV retinitis is the most common ophthalmic manifestation of both congenital CMV infection and that occurring in the context of HIV/AIDS. The clinical appearance is similar regardless of clinical context; 3 distinct variants have been described:

1. a classic or fulminant retinitis with large areas of retinal hemorrhage against a background of whitened, edematous, or necrotic retina, typically appearing in the posterior pole, from the disc to the vascular arcades, in the distribution of the nerve fiber layer, and associated with blood vessels (Fig 8-8)
2. a granular or indolent form found more often in the retinal periphery, characterized by little or no retinal edema, hemorrhage, or vascular sheathing, with active retinitis progressing from the borders of the lesion (Fig 8-9)
3. a perivascular CMV form often described as a variant of frosted branch angiitis, an idiopathic retinal perivasculitis initially described in immunocompetent children (Fig 8-10)

Early CMV retinitis may present as a small white retinal infiltrate masquerading as a cotton-wool spot, commonly seen as part of HIV-related microvasculopathy, and distinguished from the latter by its inevitable progression without treatment. In rare instances, immunocompetent adults may present with an anterior uveitis associated with ocular hypertension and sectoral iris atrophy due to intraocular CMV infection. This entity is clinically identical to HSV-associated or VZV-associated anterior uveitis. Diagnosis can be made with PCR evaluation of the aqueous.

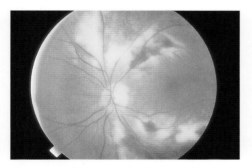

Figure 8-8 Cytomegalovirus retinitis. *(Courtesy of E. Mitchel Opremcak, MD.)*

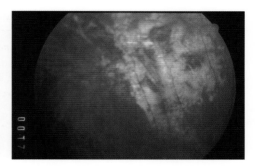

Figure 8-9 Granular CMV retinitis. *(Courtesy of Careen Lowder, MD.)*

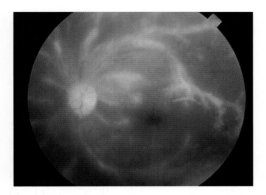

Figure 8-10 "Frosted branch" CMV perivasculitis. *(Courtesy of Albert T. Vitale, MD.)*

The diagnosis of congenital disease is suggested by the clinical appearance of the lesions, coupled with the findings of viral inclusion bodies in urine, saliva, and subretinal fluid, and associated systemic disease findings. The complement-fixation test for cytomegalic inclusion disease is of value 5–24 months after the loss of the maternal antibodies transferred during pregnancy. Likewise, the diagnosis of CMV retinitis in the setting of HIV/AIDS or iatrogenic immunomodulation is essentially clinical, based on the features just described. In patients with atypical lesions or those not responding to anti-CMV therapy, PCR-based analysis of the aqueous or vitreous samples may provide critical diagnostic information of high sensitivity and specificity that allows the clinician to differentiate CMV from other herpetic causes of necrotizing retinitis and from toxoplasmic retinochoroiditis in immunocompromised patients.

CMV reaches the eye hematogenously, with passage of the virus across the blood–ocular barrier, infection of retinal vascular endothelial cells, and cell-to-cell transmission of the virus within the retina. The histopathologic features of both congenital and acquired disease include a primary, full-thickness, coagulative necrotizing retinitis and secondary diffuse choroiditis. Infected retinal cells show pathognomonic cytomegalic changes consisting of large eosinophilic intranuclear inclusions and small multiple basophilic cytoplasmic inclusions (Fig 8-11A). Viral inclusions may also be seen in the RPE and vascular

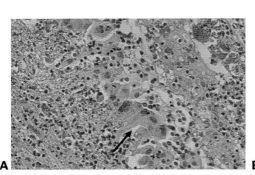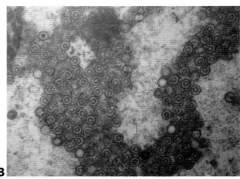

Figure 8-11 **A,** Photomicrograph of a retinal biopsy specimen demonstrating a necrotic retina and giant (megalo) cells with eosinophilic intracytoplasmic inclusions *(arrow)* consistent with CMV retinitis (H&E). **B,** Electron photomicrograph of the same specimen showing intranuclear inclusions containing scattered nucleocapsids, relative electron lucency of the central core *(arrow)*, and the typical envelope consistent with CMV. *(Part A courtesy of Careen Lowder, MD; part B reproduced with permission from Spaide RF, Vitale AT, Toth IR, et al. Frosted branch angiitis associated with cytomegalovirus retinitis. Am J Ophthalmol. 1992;113:524–525, Figs 5, 6; part B photograph courtesy of Albert T. Vitale, MD.)*

endothelium. Electron microscopy of infected retinal tissue reveals viral particles with the typical morphology of the herpes family of viruses (Fig 8-11B).

Congenital CMV retinitis is usually associated with other systemic manifestations of disseminated infection, including fever, thrombocytopenia, anemia, pneumonitis, and hepatosplenomegaly, with a reported prevalence between 11% and 22%. However, CMV retinitis has been reported to occur later in life among children with no discernible lesions ophthalmoscopically and no evidence of systemic disease reactivation. This suggests that even asymptomatic children with evidence of congenital CMV infection should be followed at regular intervals for potential ocular involvement later into childhood. Resolution of the retinitis leaves both pigmented and atrophic lesions, with retinal detachment occurring in up to one third of children. Optic atrophy and cataract formation are not uncommon sequelae.

Prior to the introduction of HAART, an estimated 30% of patients with HIV/AIDS (typically, profoundly immunomodulated individuals with $CD4^+$ T lymphocytes ≤ 50 cells/μL) developed CMV retinitis at some point during their disease course. Rhegmatogenous retinal detachments with multiple breaks, particularly in areas of peripheral retinal necrosis, occurred at a rate of approximately 33% per eye per year. The availability of HAART in the industrialized world has resulted not only in a significant decline in HIV/AIDS–associated mortality, but also in an 80% annual decline in new cases of CMV retinitis and its associated complications, including retinal detachment, itself associated with CMV lesion size. This decrease appears to have stabilized, and new cases of CMV retinitis continue to occur among HAART failures and those who may experience immune reconstitution but fail to develop CMV-specific immunity.

Successful management of CMV retinitis requires not only HAART but also appropriate anti-CMV therapy. This is particularly important given that CMV retinitis itself—independent of CD4 count, HIV viral load, and antiretroviral therapy—is associated with a 1.6-fold increase in mortality, and a clear mortality benefit is associated with systemic anti-CMV therapy. Therapeutic options for systemic coverage include ganciclovir, foscarnet, and cidofovir administered intravenously and valganciclovir (a bioavailable pro-drug of ganciclovir) administered orally. Intravitreal injection of ganciclovir or foscarnet or the ganciclovir implant, although highly effective in treating intraocular disease, fails to cover extraocular systemic CMV. In patients with CMV retinitis on HAART who experience sustained immune recovery (an increase in CD4$^+$ T lymphocytes $\geq$100 cells/μL for $\geq$3–6 months), systemic anti-CMV maintenance therapy may be safely discontinued. Moreover, aggressive anti-CMV therapy initiated at the same time as HAART may decrease the incidence of immune recovery uveitis. The management of CMV retinitis and its complications are discussed in more detail in Chapter 12.

Boppana S, Amos C, Britt WJ, Stagno S, Alford C, Pass R. Late onset and reactivation of chorioretinitis in children with congenital cytomegalovirus infection. *Pediatr Infect Dis J.* 1994;13:1139–1142.

Coats DK, Demmler GJ, Paysse EA, Du LT, Libby C. Ophthalmologic findings in children with congenital cytomegalovirus infection. *J AAPOS.* 2000;4:110–116.

Hoover DR, Peng Y, Saah A, et al. Occurrence of cytomegalovirus retinitis after human immunodeficiency virus immunosuppression. *Arch Ophthalmol.* 1996;114:821–827.

Istas AS, Demmler GJ, Dobbins JG, Stewart JA. Surveillance for congenital cytomegalovirus disease: a report from the National Congenital Cytomegalovirus Disease Registry. *Clin Infect Dis.* 1995;20:665–670.

Jabs DA, Holbrook JT, Van Natta ML, et al. Risk factors for mortality in patients with AIDS in the era of highly active antiretroviral therapy. *Ophthalmology.* 2005;112:771–779.

Jacobson NA, Stanley H, Holtzer C, Margolis TP, Cunningham ET. Natural history and outcome of new AIDS-related cytomegalovirus retinitis diagnosed in the era of highly active antiretroviral therapy. *Clin Infect Dis.* 2000;30:231–233.

Kempen JH, Jabs DA. Ocular complications of human immunodeficiency virus infection. In: Johnson GJ, Minassian DC, Weale RA, and West SK, eds. *The Epidemiology of Eye Disease.* 2nd ed. London: Hodder Arnold; 2003:318–340.

Kempen JH, Jabs DA, Wilson LA, Dunn JP, West SK, Tonascia J. Mortality risk for patients with cytomegalovirus retinitis and acquired immune deficiency syndrome. *Clin Infect Dis.* 2003;37:1365–1373.

Markomichelakis NN, Canakis C, Zafirakis P, Marakis T, Mallias I, Theodossiadis G. Cytomegalovirus as a cause of anterior uveitis with sectoral iris atrophy. *Ophthalmology.* 2002;109:879–882.

Palella FJ Jr, Delaney KM, Moormon AC, et al. Declining morbidity and mortality among patients with advanced human immunodeficiency virus infection. HIV Outpatient Study Investigators. *N Engl J Med.* 1998;338:853–860.

Epstein-Barr virus

Epstein-Barr virus (EBV) is a ubiquitous double-stranded DNA virus with a complex capsid and envelope belonging to the subfamily Gammaherpesvirinae. It is the viral agent commonly associated with infectious mononucleosis (IM), a systemic syndrome predominantly affecting adolescents between the ages of 14 and 18 years of age. By adulthood, the prevalence of seropositivity for EBV approaches 90%. EBV has a tropism for B lymphocytes, as these are the only cells known to have surface receptors for the virus. EBV has also been implicated in the pathogenesis of Burkitt lymphoma, especially among African children and those with nasopharyngeal carcinoma, Hodgkin disease, and Sjögren syndrome.

Ocular manifestations of EBV may arise as a consequence of either congenital infection or, much more commonly, primary infection in the context of IM. Cataract has been reported in association with congenital EBV infection; a mild, self-limiting follicular conjunctivitis, usually appearing early in the course of the disease, is most common with acquired IM. Other, less frequently reported anterior ocular manifestations of acquired IM include epithelial or stromal keratitis; episcleritis; bilateral, granulomatous iridocyclitis; dacryoadenitis; and, less frequently, cranial nerve palsies and Parinaud oculoglandular syndrome.

A variety of posterior segment manifestations have been reported in association with EBV infection, including isolated optic disc edema and optic neuritis, macular edema, retinal hemorrhages, retinitis, punctate outer retinitis, choroiditis, multifocal choroiditis and panuveitis (MCP), pars planitis and vitritis, progressive subretinal fibrosis, uveitis, and secondary choroidal neovascularization (CNV; Fig 8-12). The relevance of positive EBV serologies in patients with these diseases is unknown, and the evidence for these ocular associations is not well established.

The diagnosis is suggested by the aforementioned ocular findings arising during the course of IM or by the serologic evidence of antibodies against a variety of EBV-specific capsid antigens that are indicative of active or persistent EBV infection. During IM, the EBV viral capsid antigen (VCA) IgM antibody, followed by the VCA IgG titers, rise in a parallel fashion during viral incubation, 4–5 weeks after exposure to the virus. The early antigen (EA) rises with the onset of clinical disease, usually within 5–10 weeks of exposure, reaches a maximum, and then falls to undetectable levels 6–12 months after resolution of the infection. The EBV nuclear antigen (NA) antibody appears slowly, within 2 months, and persists for life, whereas the VCA IgM titer falls to undetectable levels after the infection has been resolved. The diagnosis of chronic EBV infection is best supported by abnormally elevated anti-VCA IgM and anti-EA antibody levels.

Most ocular disease is self-limiting and does not require treatment; however, the presence of iridocyclitis may necessitate the use of topical corticosteroids and cycloplegia; systemic corticosteroids may be required to treat posterior segment inflammation. The efficacy of systemic antiviral therapy for EBV infection has not been established.

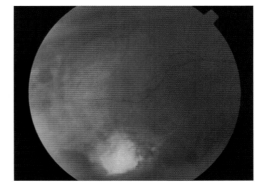

Figure 8-12 Epstein-Barr virus–related retinitis and vasculitis. *(Reproduced with permission from Vitale AT, Foster CS. Uveitis infecting infants and children: infectious. In: Hartnett ME, Trese M, Capone A, Steidl SM, Keats B. Pediatric Retina: Medical and Surgical Approaches. Philadelphia: Lippincott Williams & Wilkins; 2004:269, Fig 16-7. Photograph courtesy of Albert T. Vitale, MD.)*

Kelly ST, Rosenthal AR, Nicholson KG, Woodward CG. Retinochoroiditis in acute Epstein-Barr virus infection. *Br J Ophthalmol.* 1989;73:1002–1003.

Matoba AY. Ocular disease associated with Epstein-Barr virus infection. *Surv Ophthalmol.* 1990;35:145–149.

Raymond LA, Wilson CA, Linnemann CC Jr, Ward MA, Bernstein DI, Love DC. Punctate outer retinitis in acute Epstein-Barr virus infection. *Am J Ophthalmol.* 1987;104:424–426.

Spaide RS, Sugin S, Yannuzzi LA, DeRosa JT. Epstein-Barr virus antibodies in multifocal choroiditis and panuveitis. *Am J Ophthalmol.* 1991;112:410–413.

Usui M, Sakai J. Three cases of EB virus-associated uveitis. *Int Ophthalmol.* 1990;14:371–376.

Rubella

Rubella is the prototypical teratogenic viral agent. It consists of single-stranded RNA surrounded by a lipid envelope, or "toga," hence its inclusion in the Togaviridae family. Although rubella is still an important cause of blindness in developing nations, the epidemic pattern of the disease was interrupted in the United States by the introduction of a vaccine in 1969. The peak age incidence shifted from 5–9 years (young children) in the prevaccine era to 15–19 years (older children) and 20–24 years (young adults). Approximately 5%–25% of women of childbearing age who lack rubella antibodies are susceptible to primary infection. Rubella may involve the retina as a part of the congenital rubella syndrome (CRS) or during acquired infection (German measles).

The fetus is infected with the rubella virus transplacentally, secondary to maternal viremia during the course of primary infection. The frequency of fetal infection is highest during the first 10 weeks and during the final month of pregnancy, with the rate of congenital defects varying inversely with gestational age. Although obvious maternal infection during the first trimester of pregnancy may end in spontaneous abortion, stillbirth, or severe fetal malformations, seropositive, asymptomatic maternal rubella may also result in severe fetal disease.

The classic features of the CRS include cardiac malformations (patent ductus arteriosus, interventricular septal defects, and pulmonic stenosis), ocular findings (chorioretinitis, cataract, corneal clouding, microphthalmia, strabismus, and glaucoma), and deafness (Fig 8-13). Hearing loss is the most common systemic finding. Individuals with CRS are at greater risk for developing diabetes mellitus and subsequent diabetic retinopathy later in life.

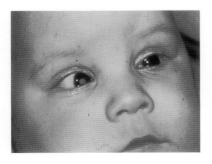

Figure 8-13 Congenital rubella syndrome patient with cataract, esotropia, mental retardation, congenital heart disease, and deafness. *(Courtesy of John D. Sheppard, Jr, MD.)*

A unilateral or bilateral pigmentary retinopathy is the most common ocular manifestation of CRS (25%–50%), followed by cataract (15%) and glaucoma (10%). The pigmentary disturbance, often described as "salt and pepper" ("salt-and-pepper fundus"), shows considerable variation, ranging from finely stippled, bone spicule–like, small black irregular masses to gross pigmentary irregularities with coarse, blotchy mottling (Fig 8-14). It can be stationary or progressive. Despite loss of the foveal light reflex and prominent pigmentary changes, neither vision nor the electroretinogram (ERG) is typically affected. Congenital (nuclear) cataracts and microphthalmia are the most frequent causes of poor visual acuity and, rarely, CNV. Unless otherwise compromised by glaucoma, the optic nerve and the retinal vessels are typically normal in appearance.

Histopathologic studies of the lens reveal retained cell nuclei in the embryonic nucleus as well as anterior and posterior cortical degeneration. Poor development of the dilator muscle, necrosis of the iris pigment epithelium, and chronic nongranulomatous inflammation are present in the iris. The RPE displays alternating areas of atrophy and hypertrophy. The anterior chamber angle appears similar to that in congenital glaucoma. Although the mechanism of rubella embryopathy is not known at a cellular level, it is thought that the virus inhibits cellular multiplication and establishes a chronic, persistent infection during organogenesis. The persistence of viral replication after birth, with ongoing tissue damage, is central to the pathogenesis of CRS and may explain the appearance of hearing and neurologic and/or ocular deficits long after birth.

Acquired infection (German measles) presents with a prodrome of malaise and fever in adolescents and adults prior to the onset of the rubella exanthem. An erythematous, maculopapular rash appears first on the face, spreads toward the hands and feet, involves the entire body within 24 hours, and disappears by the third day. Although the rash is not always prominent and the occurrence of fever is variable, lymphadenopathy is invariably present.

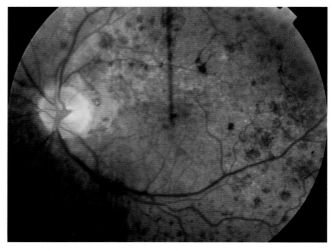

Figure 8-14 Congenital rubella syndrome with diffuse retinal pigment epithelial mottling with salt-and-pepper appearance. *(Courtesy of Albert T. Vitale, MD.)*

The most frequent ocular complication of acquired rubella infection is conjunctivitis (70%), followed by the infrequent occurrence of epithelial keratitis and retinitis. Acquired rubella retinitis has been described in adults presenting with acute onset of decreased vision and multifocal chorioretinitis, with large areas of bullous neurosensory detachment, underlying pigment epithelial detachment involving the entire posterior pole, anterior chamber and preretinal vitreous cells, dark gray atrophic lesions of the retinal pigment epithelium, normal retinal vessels and optic nerve, and the absence of retinal hemorrhage. The neurosensory detachments resolve spontaneously and visual acuity returns to normal. Most recently, chronic rubella virus infection has been implicated in the pathogenesis of Fuchs heterochromic iridocyclitis, as evidenced by the presence of rubella-specific intraocular antibody production and intraocular persistence of the virus.

The pathognomonic retinal findings, associated systemic findings, and a history of maternal exposure to rubella suggest the diagnosis of CRS. Serologic criteria for rubella infection include a fourfold increase in rubella-specific IgG in paired sera 1–2 weeks apart or the new appearance of rubella-specific IgM. Because the fetus is capable of mounting an immune response to rubella virus, specific IgM or IgA antibodies to rubella in the cord blood confirms the diagnosis.

The differential diagnosis of congenital rubella retinitis consists of those entities comprising the TORCHES syndrome (*to*xoplasmosis; *r*ubella; *c*ytomegalic inclusion disease; *h*erpesviruses, including *E*pstein-Barr; and *s*yphilis). See also BCSC Section 6, *Pediatric Ophthalmology and Strabismus*. Other viral infections, such as HSV, VZV, CMV, mumps, roseola, and vaccinoencephalitis, should be considered and ruled out by appropriate serologic tests. There is no specific antiviral therapy for congenital rubella and treatment is supportive. Similarly, uncomplicated acquired rubella does not require specific therapy; however, rubella retinitis and postvaccination optic neuritis may respond well to systemic corticosteroids.

Arnold J, McIntosh ED, Martin FJ, Menser MA. A 50-year follow up of ocular defects in congenital rubella: late ocular manifestations. *Aust N Z J Ophthalmol.* 1994;221:1–6.

Givens KT, Lee DA, Jones T, Ilstrup DM. Congenital rubella syndrome: ophthalmic manifestations and associated systemic disorders. *Br J Ophthalmol.* 1993;77:358–363.

Hayashi M, Yoshimura N, Kondo T. Acute rubella retinal pigment epitheliitis in an adult. *Am J Ophthalmol.* 1982;93:285–288.

McEvoy RC, Fedun B, Cooper LZ, et al. Children at high risk of diabetes mellitus: New York studies of families with diabetes in children with congenital rubella syndrome. *Adv Exp Med Biol.* 1988;246:221–227.

Quentin CD, Reiber H. Fuchs heterochromic cyclitis: rubella virus antibodies and genome in aqueous humor. *Am J Ophthalmol.* 2004;138:46–54.

Lymphocytic Choriomeningitis Virus

Lymphocytic choriomeningitis virus (LCMV) is an underrecognized fetal teratogen that should probably be listed among "others" in the TORCHES group of congenital infections. The microbe is a single-stranded RNA virus of the Arenaviridae family; rodents are the natural hosts and reservoirs for the virus. Transmission is thought to be airborne, from contamination of food by infected rodent excreta or possibly from the bite of an infected animal. Symptomatic maternal illness occurs in approximately two thirds of cases, with vertical transmission to the fetus occurring during episodes of maternal viremia. As with other congenital infections, transmission earlier in gestation results in more serious sequelae.

Systemic findings include macrocephaly, hydrocephalus, and intracranial calcifications. Neurologic abnormalities, seizures, and mild mental retardation are not uncommon. Ocular findings include both macular and chorioretinal peripheral scarring, similar in morphology and distribution to those seen in congenital toxoplasmosis. Other findings include optic atrophy, strabismus, and nystagmus.

The differentiation from congenital toxoplasmosis is made by serologic testing of both the mother and the infant and by the pattern of intracerebral calcifications, which in toxoplasmosis tend to be diffuse and in congenital LCMV are distributed in a periventricular fashion. Immunofluorescent antibody (IFA) tests, Western blot, and ELISA are available for detecting both the IgM and IgG antibodies that, together with the clinical findings, establish the diagnosis.

Mets MB, Barton LL, Khan AS, Ksiazek TG. Lymphocytic choriomeningitis virus: an underdiagnosed cause of congenital chorioretinitis. *Am J Ophthalmol.* 2000;130:209–215.

Measles (Rubeola)

Congenital and acquired measles infection is caused by a single-stranded RNA virus of the genus *Morbillivirus* in the Paramyxoviridae family. The virus is highly contagious and is transmitted either directly or via aerosolization of nasopharyngeal secretions to the mucous membranes of the conjunctiva or respiratory tract of susceptible individuals or from a pregnant woman to her fetus transplacentally.

Despite the existence of a safe, effective, and inexpensive vaccine for over 40 years, measles remains the fifth leading cause of mortality worldwide among children younger than 5 years of age; in the United States, measles is now quite rare.

Ocular manifestations of congenital measles infection include cataract, optic nerve head drusen, and bilateral diffuse pigmentary retinopathy involving both the posterior pole and retinal periphery. The retinopathy may also be associated with either normal or attenuated retinal vessels, retinal edema, and macular star formation. The ERG and visual acuity are typically normal.

The most common ocular complications of measles are keratitis and a mild, papillary, nonpurulent conjunctivitis. Although both keratitis and conjunctivitis resolve without sequelae in the vast majority of cases in the United States, postmeasles blindness, a severe visual impairment arising specifically as a consequence of the corneal complications of the disease, is a significant problem worldwide. Measles retinopathy is more common in acquired than in congenital disease, presenting with profound visual loss 6–12 days after the appearance of the characteristic exanthem, and may or may not be accompanied by encephalitis. It is characterized by attenuated arterioles, diffuse retinal edema, macular star formation, scattered retinal hemorrhages, blurred disc margins, and a clear media. With resolution of systemic symptoms and of the acute retinopathy, arteriolar attenuation with or without perivascular sheathing, optic disc pallor, and a secondary pigmentary retinopathy with either a bone spicule or salt-and-pepper appearance may evolve.

The ERG is usually extinguished during the acute phase of measles retinopathy but may show a return of activity with visual improvement as the inflammation resolves. Visual field testing may reveal severe constriction, ring scotomata, or small peripheral islands of vision. Resolution of acquired measles retinopathy over a period of weeks to months is usually associated with a return of useful vision; however, the extended visual prognosis is guarded due to the possibility of permanent visual field constriction.

The differential diagnosis of congenital measles retinopathy includes entities comprising the TORCHES syndrome, atypical retinitis pigmentosa, and neuroretinitis; that of the acquired disease includes central serous chorioretinopathy, Vogt-Koyanagi-Harada (VKH) disease, toxoplasmic retinochoroiditis, retinitis pigmentosa, neuroretinitis, and other viral retinopathies.

The diagnosis of measles and its attendant ocular sequelae and its differentiation from the aforementioned entities are made clinically by an accurate history and review of systems; observation of the sequence of signs, symptoms, and lesion progression; and serologic testing. The virus may be recovered from the nasopharynx, conjunctiva, lymphoid tissues, respiratory mucous membranes, urine, and blood for a few days prior to and several days after the rash. Leukopenia is frequently seen during the prodromal phase. A variety of tests are available for serologic confirmation of measles infection, including complement fixation, ELISA, and immunofluorescent and hemagglutination inhibition assays.

Supportive treatment of the systemic manifestations of measles is usually sufficient because the disease is usually self-limiting. In certain high-risk populations, including pregnant women, children younger than 1 year of age, and immunomodulated individuals, infection may be prevented by prophylactic treatment with gammaglobulin, 0.25 mL/kg of body weight, administered within 5 days of exposure. Likewise, the ocular manifestations of measles are treated symptomatically, with topical antivirals or antibiotics to prevent secondary infections in patients with keratitis or conjunctivitis. Consideration should be given to the use of systemic corticosteroids for cases of acute measles retinopathy.

Foxman SG, Heckenlively JR, Sinclair SH. Rubeola retinopathy and pigmented paravenous retinochoroidal atrophy. *Am J Ophthalmol.* 1998;99:605–606.

Yoser SL, Forster DJ, Rao NA. Systemic viral infections and their retinal and choroidal manifestations. *Surv Ophthalmol.* 1993;37:313–352.

Subacute sclerosing panencephalitis virus

Subacute sclerosing panencephalitis (SSPE) virus is a rare, late complication of acquired measles infection most often arising in unvaccinated children 6–8 years following primary infection. Children infected with measles before the age of 1 carry a 16 times greater risk than those infected at age 5 or later. Onset is usually in late childhood or adolescence and is characterized by the insidious onset of visual impairment, behavioral disturbances, and memory impairment, followed by myoclonus and progression to spastic paresis, dementia, and death within 1–3 years.

Ocular findings are reported in 10%–50% of patients and may precede the neurologic manifestations by several weeks to 2 years. The most consistent finding is a maculopathy, consisting of focal retinitis and RPE changes, occurring in 36% of patients (Fig 8-15). Retinitis may progress within several days to involve the posterior pole and peripheral retina.

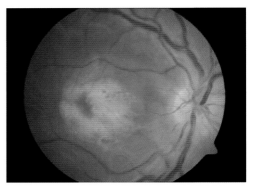

Figure 8-15 Subacute sclerosing panencephalitis macular retinitis. *(Courtesy of Emad B. Abboud, MD.)*

Other ophthalmoscopic findings include disc swelling and papilledema, optic atrophy, macular edema, macular pigment epithelial disturbances, small intraretinal hemorrhages, gliotic scar, whitish retinal infiltrates, serous macular detachment, drusen, preretinal membranes, macular hole, cortical blindness, hemianopsia, horizontal nystagmus, and ptosis. Characteristically, there is little, if any, vitritis with mottling and scarring of the RPE as the retinitis resolves.

The diagnosis is made based on clinical manifestations; the presence of characteristic, periodic electroencephalographic (EEG) discharges; the demonstration of raised IgG antibody titer against measles in the plasma and cerebrospinal fluid; and/or histopathology suggestive of panencephalitis on brain biopsy.

The differential diagnosis of the posterior segment findings associated with SSPE include those seen with necrotizing viral retinitis due to HSV, VZV, and CMV, as well as those with multiple sclerosis (MS). In contrast to SSPE, MS is not a panencephalitis; MRI imaging shows focal periventricular white matter lesions in the latter. Furthermore, CME and retinal vasculitis are prominent features of MS but have not been seen in patients with SSPE.

Definitive treatment of SSPE is undetermined. A combination of oral inosiplex (Isoprinosine) and intraventricular interferon alpha appears to be the most effective treatment; patients who respond to this regimen require lifelong therapy.

Garg RK. Subacute sclerosing panencephalitis. *Postgrad Med J.* 2002;78:63–70.

Robb RM, Watters GV. Ophthalmic manifestations of subacute sclerosing panencephalitis. *Arch Ophthalmol.* 1970;83:426–435.

West Nile Virus

West Nile virus (WNV) is a single-stranded RNA virus of the family Flaviviridae, first isolated in 1937 in the West Nile district of Uganda. It belongs to the Japanese encephalitis virus serocomplex and is endemic to Europe, Australia, Asia, and Africa. WNV first appeared in the United States in 1999 during an outbreak in New York City and has subsequently spread throughout the country; a total of 2799 cases and 102 deaths had been reported to the Centers for Disease Control and Prevention (CDC) as of December 2005.

West Nile virus is maintained in an enzootic cycle mainly involving the *Culex* genus of mosquitoes and birds. Birds are the natural host of the virus, which is transmitted from them to humans and other vertebrates through the bite of an infected mosquito. The peak onset of the disease occurs in late summer, but onset can occur anytime between July and December. The virus's incubation period ranges from 3 to 14 days, with only 20% of infections in humans becoming symptomatic and only 1 in 150 infections resulting in meningitis or encephalitis. The clinical presentation is marked by the acute onset of a febrile illness, often accompanied by myalgias, arthralgias, headache, conjunctivitis, lymphadenopathy, and a maculopapular or roseolar rash that arises in approximately 20% of infections.

Since the first description of intraocular involvement secondary to West Nile virus in 2003, multiple ophthalmic sequelae have been recognized. Presenting ocular symptoms include ocular pain, photophobia, conjunctival hyperemia, and blurred vision. A characteristic multifocal chorioretinitis is seen in the majority of patients, together with non-granulomatous anterior uveitis and vitreous cellular infiltration. Chorioretinal lesions are distributed most often in the retinal periphery in a random distribution or in linear arrays, following the course of the choroidal blood vessels, or, less frequently, in the posterior pole (Fig 8-16). During the active phase of the disease, the lesions appear whitish to yellow in color; are flat and deep, with a diameter ranging from 200 µm to 1000 µm; and evolve with varying degrees of pigmentation. Fluorescein angiography reveals hyperfluorescence and late leakage of active lesions; and early hyperfluorescence with late staining of inactive lesions. Many lesions exhibit a target-like appearance angiographically, with central hypofluorescence due to blockage from pigment (Fig 8-17). Other findings include intraretinal hemorrhages, optic disc swelling, and, less commonly, focal retinal vascular sheathing. Congenital WNV has been reported in an infant presenting without intraocular inflammation but with chorioretinal scarring in each eye.

Although the long-term natural history of WNV-associated intraocular inflammation and the risk factors for developing ocular disease are unknown, the majority of patients experience a self-limiting course, with a return of visual acuity to baseline after several months. Diabetes has been implicated as a risk factor for WNV-related death and has been observed with significantly increased frequency, together with nonproliferative retinopathy, among patients with WNV-associated ocular involvement.

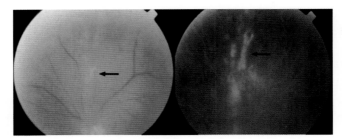

Figure 8-16 West Nile virus chorioretinitis. Fundus photograph with corresponding fluorescein angiogram of active chorioretinitis with lesions distributed in a linear array *(arrows)*. *(Reproduced with permission from Garg S, Jampol LM. Systemic and intraocular manifestations of West Nile virus infection. Surv Ophthalmol. 2005;50:8, Fig 1.)*

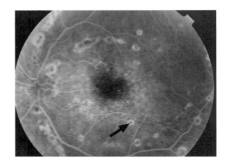

Figure 8-17 West Nile virus chorioretinitis. Midphase fluorescein angiogram showing chorioretinal lesions with central hypofluorescence and peripheral hyperfluorescence *(arrow)*. Capillary leakage is present from underlying diabetic maculopathy. *(Reproduced with permission from Khairallah M, Yahia SB, Ladjimi A, et al. Chorioretinal involvement in patients with West Nile virus infection.* Ophthalmology. *2004;111:2068, Fig 2B.)*

The presence of the unique pattern of multifocal chorioretinal lesions in patients with systemic symptoms suggestive of WNV can help to establish the diagnosis while serologic testing is pending. Conversely, a systemic ocular evaluation, including dilated funduscopy and fluorescein angiography, may be very helpful in suggesting the diagnosis of WNV infection in patients presenting with meningoencephalitis.

The most commonly used laboratory method for diagnosis is a demonstration of IgM antibody to the virus using the IgM antibody-capture enzyme-linked immunosorbent assay (MAC-ELISA), which can be confirmed by plaque reduction neutralization testing (PRNT). The differential diagnosis includes syphilis, MCP, histoplasmosis, sarcoid, and tuberculosis, all of which may be distinguished on the basis of history, systemic signs and symptoms, serology, and the pattern of chorioretinitis.

There is no currently proven treatment for WNV infection. Antiviral agents such as ribavirin and interferon alfa-2B have been found to be active against WNV in vitro but are clinically ineffective. Treatment of anterior uveitis with topical corticosteroids is certainly indicated, but the efficacy of systemic and periocular corticosteroids is unknown for the chorioretinal manifestations of WNV infection.

Garg S, Jampol LM. Systemic and intraocular manifestations of West Nile virus infection. *Surv Ophthalmol.* 2005;50:3–13.

Khairallah M, Ben Yahia S, Ladjimi A, et al. Chorioretinal involvement in patients with West Nile virus infection. *Ophthalmology.* 2004;111:2065–2070.

Other Viral Diseases

Acute iritis may occur in other infectious entities. The iritis in influenza, adenovirus, and infectious mononucleosis is mild and transient. Synechiae and ocular damage seldom occur. Iritis with adenovirus is usually secondary to corneal disease (see BCSC Section 8, *External Disease and Cornea*). Human T-lymphotropic virus type 1 (HTLV-1), a retrovirus endemic in the Caribbean islands, is a cause of iritis. Patients with HTLV-1 may also develop cotton-wool spots and intraretinal hemorrhages. Rarely, retinal periphlebitis may be seen in mononucleosis. Treatment beyond cycloplegia may not be necessary, although topical corticosteroids can be used. Iritis is unusual in mumps, although it may occur 4–14 days after onset. Papillitis or neuroretinitis appears 2–4 weeks after onset and lasts 2–3 weeks.

Fungal Uveitis

Ocular Histoplasmosis Syndrome

Ocular histoplasmosis syndrome (OHS) is a multifocal chorioretinitis presumed to be due to infection with *Histoplasma capsulatum,* a dimorphic fungus with both yeast and filamentous forms early in life. The yeast form is the cause of both systemic and ocular disease; primary infection occurs after inhalation of the fungal spores into the lungs. Ocular disease is thought to arise as a consequence of hematogenous dissemination of the organism to the spleen, liver, and choroid following the initial pulmonary infection. Acquired histoplasmosis is usually asymptomatic or may result in a benign illness, typically during childhood.

Ocular histoplasmosis syndrome is most frequently found in endemic areas of the United States such as the Ohio–Mississippi River valleys, where 60% of individuals react positively to histoplasmin skin testing. However, OHS has also been reported in nonendemic areas in this country (Maryland) and sporadically throughout Europe (United Kingdom and Netherlands). Although no serologic confirmation of histoplasmosis infection in patients with OHS has been reported, a causal relationship is strongly suggested by epidemiologic evidence linking an increased prevalence of ocular disease among patients who live or formerly resided in endemic areas. Furthermore, *H capsulatum* DNA has been detected in chronic choroidal lesions of a patient with OHS, and individuals with disciform scars are more likely than controls to react positively to histoplasmin skin testing. Men and women are affected equally, and the vast majority of patients are of northern European extraction.

The diagnosis of OHS is based on the clinical triad of multiple white, atrophic choroidal scars (so-called *histo spots*); peripapillary pigment changes; and a maculopathy due to CNV in the absence of vitreous cells. Histo spots may appear in the macula or periphery, are discrete and punched out (arising from a variable degree of scarring in the choroid and adjacent outer retina), and are typically asymptomatic (Fig 8-18). Approximately 1.5% of

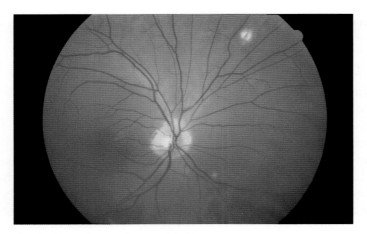

Figure 8-18 Ocular histoplasmosis, atrophic histo spots. *(Courtesy of E. Mitchel Opremcak, MD.)*

patients from endemic areas exhibit typical peripheral histo spots, first appearing during adolescence. Linear equatorial streaks can be seen in 5% of patients (Fig 8-19). In contrast, metamorphopsia and a profound reduction in central vision herald macular involvement due to CNV and bring the patient to the attention of the ophthalmologist. The mean age of patients presenting with vision-threatening maculopathy is 41 years. Funduscopy of active neovascular lesions reveals a yellow-green subretinal membrane typically surrounded by a pigment ring; overlying neurosensory detachment; and subretinal hemorrhage, frequently arising at the border of a histo scar in the disc–macula area. Cicatricial changes characterize advanced disease, with subretinal fibrosis and disciform scarring of the macula.

The pathogenesis of OHS is thought to involve a focal infection of the choroid at the time of initial systemic infection. This choroiditis may subside and leave an atrophic scar and depigmentation of the RPE, or it may result in disruption of Bruch's membrane, choriocapillaris, and RPE, with subsequent proliferation of subretinal vessels originating from the choroid. Lacking tight junctions, these neovascular complexes leak fluid, lipid, and blood, resulting in loss of macular function. The initiating stimulus for the growth of new subretinal vessels is unknown; however, immune mechanisms in patients with an underlying genetic predisposition for the development of this disease have been implicated. Human leukocyte antigen (HLA) DRw2 (HLA-DRw2) is twice as common among patients with histo spots alone, whereas both HLA-B7 and HLA-DRw2 are 2 to 4 times more common among patients with disciform scars due to OHS as compared to controls. Similarly, HLA-DR2 was found to be absent in a group of patients with MCP, a disease that simulates OHS in many respects, whereas the antigen was present among those with CNV due to OHS.

The differential diagnosis includes entities other than age-related macular degeneration (AMD) that are frequently associated with CNV, including angioid streaks, choroidal rupture, idiopathic CNV, MCP, punctate inner choroidopathy (PIC), and granulomatous fundus lesions that may mimic the scarring seen in OHS (as in toxoplasmosis, tuberculosis, coccidioidomycosis, syphilis, sarcoidosis, and toxocariasis). The atrophic spots and maculopathy of myopic degeneration and disciform scarring in AMD may also be confused with OHS.

Over time, new choroidal scars develop in more than 20% of patients; however, only 3.8% of these progress to CNV. If histo spots appear in the macular area, the patient has

Figure 8-19 Ocular histoplasmosis, linear equatorial streaks. *(Courtesy of E. Mitchel Opremcak, MD.)*

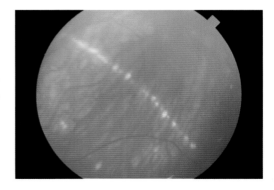

a 25% chance of developing maculopathy within 3 years; if no spots are observed, the chances fall to 2%. The risk of developing CNV in the contralateral eye is high, ranging from 8% to 24% over a 3-year period. Massive subretinal exudation and hemorrhagic retinal detachments may occur and result in permanent loss of macular function. Although some cases of spontaneous resolution with a return to normal vision have been reported, the visual prognosis of untreated OHS-associated CNV is poor, with 50%–70% of eyes reaching a final visual acuity of 20/200 or worse.

The early, acute granulomatous lesions of OHS are rarely observed but may be treated with oral or regional corticosteroids (Fig 8-20). In the early stages of the fluorescein angiogram (FA), foci of active choroiditis block the dye and appear hypofluorescent; later in the study, these lesions stain, becoming hyperfluorescent. In contrast, areas of active CNV appear hyperfluorescent early in the angiogram and leak later in the study. Choroidal neovascular membranes may arise outside the vascular arcades, but they typically do not reduce vision and may be safely observed. Clinically important CNV requiring treatment includes that with membranes located 20–200 µm from the foveal center (extrafoveal), that between 1 µm and 199 µm from the center of the foveal avascular zone (juxtafoveal), and that extending beneath the foveal center (subfoveal). Treatment options for vision-threatening CNV include thermal laser photocoagulation (Fig 8-21), photodynamic therapy (PDT) with verteporfin and/or intravitreal triamcinolone, submacular surgical membrane removal, and antivascular endothelial growth factor (anti-VEGF) therapy.

The Macular Photocoagulation Study (MPS) group conducted 2 multicenter, randomized, controlled clinical trials that showed a beneficial effect of argon blue-green and krypton-red laser photocoagulation for well-defined, classic extrafoveal, juxtafoveal, and peripapillary CNV secondary to OHS. For extrafoveal lesions, approximately 10% of treated eyes versus 40% of observed eyes had a 6-line loss of vision from baseline at 5 years. In eyes with juxtafoveal lesions, the proportion of eyes losing 6 or more lines of visual acuity from baseline over a similar period was nearly 11% in laser-treated eyes and approximately 30% in observed eyes. Persistent or recurrent CNV was observed in 26% and 33% of laser-treated eyes with extrafoveal and juxtafoveal lesions, respectively, as compared to 7% and 2% of eyes similarly assigned to observation. Given concerns regarding the potential for damage to the papillomacular bundle, a subgroup analysis was performed by the MPS group that concluded that laser photocoagulation was not contraindicated for lesions located nasal to the fovea (see Fig 8-21). Thermal laser photocoagulation is not

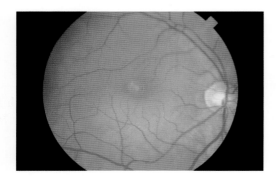

Figure 8-20 Ocular histoplasmosis, macular choroiditis with multiple yellow elevated lesions. *(Courtesy of E. Mitchel Opremcak, MD.)*

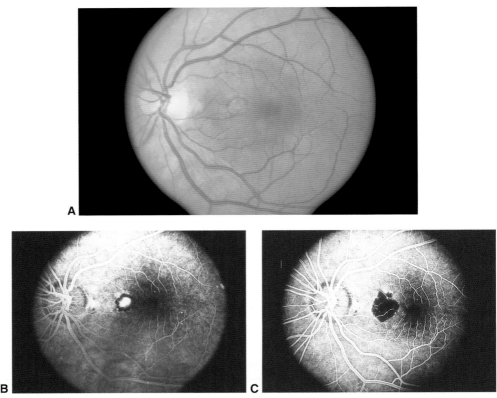

Figure 8-21 Ocular histoplasmosis. **A,** Extrafoveal subretinal neovascularization. **B,** Fluorescein angiogram of an extrafoveal subretinal neovascular membrane. **C,** Fluorescein angiogram of a subretinal neovascular membrane following laser photocoagulation. *(Courtesy of E. Mitchel Opremcak, MD.)*

used in the treatment of subfoveal CNV in the context of OHS given the profound and immediate loss of central vision that results from the destructive effects of this modality.

Photodynamic therapy with verteporfin has been advocated for the treatment of subfoveal OHS-associated CNV based on small, prospective, uncontrolled case series. The Verteporfin in Ocular Histoplasmosis study recently reported 2-year results showing a mean improvement in visual acuity score of 6 letters from baseline, an increase in the median contrast sensitivity score by 3.5 letters, and an absence of serious adverse events. Similarly, intravitreal triamcinolone has been shown to be relatively safe, with favorable visual outcomes for juxtafoveal and subfoveal CNV in small retrospective case studies.

A number of anti-VEGF agents are currently being used or are in development for the treatment of neovascular AMD, including the ribonucleic acid aptamer pegaptanib (Macugen, Eyetech/Pfizer, New York), approved by the Food and Drug Administration (FDA) in December 2004; ranibizumab (Lucentis, Genentech, San Francisco); the active fragment of a humanized anti-VEGF monoclonal antibody, currently in phase 3 trials; and the off-label use of the related full-length molecule, bevacizumab (Avastin, Genentech, San Francisco), approved by the FDA for the treatment of metastatic colon cancer. The results of 2 concurrent, prospective, randomized, double-masked, multicenter, dose-ranging trials with broad entry criteria demonstrated the safety and efficacy of pegaptanib in preserving visual acuity in patients with neovascular AMD. Early studies demonstrating the efficacy of ranibizumab are also very promising, with a vast majority of patients achieving stable vision and a significant percentage experiencing an improvement in visual function. With such encouraging results, further evaluation of anti-VEGF agents will almost certainly examine less common causes of CNV, including OHS. As with neovascular AMD, combination therapeutic approaches with PDT and intravitreal corticosteroid or anti-VEGF agents may prove fruitful, especially in treating entities with an underlying inflammatory etiology.

Patients with an active subretinal neovascular membrane located under the foveal avascular zone may benefit from submacular surgery and removal of the membrane (Fig 8-22). However, although early short-term visual outcomes were initially encouraging, longer follow-up and the recent publication of the Submacular Surgery Trials (SST) group H results showing a high recurrence rate of CNV following surgery has muted the enthusiasm for this approach. The SST was a multicenter, randomized clinical trial designed to compare vision and quality-of-life outcomes in patients with OHS; the patients were randomly assigned to surgery or observation. Despite the fact that at 2 years, 20% more eyes treated with surgery as compared with controls had visual acuity that was better or about the same as baseline, the overall benefit of surgery could not be confirmed except in a subgroup of patients with visual acuity worse than 20/100 at baseline. Among these patients, 76% of eyes undergoing surgery had a visual acuity better than or nearly the same as baseline compared to 50% in the observation group. In addition, vision-targeted quality-of-life measures improved more following surgery than with observation. Submacular surgery may be considered in patients with OHS-associated subfoveal CNV although this decision must be tailored to patients, taking into consideration the not-infrequent occurrence of complications, including intraoperative retinal breaks (12.5% peripheral and 2% posterior pole), cataract (39%), retinal detachment (4.5%), and CNV recurrence rates approaching 50% within the first 12 months following surgery.

Thermal laser, PDT, anti-VEGF agents, intravitreal corticosteroids, and submacular surgery for the treatment of CNV are discussed in greater detail in BCSC Section 12, *Retina and Vitreous.*

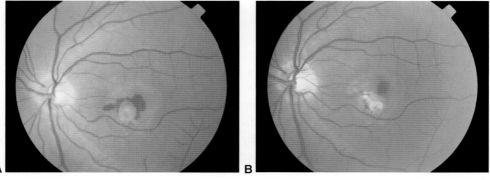

Figure 8-22 Ocular histoplasmosis. **A,** Subfoveal neovascularization. **B,** Subfoveal neovascular membrane following submacular surgical removal. *(Courtesy of E. Mitchel Opremcak, MD.)*

Five-year follow-up of fellow eyes of individuals with ocular histoplasmosis and unilateral extrafoveal or juxtafoveal choroidal neovascularization. Macular Photocoagulation Study Group. *Arch Ophthalmol.* 1996;114:677–688.

Gragoudas ES, Adamis AP, Cunningham ET Jr, et al. Pegaptanib for neovascular age-related macular degeneration. *N Engl J Med.* 2004;351:2805–2816.

Hawkins BS, Bressler NM, Bressler SB, et al. Surgical removal vs observation for subfoveal choroidal neovascularization, either associated with the ocular histoplasmosis syndrome or idiopathic: I. Ophthalmic findings from a randomized clinical trial. Submacular Surgery Trials (SST) Group H trial. SST report no. 9. *Arch Ophthalmol.* 2004;122:1597–1612.

Kleiner RC, Ratner CM, Enger C, Fine SL. Subfoveal neovascularization in the ocular histoplasmosis syndrome. A natural history study. *Retina.* 1988;8:225–229.

Melberg NS, Thomas MA, Dickinson JD, Valluri S. Managing recurrent neovascularization after subfoveal surgery in presumed ocular histoplasmosis syndrome. *Ophthalmology.* 1996;103:1064–1067.

Meredith TA, Smith RE, Braley RE, Witkowski JA, Koethe SM. The prevalence of HLA-B7 in presumed ocular histoplasmosis in patients with peripheral atrophic scars. *Am J Ophthalmol.* 1978;86:325–328.

Meredith TA, Smith RE, Duquesnoy RJ. Association of HLA-DRw2 with presumed ocular histoplasmosis. *Am J Ophthalmol.* 1980;89:70–76.

Rechtman E, Allen VD, Danis RP, Pratt LM, Harris A, Speicher MA. Intravitreal triamcinolone for choroidal neovascularization in ocular histoplasmosis syndrome. *Am J Ophthalmol.* 2003;136:739–741.

Rosenfeld PJ, Saperstein DA, Bressler NM, et al. Photodynamic therapy with verteporfin in ocular histoplasmosis: uncontrolled, open-label 2-year study. *Ophthalmology.* 2004;111:1725–1733.

Spencer WH, Chan CC, Shen DF, Rao NA. Detection of *Histoplasma capsulatum* DNA in lesions of chronic ocular histoplasmosis syndrome. *Arch Ophthalmol.* 2003;121:1551–1555.

Candidiasis

Candida species are an important cause of nosocomial infections and the most common fungal organisms, causing endogenous infections of the retina, choroid, and vitreous in both the pediatric and adult populations. Although *Candida albicans* remains the most common etiology, non-*albicans* species have been identified as pathogens in patients developing ocular disease. In patients with candidemia, the prevalence rates of intraocular candidiasis vary widely, ranging between 9% and 78%. However, when strict criteria are applied for the classification of chorioretinitis and endophthalmitis, these numbers drop precipitously, with only 9% of patients having chorioretinitis and no patients having endophthalmitis, as observed in one series when patients were examined within 72 hours of a positive blood culture. Predisposing conditions associated with candidemia and the development of intraocular infection include hospitalization with a history of recent major gastrointestinal (GI) surgery, bacteria sepsis, systemic antibiotic use, indwelling catheters, hyperalimentation, debilitating diseases (eg, diabetes mellitus), immunomodulation, prolonged neutropenia, organ transplantation, or a combination of these. Hospitalized neonates and intravenous drug abusers are also at risk. Immunodeficiency per se does not appear to be a prominent predisposing factor, attested to by the paucity of reported cases of *Candida* chorioretinitis or endophthalmitis among patients with HIV/AIDS. (See also Chapter 9, Endophthalmitis.)

Patients may present with blurred or decreased vision due to macular chorioretinal involvement or pain arising from anterior uveitis, which may be severe. Typically, *Candida* chorioretinitis is characterized by multiple, bilateral, white, well-circumscribed lesions less than 1 mm in diameter, distributed throughout the postequatorial fundus and associated with overlying vitreous cellular inflammation (Fig 8-23). The chorioretinal lesions may be associated with vascular sheathing and intraretinal hemorrhages; the vitreous exudates may assume a "string-of-pearls" appearance.

Histopathologically, *Candida* species are recognized as budding yeast with a characteristic pseudohyphate appearance (Fig 8-24). The organisms reach the eye hematogenously through metastasis to the choroid. Fungi may then break through Bruch's membrane, form subretinal abscesses, and secondarily involve the retina and vitreous.

The diagnosis of ocular candidiasis is suggested by the presence of chorioretinitis or endophthalmitis in the appropriate clinical context and confirmed by either positive blood or vitreous cultures. Because earlier treatment of candidal endophthalmitis has been shown to be associated with better visual outcomes, and patients with ocular lesions are likely to have infection involving a greater number of organ systems than those without eye lesions, it has been suggested that all patients with candidemia have baseline dilated funduscopic examinations and that these patients be followed for the development of metastatic ocular candidiasis for at least 2 weeks following an initial eye examination.

Treatment of intraocular candidiasis includes intravenous and intravitreal administration of antifungal agents. Chorioretinal lesions not yet involving the vitreous body may be effectively treated with oral triazole antifungal agents fluconazole and voriconazole, a newer agent (200 mg bid for 2–4 weeks), with vigilant monitoring for evidence of progression. Voriconazole has good oral bioavailability, achieving therapeutic intravitreal levels with a broad spectrum of antifungal activity. Intravitreal injection of antifungal agents (amphotericin B 5–10 µg/0.1 mL or voriconazole 100 µg/0.1 mL, with or without dexamethasone 0.4 mg/0.1 mL) should be considered when the vitreous body is involved,

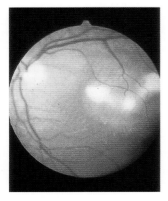

Figure 8-23 *Candida* retinitis.

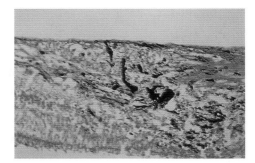

Figure 8-24 Pathology of *Candida* retinitis. Note fungi *(black)* in Gomori methenamine silver stain of retina.

usually in conjunction with pars plana vitrectomy. This approach may be useful diagnostically, allowing for the analysis of intraocular fluid by both microbiologic and molecular techniques, and therapeutically, by debulking the pathogen load. More severe infections may require intravenous amphotericin B with or without flucytosine. Significant dose-limiting toxicities (renal, cardiac, and neurologic) associated with conventional amphotericin B therapy have been significantly reduced with the development of liposomal lipid complex formulations of amphotericin B. Finally, intravenously administered caspofungin, a novel antifungal of the echinocandin class of cell wall inhibitors with activity against both *Candida* and *Aspergillus,* has been successfully employed in a small number of patients with *Candida* endophthalmitis; however, some treatment failures have also been reported with this agent. Prompt treatment of both peripherally located lesions and those not involving the macular center may salvage useful vision. Consultation with an infectious disease specialist may be extremely helpful.

Breit SM, Hariprasad SM, Mieler WF, Shah GK, Mills MD, Grand MG. Management of endogenous fungal endophthalmitis with voriconazole and caspofungin. *Am J Ophthalmol.* 2005;139:135–140.

Donahue SP, Greven CM, Zuravleff JJ, et al. Intraocular candidiasis in patients with candidemia. Clinical implications derived from a prospective multicenter study. *Ophthalmology.* 1994;101:1302–1309.

Krishna R, Amuh D, Lowder CY, Gordon SM, Adal KA, Hall G. Should all patients with candidemia have an ophthalmic examination to rule out ocular candidiasis? *Eye.* 2000;14:30–34.

McDonnell PJ, McDonnell JN, Brown RH, Green WR. Ocular involvement in patients with fungal infections. *Ophthalmology.* 1985;92:706–709.

Park DW 2nd , Jones DB, Gentry LO. Endogenous endophthalmitis among patients with candidemia. *Ophthalmology.* 1982;89:789–796.

Aspergillosis

Aspergillosis is caused by *Aspergillus* species, a ubiquitous mold found in the environment, frequently among decaying vegetable matter. It is the second most common fungus after *C albicans* to infect the retina and choroid. Individuals at risk for ocular infection include those with debilitating diseases, especially chronic pulmonary disease, endocarditis, and cancer, and intravenous drug abusers. Disseminated infection most commonly involves the lung, with the eye being the second most common site of infection. *A fumigatus* and *A flavus* are the species most frequently isolated from patients with intraocular infection. See also Chapter 9, Endophthalmitis.

Aspergillus infection of the eye presents with unilateral or bilateral vitritis, fluffy vitreous exudates, and yellow-white subretinal and retinal infiltrates similar to those seen with candidal infections, frequently involving the posterior pole and macula (Fig 8-25A). *Aspergillus* species endophthalmitis may progress rapidly, with severe inflammation, retinal hemorrhage, and significant visual loss. In contrast to the lesions associated with *Candida* chorioretinitis and endophthalmitis, those produced by *Aspergillus* species are larger and more likely to be hemorrhagic, and they commonly invade the retinal and choroidal vessels, which may result in broad areas of ischemic infarction. Histopathologically, these lesions are angiocentric, with mixed acute (polymorphonuclear leukocytes) and chronic

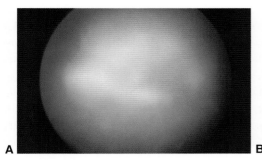 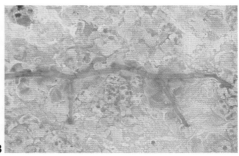

Figure 8-25 **A,** Subhyaloidal hypopyon due to endogenous *Aspergillus* endophthalmitis in an immunocompetent patient. **B,** Light micrograph shows branching hyphae of *Aspergillus fumigatus* (periodic acid–Schiff × 220). *(Reprinted with permission from Valluri S, Moorthy RS, Liggett PE, et al. Endogenous* Aspergillus *endophthalmitis in an immunocompetent individual.* Int Ophthalmol. *1993;17:131–135.)*

(lymphocytes and plasma cells) inflammatory infiltrates throughout the retina and choroid and hemorrhage present in all retinal layers. Granulomas contain rare giant cells. Branching fungal hyphae (Fig 8-25B) may be observed spreading on the surface of an intact Bruch's membrane without penetration or within the vitreous cavity, surrounded by macrophages and lymphocytes, with abscess formation.

The diagnosis requires a high degree of suspicion within the correct clinical context and is confirmed by the demonstration of septate, dichotomously branching hyphae on analysis of vitreous fluid specimens. *Aspergillus* may be difficult to culture from the blood.

As with other cases of endogenous endophthalmitis, therapy requires both systemic and intraocular antifungal therapy, together with diagnostic and therapeutic pars plana vitrectomy. Amphotericin B, with or without flucytosine, remains the treatment of choice for severe disease; however, voriconazole is being increasingly used to treat invasive aspergillosis. Voriconazole may be especially advantageous in obviating the toxicity associated with systemic amphotericin administration, given its high bioavailability and good intraocular penetration after oral administration. As in the treatment of *Candida* endophthalmitis, intravitreous injections of 100 µg of voriconazole appear to be safe in humans.

Hariprasad SM, Mieler WF, Holtz ER, et al. Determination of vitreous, aqueous, and plasmic concentration of orally administered voriconazole in humans. *Arch Ophthalmol.* 2004;122:42–47.

Rao NA, Hidayat AA. Endogenous micotic endophthalmitis: variations in clinical and histopathologic changes in candidiasis compared with aspergillosis. *Am J Ophthalmol.* 2001;132:244–251.

Cryptococcosis

Cryptococcus neoformans is yeast that is found in contaminated soil and in pigeon feces in high concentrations worldwide. Infection is acquired through inhalation of the aerosolized fungus. It has a predilection for the central nervous system and may produce severe disseminated disease among immunomodulated or debilitated patients. Although overall it remains an uncommon disease, cryptococcosis is the most common cause of fungal meningitis, as well as the most frequent fungal eye infection in patients with HIV/AIDS.

The fungus probably reaches the eye hematogenously; however, the frequent association of ocular cryptococcosis with meningitis suggests that ocular infection may result from a direct extension from the optic nerve. Ocular infections may occur months after the onset of meningitis or, in rare instances, before the onset of clinically apparent central nervous system disease.

The most frequent presentation of ocular cryptococcosis is multifocal chorioretinitis, which appears as solitary or multiple discrete yellow-white lesions varying markedly in size in the postequatorial fundus. Associated findings include variable degrees of vitritis, vascular sheathing, exudative retinal detachment, papilledema, and granulomatous anterior cellular inflammation. It has been hypothesized that infection begins as a focus in the choroid with subsequent extension and secondary involvement of overlying tissues. Severe intraocular infection progressing to endophthalmitis may be observed in the absence of meningitis or clinically apparent systemic disease.

The clinical diagnosis requires a high degree of suspicion and is supported by demonstration of the organism with India ink stains or by culture of the fungus from cerebrospinal fluid. Intravenous amphotericin B and oral flucytosine are required to halt disease progression. With optic nerve or macular involvement, the prognosis is poor for visual recovery.

Sheu SJ, Chen YC, Kuo NW, Wang JH, Chen CJ. Endogenous cryptococcal endophthalmitis. *Ophthalmology.* 1998;105:377–381.

Shields JA, Wright DM, Augsburger JJ, Wolkowicz MI. Cryptococcal chorioretinitis. *Am J Ophthalmol.* 1990;89:210–217.

Coccidioidomycosis

Coccidioidomycosis is a disease produced by the dimorphic soil fungus *Coccidioides immitis,* which is endemic to the San Joaquin Valley of central California, certain parts of the southwestern United States, and parts of Central and South America. Infection follows inhalation of dustborne arthrospores, most commonly resulting in pulmonary infection and secondary dissemination to the central nervous system, skin, and eyes. Approximately 40% of infected patients are symptomatic; the vast majority presents with a mild upper respiratory tract infection or pneumonitis approximately 3 weeks after exposure to the organism. Erythema nodosum or multiforme may appear from 3 days to 3 weeks following the onset of symptoms; disseminated infection is rare, occurring in less than 1% of patients with pulmonary coccidioidomycosis.

Ocular coccidioidomycosis is likewise uncommon, even with disseminated disease. Disseminated disease more commonly results in blepharitis, keratoconjunctivitis, phlyctenular and granulomatous conjunctivitis, episcleritis and scleritis, and extraocular nerve palsies and orbital infection. Uveal involvement is still rarer, with fewer than 20 pathologically verified cases having been reported. The anterior segment and posterior segment are equally involved. Intraocular manifestations include unilateral or bilateral granulomatous iridocyclitis, iris granulomas (Fig 8-26), and a multifocal chorioretinitis characterized by multiple, discrete, yellow-white lesions usually less than 1 disc diameter in size located in the postequatorial fundus. Vitreous cellular infiltration, vascular sheathing, retinal hemorrhage, serous retinal detachment, and involvement of the optic nerve have

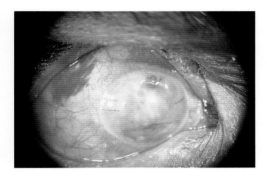

Figure 8-26 Coccidioidal iris granuloma in the pupil. This granuloma was biopsied and a peripheral iridectomy had just been performed because it was causing pupillary block and angle-closure glaucoma. *(Courtesy of Ramana S. Moorthy, MD.)*

also been reported. These choroidal granulomas may resolve, leaving punched-out chorioretinal scars.

Serologic testing for anticoccidioidal antibodies in the serum, cerebral spinal fluid, vitreous, and aqueous, as well as skin testing for exposure to coccidioidin, establishes the diagnosis in the correct clinical context. One half of patients with ocular involvement have systemic disease, and complement-fixation titers are often elevated (>1:32). With isolated anterior segment involvement, an anterior chamber tap may be useful. Culturing for the organism may delay diagnosis. The material from the anterior chamber tap may also be directly examined for coccidioidal organisms using the Papanicolaou stain.

Histopathologically, *C immitis* evokes pyogenic, granulomatous, and mixed reactions. Intraocular lesions from the anterior segment usually demonstrate zonal granulomatous inflammation that involves the uvea and angle structure, and *Coccidioides* organisms are usually seen.

The differential diagnosis of coccidioidal uveitis includes *Candida, Aspergillus,* and *Histoplasma* endophthalmitis and tuberculous uveitis. Coccidioidal uveitis should be considered in the differential diagnosis of any patient with apparent idiopathic granulomatous iritis who has lived or traveled through endemic areas of the southwestern United States, southern California and the San Joaquin Valley, northern Mexico, and Argentina.

Amphotericin B is the most effective therapy for active infection. However, the triazoles fluconazole, intraconazole, and voriconazole may also be effective and have the advantage of oral administration and less toxicity. The visual prognosis is variable and determined in large part by the location of the chorioretinal lesions with respect to the optic nerve and foveal center. Surgical debulking of anterior chamber granulomas, pars plana vitrectomy, and intraocular injections of amphotericin and voriconazole may be required. With systemic disease, much higher doses and a longer duration of intravenous amphotericin therapy or oral voriconazole therapy may be needed. An infectious disease specialist is essential in the management of coccidioidomycosis.

Despite aggressive treatment, ocular coccidioidomycosis carries a poor visual prognosis, with most eyes requiring enucleation because of pain and blindness.

Glasgow BJ, Brown HH, Foos RY. Miliary retinitis in coccidioidomycosis. *Am J Ophthalmol.* 1987;104:24–27.

Moorthy RS, Rao NA, Sidikaro Y, Foos RY. Coccidioidomycosis iridocyclitis. *Ophthalmology.* 1994;101:1923–1928.

Rodenbiker HT, Ganley JP. Ocular coccidioidomycosis. *Surv Ophthalmol.* 1980;24:263–290.

Protozoal Uveitis

Toxoplasmosis

Toxoplasmosis is the most common cause of infectious retinochoroiditis in both adults and children. It is caused by the parasite *Toxoplasma gondii,* a single-cell obligate intracellular protozoan parasite with a worldwide distribution (Fig 8-27). Cats are the definitive hosts of *T gondii,* and humans and a variety of other animals serve as intermediate hosts. *T gondii* has a complex life cycle and exists in 3 major forms:

1. the oocyst, or soil form (10–12 μm)
2. the tachyzoite, or infectious form (4–8 μm; Fig 8-28)
3. the tissue cyst, or latent form (10–200 μm), which contains as many as 3000 bradyzoites

Transmission of *T gondii* to humans and other animals may occur with all 3 forms of the parasite through a variety of vectors. The oocysts, which reproduce sexually and are found uniquely in the intestinal mucosa of cats, are shed in the infected cats' feces in large numbers, contaminating the environment, where they undergo a sporulation process. These oocysts may then be ingested by the intermediate hosts or reingested by cats. Tachyzoites are found in the circulatory system and may invade nearly all host tissue; however, in the immunocompetent host, the replication of tachyzoites eventually ceases and most organisms are removed, although a small number remain as dormant bradyzoites within intercellular tissue cysts.

Recent studies have indicated that not all toxoplasma organisms are the same. Three distinct strains of *T gondii* have been identified (types I, II and III, plus recombinant types); these vary in their virulence but are antigenically identical. Ocular toxoplasmosis in immunocompetent patients involves type I strains predominantly, whereas that in patients

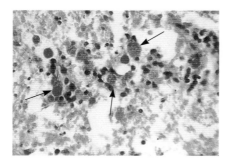

Figure 8-27 *Toxoplasma,* histopathologic view. Note the cysts *(arrows)* in the necrotic retina.

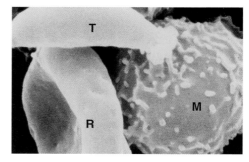

Figure 8-28 Scanning electron microscope view of toxoplasmal tachyzoite *(T)* parasitizing a macrophage *(M)* while a red blood cell *(R)* looks on. *(Courtesy of John D. Sheppard, Jr, MD.)*

with HIV/AIDS and congenital infections involves type II strains. Although antigenically identical, these 3 genotypes are unique molecularly, which allows for the possibility of molecular diagnosis from serology and the development of strategies to target strains most likely to be pathogenic in humans.

Human infection by *T gondii* may be either acquired or congenital. The principal modes of transmission include the following:

- ingestion of undercooked, infected meat containing toxoplasma cysts or contaminated water, fruit, vegetables, or unpasteurized goat milk from a chronically infected animal
- inadvertent contact with cat feces, cat litter, or soil containing oocysts
- transplacental transmission with primary infection during pregnancy
- inoculation of tachyzoites through a break in the skin
- blood transfusion or organ transplantation

Epidemics of toxoplasmosis from inhaled sporulated oocysts and contaminated municipal water supplies have been reported.

The seropositivity rates among healthy adults vary considerably throughout the world, ranging from 3% to 70% in the United States to between 50% and 80% in France. Among patients with HIV in the United States, the seroprevalence of *T gondii* varies from 15% to 40%.

It has been estimated that between 70% and 80% of women of childbearing age in the United States lack antibodies to *T gondii*, which places them at risk for contracting the disease; however, the incidence of toxoplasmosis acquired during pregnancy is only 0.2%–1%. Overall, 40% of primary maternal infections result in congenital infection, with the transplacental transmission rate being greatest during the third trimester of pregnancy. The risk of severe disease developing in the fetus is inversely proportional to gestational age: disease acquired early in pregnancy often results in spontaneous abortion, stillbirth, or severe congenital disease, whereas that acquired later in gestation may produce an asymptomatic, normal-appearing infant with latent infection. Chronic or recurrent maternal infection during pregnancy is not thought to confer a risk of congenital toxoplasmosis because maternal immunity protects against fetal transmission. Nonimmune pregnant women without serologic evidence of prior exposure to the disease should take sanitary precautions when cleaning up after cats and avoid undercooked meats.

The classic presentation of congenital toxoplasmosis is that of chorioretinitis, hydrocephalus, and intracranial calcification. Retinochoroiditis, which occurs in up to 80% of cases, is the most common abnormality in patients with congenital infections and is bilateral in approximately 85% of affected individuals, with a predilection for the posterior pole and macula (Fig 8-29). In children with mild infection, posterior segment involvement may be subclinical and chronic, and as many as 85% develop chorioretinitis after 3.7 years, with 25% of these becoming blind in 1 or both eyes. It is now the standard of care to treat newborns with toxoplasmosis with antiparasitic therapy for the first year of life to reduce the rate and severity of ocular involvement. BCSC Section 6, *Pediatric Ophthalmology and Strabismus,* discusses maternal transmission of toxoplasmosis and congenital toxoplasmosis in greater detail.

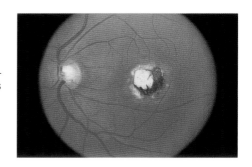

Figure 8-29 Congenital quiescent, mature, hyperpigmented toxoplasmal macular scar. Patient has 20/400 acuity. *(Courtesy of John D. Sheppard, Jr, MD.)*

Although once considered to be exclusively the result of reactivation of congenital disease, acquired infection is now thought to play an important role in the development of ocular toxoplasmosis in children and adults. In one study, acquired postnatal infection was thought to represent up to two thirds of ocular disease. This has significant public health implications with respect to primary prevention strategies that target not only pregnant women but also children and adults who are at risk for acquiring the disease. In the United States, previous studies indicate that toxoplasmosis may account for up to 38% of all cases of posterior uveitis, although this figure appears to be decreasing and varies with geography and referral bias.

Presenting symptoms, although dependent on the location of the lesion, frequently include unilateral blurred or hazy vision and floaters. A mild to moderate granulomatous anterior uveitis is frequently observed, and 10%–20% of patients have an acutely elevated IOP at presentation. Classically, ocular toxoplasmosis appears as a focal, white retinitis with overlying moderate vitreous inflammation ("headlight in the fog"), often adjacent to a pigmented chorioretinal scar (Figs 8-30, 8-31). These lesions occur more commonly in the posterior pole but may occasionally be seen immediately adjacent to or directly involving the optic nerve; they are sometimes mistaken for optic papillitis. Retinal vessels in the vicinity of an active lesion may show perivasculitis with diffuse venous sheathing and segmental arterial sheathing (Kyrieleis arteriolitis). Additional ocular complications include cataract, CME, serous retinal detachment, and CNV (Fig 8-32). Focal retinitis in the absence of chorioretinal scarring should raise the suspicion of acquired disease or another cause for the necrotizing retinitis (Fig 8-33). Retinochoroiditis developing in immunocompromised (HIV/AIDS) and elderly patients may present with atypical findings, including large, multiple, and/or bilateral lesions, with or without associated chorioretinal scars. Other atypical presentations include unilateral neuroretinitis, punctate outer retinal toxoplasmosis (PORT), unilateral pigmentary retinopathy simulating retinitis pigmentosa, scleritis, rhegmatogenous and serous retinal detachments, retinal vascular occlusions, and a presentation in association with Fuchs uveitis syndrome. PORT is characterized by small, multifocal lesions at the level of the deep retina that are associated with scant overlying vitreous inflammation (Fig 8-34).

Diagnosis

In most instances, the diagnosis of toxoplasmic retinochoroiditis is made clinically, on the basis of the appearance of the characteristic lesion on indirect ophthalmoscopy. Serologic

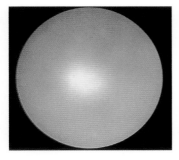

Figure 8-30 *Toxoplasma* retinochoroiditis, "headlight in the fog."

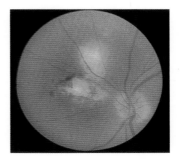

Figure 8-31 *Toxoplasma,* satellite retinitis around old scar.

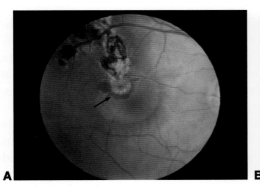

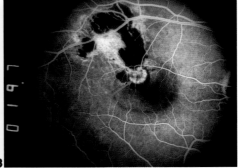

Figure 8-32 Toxoplasmic retinochoroiditis–associated choroidal neovascularization. **A,** Fundus photograph showing a choroidal neovascular membrane (CNVM) with intraretinal hemorrhage and subretinal fluid adjacent to an old toxoplasmic scar *(arrow).* **B,** Early-phase fluorescein angiogram showing blocked fluorescence associated with scar and lacy hyperfluorescence that corresponds to CNVM *(arrow). (Courtesy of Albert T. Vitale, MD.)*

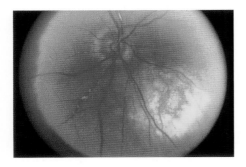

Figure 8-33 Recently acquired large, nonpigmented, inactive toxoplasmal retinal scar. *(Courtesy of John D. Sheppard, Jr, MD.)*

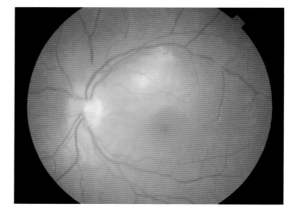

Figure 8-34 Punctate outer retinal toxoplasmosis (PORT). *(Courtesy of E. Mitchel Opremcak, MD.)*

evaluation using indirect fluorescent antibody (IFA) and ELISA tests to detect specific anti–*T gondii* antibodies is commonly used to confirm exposure to the parasite. IgG antibodies appear within the first 2 weeks following infection, typically remain positive for life, albeit at low levels, and may cross the placenta. IgM antibodies, however, rise early during the acute phase of the infection, typically remain positive for less than 1 year, and do not cross the placenta. The presence of IgG antibodies supports the diagnosis of toxoplasmic retinochoroiditis in the appropriate clinical context, whereas a negative antibody titer essentially rules out the diagnosis. The presence of IgM in newborns confirms congenital infection and is indicative of acquired disease when present in adults. IgA antibody titers may also be useful in a diagnosis of congenital toxoplasmosis in a fetus or newborn, because IgM production is often weak during this period and the presence of IgG antibodies may indicate passive transfer of maternal antibodies in utero. IgA antibodies, however, usually disappear by 7 months. Intraocular production of specific anti-*Toxoplasma* antibodies may be computed using the Goldmann-Witmer quotient: the ratio of specific antibody (aqueous or vitreous)/total IgG (aqueous or vitreous) to specific antibody (serum)/total IgG (serum), as measured by ELISA or radioimmunoassay. A ratio of greater than 4 is considered diagnostic of local antibody production. More recently, highly sensitive and specific PCR-based techniques have been used to detect *T gondii* DNA in both the aqueous humor and vitreous fluid of patients with ocular toxoplasmosis; these techniques are of particular value in cases with atypical presentations.

Treatment

Ocular toxoplasmosis is a progressive and recurrent disease, with new lesions occurring at the margins of old scars as well as elsewhere in the fundus. In the immunocompetent patient, the disease has a self-limiting course; the borders of the lesions become sharper and less edematous over a 6–8 week period without treatment, and RPE hypertrophy occurs gradually over a period of months. In the immunomodulated patient, the disease tends to be more severe and progressive. Treatment is aimed at shortening the duration of the parasitic replication, which leads to more rapid cicatrization of the lesions and thereby limits chorioretinal scarring and progression, reduces the frequency of inflammatory recurrences, and minimizes structural complications associated with intraocular inflammation.

Numerous agents have been used to treat toxoplasmosis over the years, but no single drug combination can be applied categorically to every patient, and there is no consensus as to the most efficacious regimen. There is, in fact, little firm evidence that antimicrobial therapy alters the natural history of toxoplasmic retinochoroiditis in nonimmunocompromised patients. In this setting, the decision to treat is influenced by the number, size, and location of the lesions relative to the macula and optic disc, as well as to the severity and duration of the vitreous inflammation. Some clinicians may elect to observe small lesions in the retinal periphery that are not associated with a significant decrease in vision or vitritis; others treat virtually all patients in an effort to reduce the number of subsequent recurrences. Relative treatment indications include

- lesions threatening the optic nerve or fovea
- decreased visual acuity
- lesions associated with moderate to severe vitreous inflammation
- lesions greater than 1 disc diameter in size
- persistence of the disease for more than 1 month
- the presence of multiple active lesions

Treatment is almost always indicated in immunocompromised patients (those with HIV/AIDS, neoplastic disease, and iatrogenic immunomodulation), patients with congenital toxoplasmosis, and pregnant women with acquired disease.

The classic regimen for the treatment of ocular toxoplasmosis consists of "triple therapy": pyrimethamine (loading dose: 50–100 mg; treatment dose: 25–50 mg daily), sulfadiazine (loading dose: 2–4 g; treatment dose: 1.0 g 4 times daily), and prednisone (treatment dose: 0.5–1.0 mg/kg/day, depending on the severity of the inflammation). Because sulfonamides and pyrimethamine inhibit folic acid metabolism, folinic acid (5 mg every other day) is added to this regimen to try to prevent the leukopenia and thrombocytopenia that may result from the pyrimethamine therapy. Leukocyte and platelet counts should be monitored weekly. Potential side effects of sulfa compounds include skin rash, kidney stones, and Stevens-Johnson syndrome. Some clinicians advocate adding clindamycin (300 mg 4 times daily) to this regimen as "quadruple" therapy or in the instance of sulfa allergy. Clindamycin, either alone or in combination with other agents, has been effective in managing acute lesions, but pseudomembranous colitis is a potential complication of its use.

Systemic corticosteroids are generally begun either at the time of antimicrobial therapy or within 48 hours in immunocompetent patients. The use of systemic corticosteroids without appropriate antimicrobial cover or the use of long-acting periocular and intraocular corticosteroid formulations such as triamcinolone acetonide (Kenalog) is contraindicated because these agents have been associated with severe, uncontrollable intraocular inflammation and loss of the eye (Fig 8-35). Topical corticosteroids, however, are used liberally in the presence of prominent anterior segment inflammation. In general, the duration of treatment varies between 4 and 6 weeks, at which time inflammation begins to subside and the retinal lesion shows signs of consolidation. This period may be extended with persistent disease activity.

Many ophthalmologists have begun to use trimethoprim/sulfamethoxazole (treatment dose: 160 mg/80 mg twice daily) and prednisone as an alternative to classic therapy

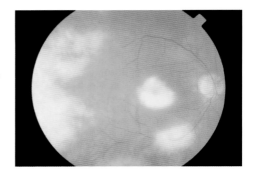

Figure 8-35 Toxoplasmosis, acute retinal necrosis following periocular corticosteroid injection. *(Courtesy of E. Mitchel Opremcak, MD.)*

for reasons of cost, the frequent unavailability of sulfadiazine, and the presumption that trimethoprim/sulfamethoxazole has a better safety profile. However, a recent prospective randomized trial of trimethoprim/sulfamethoxazole versus pyrimethamine and sulfadiazine in the treatment of ocular toxoplasmosis showed no major differences in efficacy between these 2 regimens and did not convincingly demonstrate that trimethoprim/sulfamethoxazole had a superior safety profile. Azithromycin (250 mg daily) has been used successfully to treat ocular toxoplasmosis in immunocompetent patients alone and in combination with pyrimethamine (50 mg daily), demonstrating efficacy similar to that of the standard treatment of pyrimethamine and sulfadiazine. The treatment combination of azithromycin and pyrimethamine may be better tolerated and have fewer side effects.

Newborns with congenital toxoplasmosis are commonly treated with pyrimethamine and sulfonamides for a year, in consultation with a pediatric infectious disease specialist.

In cases of newly acquired toxoplasmosis during pregnancy, treatment is given to prevent infection of the fetus and to limit fetal damage if infection has already occurred, as well as to limit the destructive sequelae of intraocular disease in the mother. Spiramycin (treatment dose: 400 mg 3 times daily) may be used safely without undue risk of teratogenicity and may reduce the rate of tachyzoite transmission to the fetus. Because this agent is commonly unavailable in the United States, alternative medications may be needed; these include azithromycin, clindamycin, and atovaquone (treatment dose: 750 mg every 6 hours). Sulfonamides may be used safely in the first 2 trimesters of pregnancy. Alternatively, local treatment involving intraocular injections of clindamycin and short-acting periocular corticosteroids (dexamethasone) has been advocated in pregnant women in an effort to reduce systemic side effects and the risk of teratogenicity.

Patients with HIV/AIDS require extended systemic treatment given the frequent association of ocular disease with cerebral involvement (56%) and the frequency of recurrent ocular disease when antitoxoplasmic medication is discontinued (Fig 8-36). The best regimen for secondary prophylaxis remains to be determined; however, atovaquone acts synergistically with pyrimethamine and sulfadiazine and may be useful in reducing the dose and toxicity of these drugs in the treatment of patients with AIDS and toxoplasmosis. The management of ocular toxoplasmosis in association with HIV/AIDS is covered in more detail in Chapter 12.

Recently, the use of long-term intermittent trimethoprim/sulfamethoxazole (1 tablet taken every 3 days) has been shown to decrease the risk of reactivation among patients with

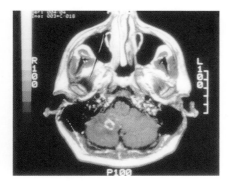

Figure 8-36 CNS toxoplasmosis presenting with ataxia in a patient with AIDS: cerebellar lesion in enhanced CT scan. *(Courtesy of John D. Sheppard, Jr, MD.)*

recurrent toxoplasmic retinochoroiditis followed for a 20-month period. A similar strategy may be useful as prophylaxis in patients with ocular toxoplasmosis and HIV/AIDS.

Similarly, the utility of prophylactic antimicrobial treatment shortly before and after intraocular surgery in patients with inactive toxoplasmic scars, particularly those that threaten the optic disc or fovea, has been raised by a recent report describing an association between cataract surgery and an increased risk of reactivation of otherwise inactive toxoplasmic retinochoroiditis. There is, however, no consensus with respect to this treatment approach or to the optimal antibiotic regimen in this clinical situation.

Bosch-Driessen LE, Berendschot TT, Ongkosuwito JV, Rothova A. Ocular toxoplasmosis: clinical features and prognosis of 154 patients. *Ophthalmology.* 2002;109:869–878.

Bosch-Driessen LH, Plaisier MB, Stilma JS, van der Lelij A, Rothova A. Reactivations of ocular toxoplasmosis after cataract extraction. *Ophthalmology.* 2002;109:41–45.

Grigg ME, Ganatra J, Boothroyd JC, Margolis TP. Unusual abundance of atypical strains associated with human ocular toxoplasmosis. *J Infect Dis.* 2001;184:633–639.

Holland GN. Ocular toxoplasmosis: a global reassessment. Part I: epidemiology and course of disease. *Am J Ophthalmol.* 2003;136:973–988.

Holland GN, Engstrom RE Jr, Glasgow BJ, et al. Ocular toxoplasmosis in patients with the acquired immunodeficiency syndrome. *Am J Ophthalmol.* 1988;106:653–667.

Holland GN, Lewis KG. An update on current practices in the management of ocular toxoplasmosis. *Am J Ophthalmol.* 2002;134:102–114.

Kishore K, Conway MD, Peyman GA. Intravitreal clindamycin and dexamethasone for toxoplasmic retinochoroiditis. *Ophthalmic Surg Laser.* 2001;32:183–192.

Kump LI, Androudi SN, Foster CS. Ocular toxoplasmosis in pregnancy. *Clin Experiment Ophthalmol.* 2005;33:455–460.

Montoya JG, Parmley S, Liesenfeld O, Jaffe GJ, Remington JS. Use of polymerase chain reaction for diagnosis of ocular toxoplasmosis. *Ophthalmology.* 1999;106:1554–1563.

Rothova A. Ocular manifestations of toxoplasmosis. *Curr Opin Ophthalmol.* 2003;14:384–388.

Silveira C, Belfort R Jr, Muccioli C, et al. The effect of long-term intermittent trimethoprim/sulfamethoxazole treatment on recurrences of toxoplasmic retinochoroiditis. *Am J Ophthalmol.* 2002;134:41–46.

Smith JR, Cunningham ET Jr. Atypical presentations of ocular toxoplasmosis. *Curr Opin Ophthalmol.* 2002;13:387–392.

Soheilian M, Sadoughi MM, Ghajarnia M, et al. Prospective randomized trial of primethoprim/ sulfamethoxazole versus pyrimethamine and sulfadiazine in the treatment of ocular toxoplasmosis. *Ophthalmology.* 2005;112:1876–1882.

Stanford MR, Gilbert RE, Jones LV, Gilbert RE. Antibiotics for toxoplasmic retinochoroiditis: an evidence-based systematic review. *Ophthalmology.* 2003;110:926–931.

Helminthic Uveitis

Toxocariasis

Ocular toxocariasis is an uncommon disease of children and young adults that may produce significant visual loss. Caucasian, non-Hispanic individuals are affected most commonly; there is no sexual predisposition. Its prevalence has recently been estimated to be 1% of a large tertiary uveitic population in northern California.

Human toxocariasis results from tissue invasion by the second-stage larvae of *Toxocara canis* or *Toxocara cati,* roundworm parasites that complete their life cycles in the small intestines of dogs and cats, respectively. Transmission occurs through geophagia, ingestion of contaminated foods, or the oral-fecal route. Pica and contact with puppies or kittens are common among children with toxocariasis. The organisms grow in the small intestine, enter the portal circulation, disseminate throughout the body by hematogenous and lymphatic routes, and ultimately reside in the target tissue, including the eye. Maturation of the adult worm does not occur in humans; consequently, ova are not shed in the alimentary tract, rendering stool analysis for larvae unproductive. Ocular toxocariasis and the systemic disease visceral larvae migrans (VLM) rarely present contemporaneously or at later times in the same individual. VLM typically affects children younger than 3 years of age, possibly due to an increased rate of pica among this group, whereas ocular toxocariasis is seen most often in older children or young adults. In cases of ocular toxocariasis reported before 1970, the mean age of patients was 7.5 years, whereas the mean age reported after 1991 was 13 years or older. This upward age trend was observed in a recent report in which ocular toxocariasis occurred at a mean age of 16.5 years. Finally, there is a direct relationship between the degree of peripheral eosinophilia and the parasitic burden in the systemic disease but not in ocular toxocariasis.

Patients with ocular toxocariasis present with unilateral decreased vision that may be accompanied by pain, photophobia, floaters, strabismus, or leukocoria. Bilateral disease is exceedingly rare. The anterior segment is typically white and quiet. However, nongranulomatous anterior inflammation and posterior synechiae may be present with severe disease. Posterior segment findings include 3 recognizable ocular syndromes:

1. leukocoria resulting from moderate to severe vitreous inflammation and mimicking endophthalmitis: 25% of cases (Fig. 8-37)
2. localized macular granuloma: 25% of cases (Fig 8-38)
3. peripheral granuloma: 50% of cases (Fig 8-39)

Uncommon variants include unilateral pars planitis with diffuse peripheral inflammatory exudates and granulomas involving the optic nerve. Table 8-2 lists the characteristics of each presentation.

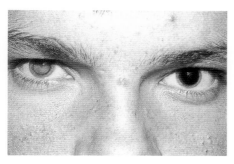

Figure 8-37 *Toxocara*, leukocoria.

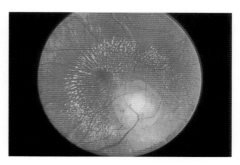

Figure 8-38 *Toxocara*, macular granuloma.

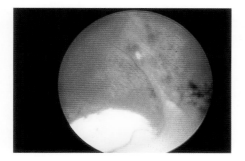

Figure 8-39 *Toxocara*, peripheral granuloma.

Table 8-2 **Ocular Toxocariasis**

Syndrome	Age of Onset	Characteristic Lesion
Chronic endophthalmitis	2–9	Chronic unilateral uveitis, cloudy vitreous cyclitic membrane
Localized granuloma	6–14	Present in the macula and peripapillary region Solitary, white, elevated in the retina: minimal reaction; 1–2 disc diameters in size
Peripheral granuloma	6–40	Peripheral hemispheric masses with dense connective tissue strands in the vitreous cavity that may connect to the disc Rarely bilateral

Determinants of the visual prognosis are multifactorial and include the degree of intraocular inflammation and the location of the inflammatory foci with respect to the foveal center; the presence or absence of CME; and the development of tractional membranes involving the optic nerve, macula, and ciliary body. In the absence of foveal involvement, vision at presentation is usually best when the granulomas are located in the posterior pole, as these eyes are less likely than those with peripheral granulomas to have macular traction. Eyes presenting with endophthalmitis have the worst vision at presentation.

The diagnosis of ocular toxocariasis is essentially clinical, based on the characteristic lesion morphology, supportive laboratory data, and imaging studies. The serum ELISA titer of 1:8 is 91% sensitive and 90% specific for prior exposure to the organism; however, any positive titer should be considered significant in the appropriate clinical context. On the other hand, the absence of serum antibodies does not rule out the diagnosis. In these latter cases, ELISA of intraocular fluids may reveal specific *T canis* antibodies and a positive Goldmann-Witmer coefficient, providing evidence of primary ocular involvement. *Toxocara* larvae have been recovered from the vitreous during pars plana vitrectomy (Fig 8-40). Finally, B-scan ultrasonography and CT are useful in the setting of media opacity and may reveal vitreous membranes and tractional retinal detachment and confirm the absence of calcium, a characteristic finding in retinoblastoma.

The most important differential diagnostic consideration is that of sporadic unilateral retinoblastoma. Factors that may be helpful in making this distinction include the distinctly younger age at presentation, the paucity of inflammatory stigmata, and the demonstration of lesion growth in children with retinoblastoma. Other differential diagnostic entities include infectious endophthalmitis, toxoplasmosis, and pars planitis, as well as congenital retinovascular abnormalities such as retinopathy of prematurity, persistent fetal vasculature, Coats disease, and familial exudative vitreoretinopathy.

Although there is no uniformly satisfactory treatment for ocular toxocariasis, medical therapy with periocular and systemic corticosteroids is aimed at reducing the inflammatory response in an effort to prevent the structural complications of the disease. The utility of antihelminthic therapy has not been established. Vitreoretinal surgical techniques have been successfully used to manage tractional and rhegmatogenous complications. Laser photocoagulation of live, motile larvae may be considered both if identified on clinical examination and in treating the rare occurrence of CNV arising in association with inactive *Toxocara* granulomas.

Stewart JM, Cubillan LD, Cunningham ET Jr. Prevalance, clinical features, and causes of vision loss among patients with ocular toxocariasis. *Retina*. 2005;25:1005–1013.

Cysticercosis

Cysticercosis is the most common ocular tapeworm infection; it occurs especially in underdeveloped areas where hygiene is poor. Human infection is caused by *Cysticercus cellulosae,*

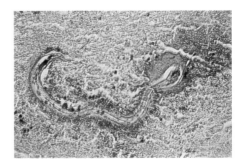

Figure 8-40 *Toxocara*, eosinophilic vitreous abscess. The organism is in the center of the abscess.

the larval form of the cystode *Taenia solium,* which is endemic to Mexico, Africa, Southeast Asia, eastern Europe, Central and South America, and India. Although the eye is more commonly affected than any other organ, neural cysticercosis is associated with significant morbidity and a mortality of 40%.

Human cysticercosis is caused by ingestion of water or foods contaminated by the pork tapeworm. The eggs mature into larvae, penetrate the intestinal mucosa, and spread hematogenously to the eye via the posterior ciliary arteries into the subretinal space in the region of the posterior pole. Larvae within the subretinal space may cause an exudative retinal detachment or may perforate the retina, causing a retinal break that may or may not be self-sealing or associated with retinal detachment, and gain access to the vitreous cavity.

Ocular cysticercosis is a disorder of the young, occurring most frequently between the ages of 10 and 30 years, without sexual predilection. Although cysticercosis may involve any structure of the eye and its adnexae (orbit, eyelid, subconjunctiva, or anterior chamber), the posterior segment is involved most often, with the subretinal space harboring the parasite more often than the vitreous body. Depending on the location of the intraocular cyst, patients may present asymptomatically with relatively good vision or may complain of floaters, moving sensations, ocular pain, photophobia, redness, and very poor visual acuity. Epileptiform seizures may be the first sign of cerebral cysticercosis, occurring in patients with concomitant ocular involvement. Biomicroscopy of the anterior segment and vitreous body reveals variable degrees of inflammatory activity, with vitreous infiltration being most pronounced during the early stages of the disease. Larvae death produces a severe inflammatory reaction that is characterized by zonal granulomatous inflammation surrounding necrotic larvae on histopathologic examination.

Larvae may be seen in the vitreous or subretinal space in 13%–46% of infected patients. The characteristic clinical appearance is that of a globular or spherical, translucent, and white cyst with a head, or scolex, that undulates in response to the examining light within the vitreous or subretinal space. The cyst itself varies in size from 1.5 to 6 disc diameters. Retinal pigment epithelial atrophy may be observed surrounding the presumptive entry site of the cysticercus into the subretinal space; retinal detachment has been observed with high frequency in some series.

The characteristic appearance of a motile anterior chamber, intravitreous, or subretinal cysticercus is pathognomonic (Figs 8-41, 8-42). Anticysticercus antibodies are detected by ELISA in approximately 80% of patients with neural cysticercosis and in 50% of patients with ocular cysticercosis. Anterior chamber paracentesis may reveal a large number of eosinophils; peripheral eosinophilia may also be present. If a patient is a definitive host, with an adult tapeworm in the gastrointestinal tract, stool examination may be positive for the eggs of *T solium.* B-scan ultrasonography may also be helpful diagnostically in the presence of intraocular cysticerci, revealing a characteristic picture of a sonolucent zone with a well-defined anterior and posterior margin. A central, echo-dense, curvilinear, highly reflective structure within the cyst is suggestive of a scolex, further narrowing the diagnosis. Computed tomography may reveal intracerebral calcification or hydrocephalus in the setting of neural cysticercosis.

The differential diagnosis includes that of leukocoria (retinoblastoma, Coats disease, retinopathy of prematurity, persistent fetal vasculature, toxocariasis, retinal

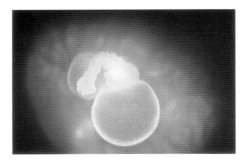

Figure 8-41 Intraocular cysticercus.

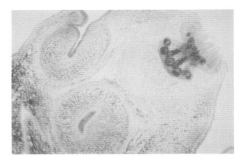

Figure 8-42 Pathology of cysticercus, showing the protoscolex, or head, of the larva.

detachment, and so on) and diffuse unilateral subacute neuroretinitis (DUSN; see the following section).

The natural history of untreated intravitreal or subretinal cysticercosis is blindness, atrophy, and phthisis within 3 to 5 years. Antihelminthic drugs such as praziquantel and albendazole have been used successfully in the medical management of active neural cysticercosis; however, these agents are generally not effective for intraocular disease. They are frequently used in combination with systemic corticosteroids, because larvae death is accompanied by worsening of the ocular disease and panuveitis. Similarly, laser photocoagulation has been advocated for small subretinal cysticerci; however, most authors report poor results when the dead parasite is allowed to remain within the eye. For this reason, early removal of the larvae from the vitreous cavity or subretinal space with vitreoretinal surgical techniques has been advocated and successfully employed.

Cardenas F, Quiroz H, Plancarte A, Meza A, Dalma A, Flisser A. Taenia solium ocular cysticercosis: findings in 30 cases. *Ann Ophthalmol.* 1992;24:25–28.

Kaliaperumal S, Rao VA, Parija SC. Cysticercosis of the eye in South India: a case series. *Indian J Med Microbiol.* 2005;23:227–230.

Kruger-Leite E, Jalkh AE, Quiroz H, Schepens CL. Intraocular cysticercosis. *Am J Ophthalmol.* 1985;99:252–257.

Diffuse Unilateral Subacute Neuroretinitis

Diffuse unilateral subacute neuroretinitis (DUSN) is an uncommon but important nematode ocular infection to consider in the differential diagnosis of posterior uveitis occurring among otherwise healthy, young patients (mean age 14 years; range 11–65 years), because early recognition and prompt treatment may preserve vision. Evidence to date suggests that DUSN is caused by a solitary nematode of 2 different sizes, apparently related to geographic region, which migrates through the subretinal space. The identity of the smaller worm, measuring 400–1000 μm in length, has been proposed to be *Ancylostoma canium* (the dog roundworm) or *T canis,* the latter being endemic to the southeastern United States, Caribbean islands, and Brazil. The larger worm is believed to be *Baylisascaris procyonis* (the raccoon roundworm), which measures 1500–2000 μm in length and has been described in the northern midwestern United States and Canada. DUSN has also been reported in Germany and China.

The clinical course of DUSN is characterized by the insidious onset of unilateral visual loss from recurrent episodes of focal, multifocal, and diffuse inflammation of the retina, RPE, and optic nerve. The early stages of the disease are marked by moderate to severe vitritis; optic disc swelling; and multiple, focal, gray-white lesions in the postequatorial fundus that vary in size from 1200 μm to 1500 μm (Fig 8-43). These lesions are evanescent and may be associated with overlying serous retinal detachment. It is at this stage that subretinal worms are most easily visualized. Differential diagnostic considerations at this phase of the disease include sarcoid-associated uveitis, MCP, acute posterior multifocal placoid pigment epitheliopathy (APMPPE), multiple evanescent white dot syndrome (MEWDS), serpiginous choroidopathy, Adamantiades-Behçet disease, ocular toxoplasmosis, OHS, nonspecific optic neuritis, and papillitis. The later stages are typified by retinal arteriolar narrowing, optic atrophy, diffuse pigment epithelial degeneration, and an abnormal electroretinogram (Fig 8-44). These findings may be confused with posttraumatic chorioretinopathy, occlusive vascular disease, toxic retinopathy, and retinitis pigmentosa. Although highly unusual, bilateral cases have been reported, as have cases of DUSN associated with neurologic disease (neural larvae migrans).

The diagnosis is made in the aforementioned clinical setting and is most strongly supported by the observation of a subretinal worm. Systemic and laboratory evaluations of patients with DUSN are typically negative. Electroretinographic abnormalities may be present even when the test is performed early in the disease course.

Direct laser photocoagulation of the subretinal worm in the early phases of the disease may be highly effective in halting progression of the disease and improving visual acuity; it has not been associated with a significant exacerbation in inflammatory activity (Fig 8-45). Medical therapy with corticosteroids may achieve transient improvement in inflammatory control, but that is followed by a recurrence of the symptoms and progression of visual loss. Initial experience with antihelminthic therapy was disappointing; however, successful treatment with oral thiabendazole (22 mg/kg twice daily for 2–4 days with a maximum dose of 3 g) has been reported in patients with moderate to severe inflammation. Treatment with albendazole (200 mg twice daily for 30 days) may be a better-tolerated alternative. Immobilization of the subretinal nematode has been observed following systemic antihelminthic therapy, and so it has been recommended that patients with DUSN in whom the worm cannot be initially identified receive a course of such therapy in order to maximize the chances of identifying and treating the offending organism. Furthermore, a second nematode, presumably

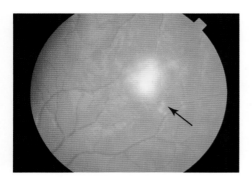

Figure 8-43 Diffuse unilateral subacute neuroretinitis. Note the multiple white retinal lesions and the S-shaped subretinal nematode *(arrow)*. *(Courtesy of E. Mitchel Opremcak, MD.)*

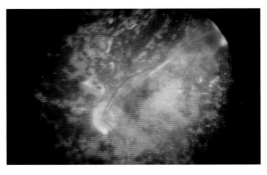

Figure 8-44 DUSN, or unilateral wipeout. *(Courtesy of E. Mitchel Opremcak, MD.)*

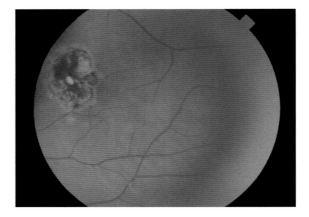

Figure 8-45 Retinal scar following laser photocoagulation of a nematode in DUSN. *(Courtesy of E. Mitchel Opremcak, MD.)*

from reinfection, may occasionally be observed in patients who have undergone successful previous photocoagulation of a subretinal worm. These patients may also benefit from a course of systemic antihelminthic therapy, particularly if inflammation does not abate promptly following laser photocoagulation.

Cortez R, Denny JP, Muci-Mendoza R, Ramirez G, Fuenmayor D, Jaffe GJ. Diffuse unilateral subacute neuroretinitis in Venezuela. *Ophthalmology.* 2005;112:2110–2114.

Onchocerciasis

One of the leading causes of blindness in the world, onchocerciasis is endemic in many areas of sub-Saharan Africa and in isolated foci in Central and South America. It is rarely seen or diagnosed in the United States. Worldwide, at least 18 million people are infected, and of these, 1–2 million are blind. In hyperendemic areas, everyone over the age of 15 is infected, and half will become blind before they die.

Humans are the only host for *Onchocerca volvulus,* the filarial parasite that causes the disease. The infective larvae of *O volvulus* are transmitted through the bite of female blackflies of the *Simulium* genus. The flies breed in fast-flowing streams; hence, the disease is commonly called *river blindness.* The larvae develop into mature adult worms that form subcutaneous nodules. The adult female releases millions of microfilariae that migrate throughout the body, particularly to the skin and the eye. Microfilariae probably reach the eye by multiple routes:

- direct invasion of the cornea from the conjunctiva
- penetration of the sclera, both directly and through the vascular bundles
- possibly by hematogenous spread

Live microfilariae are usually well tolerated, but dead microfilariae initiate a focal inflammatory response.

Anterior segment signs of onchocerciasis are common. Microfilariae can be observed swimming freely in the anterior chamber. Live microfilariae can be seen in the cornea; dead microfilariae cause a small stromal punctate inflammatory opacity that clears with time. Mild uveitis and limbitis are common, but severe anterior uveitis may occur and lead to synechiae, secondary glaucoma, and secondary cataract. Chorioretinal changes are also common and vary widely in severity. Early disruption of the RPE is typical, with pigment dispersion and focal areas of atrophy. Later, severe chorioretinal atrophy occurs, predominantly in the posterior pole. Optic atrophy is common in advanced disease.

Diagnosis is based on clinical appearance and a history of exposure in an endemic area. The diagnosis is confirmed by finding microfilariae in small skin biopsies or in the eye. Ivermectin, a macrolytic lactone, is the treatment of choice for onchocerciasis. Although not approved for sale in the United States, ivermectin is available on a compassionate basis for individual treatment. Ivermectin safely kills the microfilariae but does not have a permanent effect on the adult worms. A single oral dose of 150 µg/kg should be repeated annually, probably for 10 years. Topical corticosteroids can be used to control any anterior uveitis.

The former treatment, a course of diethylcarbamazine, was associated with many severe adverse reactions (*Mazzotti reaction*) caused by massive worm kill. This treatment has now been totally replaced by ivermectin. Although annual ivermectin treatment reduces anterior chamber microfilarial load and the development of new anterior chamber lesions, it does not reduce the macrofilarial load even at doses as high as 1600 µg/kg. Ivermectin does not appear to reduce the development of new chorioretinal lesions or to resolve existing lesions. It does appear to slow progression of visual field loss and optic atrophy, even in advanced disease. Nodules containing adult worms can be removed surgically, but this approach does not usually cure the disease because many nodules are deeply buried and cannot be found. Further research to develop more effective macrofilaricidal agents is needed to augment the beneficial effect of ivermectin in the control of onchocerciasis.

Awadzi K, Attah SK, Addy ET, Opoku NO, Quartey BT. The effects of high-dose ivermectin regimens on Onchocerca volvulus in onchocerciasis patients. *Trans R Soc Trop Med Hyg.* 1999;93:189–194.

Chan CC, Nussenblatt RB, Kim MK, Palestine AG, Awadzi K, Ottesen EA. Immunopathology of ocular onchocerciasis. 2. Anti-retinal autoantibodies in serum and ocular fluids. *Ophthalmology.* 1987;94:439–443.

Cousens SN, Cassels-Brown A, Murdoch I, et al. Impact of annual dosing with ivermectin on progression of onchocercal visual field loss. *Bull World Health Organ.* 1997;75:229–236.

Ejere H, Schwartz E, Wormald R. Ivermectin for onchocercal eye disease (river blindness). *Cochrane Database Syst Rev.* 2001;1:CD002219.

Mabey D, Whitworth JA, Eckstein M, Gilbert C, Maude G, Downham M. The effects of multiple doses of ivermectin on ocular onchocerciasis. A six-year follow-up. *Ophthalmology.* 1996;103:1001–1008.

Bacterial Uveitis

Syphilis

Syphilis is a multisystemic, chronic bacterial infection caused by the spirochete *Treponema pallidum* and is associated with multiple ocular manifestations that occur in both the acquired and congenital forms of the disease. Transmission occurs most often during sexual contact; however, transplacental infection of the fetus may occur after the tenth week of pregnancy. Having reached an all-time low in the year 2000, the incidence of syphilis is currently 2.5 cases per 100,000 population and is increasing, especially among men and African Americans, where the rate is 5.2 times greater than among non-Hispanic Caucasians. In contrast, the rate of congenital syphilis was reported to be 11.1 per 100,000 live births in 2001, reflecting sharp declines in both primary and secondary syphilis among women over the past decade.

Although syphilis is thought to be responsible for less than 1%–2% of all uveitis cases, it one of the great masqueraders of medicine and should always be considered in the differential diagnosis of any case of intraocular inflammatory disease because it is one of the few entities that can be cured with appropriate antimicrobial therapy, even in patients with HIV/AIDS. Delay in the diagnosis of syphilitic uveitis may lead not only to permanent visual loss but also to significant neurologic and cardiac morbidity that may have been averted with early treatment.

Congenital syphilis

Congenital syphilis persists in the United States largely because a significant number of women do not receive serologic testing until late in pregnancy, if at all, which in turn is related to absent or late prenatal care. Systemic findings in early congenital syphilis (2 years of age or younger) include hepatosplenomegaly, characteristic changes of the long bones on radiographic examination, abdominal distention, desquamative skin rash, low birth weight, pneumonia, and severe anemia. Late manifestations (3 years of age or older) result from scarring during early systemic disease and include Hutchinson teeth, Mulberry molars, abnormal faces, cranial nerve (CN) VIII deafness, bony changes such as saber shins and perforations of the hard palate, cutaneous lesions such as rhagades, and neurosyphilis. Cardiovascular complications are unusual in late congenital syphilis.

Ocular inflammatory disease may present at birth or decades later and includes uveitis, interstitial keratitis, optic neuritis, glaucoma, and congenital cataract. A multifocal chorioretinitis and, less commonly, retinal vasculitis are the most frequent uveitic manifestations of early congenital infection. They may result in a bilateral salt-and-pepper fundus, which affects the peripheral retina, posterior pole, or a single quadrant. These changes are not progressive and may be associated with normal vision. A less commonly described funduscopic variation is that of a bilateral secondary degeneration of the RPE, which may mimic retinitis pigmentosa with narrowing of the retinal and choroidal vessels, optic disc pallor with sharp margins, and morphologically variable deposits of pigment.

Nonulcerative stromal interstitial keratitis, often accompanied by anterior uveitis, is the most common inflammatory sign of untreated late congenital syphilis, occurring in 20%–50% of cases, most commonly in girls (Fig 8-46). Keratouveitis is thought to be an allergic response to *T pallidum* in the cornea. Symptoms include intense pain and photophobia. The cornea may be diffusely opaque, with reduced vision even to light perception. Blood vessels invade the cornea, and when they meet in the center of the visual axis after several months, the inflammation subsides and the cornea partially clears. Late stages show deep ghost (nonperfused) stromal vessels and opacities. Although the iritis accompanying interstitial keratitis may be difficult to observe due to corneal haze, secondary guttata and hyaline strands projecting into the angle provide evidence of anterior segment inflammation. Glaucoma may also occur. The constellation of interstitial keratitis, CN VIII deafness, and Hutchinson teeth is called the Hutchinson triad.

Acquired syphilis

The natural history of untreated, acquired syphilis has been well described. *Primary syphilis* follows an incubation period of approximately 3 weeks and is characterized by a chancre, a painless, solitary lesion that originates at the site of inoculation, resolving spontaneously within 3–12 weeks regardless of treatment. The central nervous system may be seeded with treponemes during this period in the absence of neurologic findings. *Secondary syphilis* occurs 6–8 weeks later and is heralded by the appearance of lymphadenopathy and a generalized maculopapular rash that may be prominent on the palms and soles. Uveitis occurs in approximately 10% of cases. This is followed by a latent period ranging from 1 year (early latency) to decades (late latency). Approximately one third of untreated patients progress to *tertiary syphilis,* which may be further subcategorized as benign tertiary syphilis (the characteristic lesion being gumma, which is most frequently found on

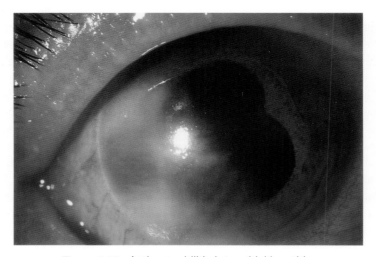

Figure 8-46   Active syphilitic interstitial keratitis.

the skin and mucous membranes but also appears in the choroid and iris), cardiovascular syphilis, and neurosyphilis. Although uveitis may occur in approximately 2.5%–5% of patients who have progressed to tertiary syphilis, it can occur in all stages of infection, including primary disease. Because the eye is an extension of the CNS, ocular syphilis is best regarded as a variant of neurosyphilis, a notion that has important diagnostic and therapeutic implications.

The ocular manifestations of syphilis are protean and affect all ocular structures, including the conjunctiva, sclera, cornea, lens, uveal tract, retina, retinal vasculature, optic nerve, cranial nerves, and pupillomotor pathways. Patients present with pain, redness, photophobia, blurred vision, and floaters. Intraocular inflammation may be granulomatous or nongranulomatous and unilateral or bilateral, and it may affect the anterior, intermediate, or posterior segments of the eye. Iridocyclitis may be associated with iris roseola, vascularized papules (iris papulosa), larger red nodules (iris nodosa), and gummata. Interstitial keratitis, posterior synechiae, lens dislocation, and iris atrophy are additional anterior segment findings seen in association with acquired syphilitic uveitis.

Posterior segment findings of acquired syphilis include vitritis, chorioretinitis, focal retinitis, necrotizing retinitis, retinal vasculitis, exudative retinal detachment, isolated papillitis, and neuroretinitis. A focal or multifocal chorioretinitis, usually associated with a variable degree of vitritis, is the most common manifestation (Fig 8-47). These lesions are typically small, grayish yellow in color, and located in the postequatorial fundus, but they may become confluent. Retinal vasculitis and disc edema, with exudates appearing around the disc and the retinal arterioles, together with serous retinal detachment, may accompany the chorioretinitis. A syphilitic posterior placoid chorioretinitis has been described, the clinical appearance and angiographic characteristics of which are thought to be pathognomonic of secondary syphilis (Fig 8-48). Solitary or multifocal, macular or papillary, placoid, yellowish gray lesions at the level of the RPE, often with accompanying vitritis, display corresponding early hypofluorescence and late staining, along with retinal perivenous staining on fluorescein angiography.

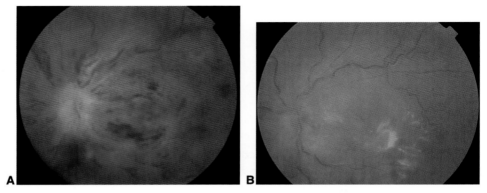

Figure 8-47 **A,** Acute syphilitic chorioretinitis. Note the diffuse disc edema, retinal edema, and choroidal edema in the posterior pole. **B,** Healed chorioretinitis after 2 weeks of intravenous penicillin therapy. Note the subretinal hard exudate that is organizing, as well as the reduction in disc edema and choroidal inflammation. *(Courtesy of Ramana S. Moorthy, MD.)*

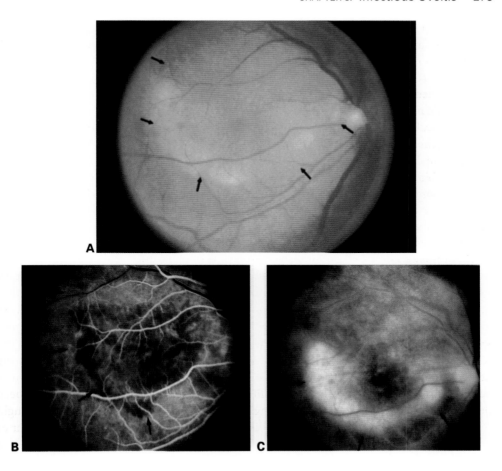

Figure 8-48 Syphilitic posterior placoid chorioretinitis. **A,** Fundus photograph of the right eye showing a large, geographic lesion involving the central macula *(arrows)*. **B,** Fluorescein angiogram disclosing early, irregular hypofluorescence *(arrows)* followed by **(C)** late staining at the level of the pigment epithelium *(arrows)*. *(Reproduced with permission from Gass JDM, Braunstein RA, Chenoweth RG. Acute syphilitic posterior placoid chorioretinitis. Ophthalmology. 1990;97:1289–1290, Figs 1, 2.)*

Less common posterior segment involvement includes focal retinitis, periphlebitis, and, infrequently, exudative retinal detachment. Syphilis may present as a focal retinitis (Fig 8-49) or as a peripheral necrotizing retinitis that may resemble that of ARN or PORN (Fig 8-50). Although foci of retinitis may become confluent and are frequently associated with retinal vasculitis, syphilitic retinitis is more slowly progressive and responds dramatically to therapy with intravenous penicillin, often with a good visual outcome. Isolated retinal vasculitis that affects the retinal arterioles, capillaries, larger arteries and veins, or both, is another feature of syphilitic intraocular inflammation that may best be appreciated on fluorescein angiography. Focal retinal vasculitis may masquerade as a branch retinal vein occlusion.

Syphilis is an important entity to consider in the differential diagnosis of neuroretinitis and papillitis that present with macular star formation. Patients with syphilis who

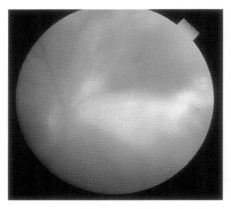

Figure 8-49 Acute syphilitic retinitis.

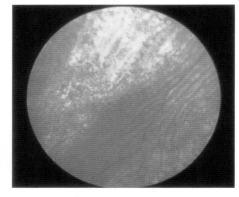

Figure 8-50 Syphilitic uveitis, acute retinitis.

are immunocompromised or who have HIV/AIDS may have atypical or more fulminant ocular disease patterns. Optic neuritis and neuroretinitis are more common in the initial presentation of these patients, and disease recurrences are noted even after appropriate antibacterial therapy.

Neuro-ophthalmic manifestations of syphilis include the Argyll-Robertson pupil, ocular motor nerve palsies, optic neuropathy, and retrobulbar optic neuritis, which all appear most often in tertiary syphilis or in neurosyphilis (see BCSC Section 5, *Neuro-Ophthalmology*, for a more complete discussion).

Diagnosis

The diagnosis of syphilitic uveitis is usually based on the history and clinical presentation and is supported by serologic testing. Primary syphilis may be diagnosed by direct visualization of spirochetes with dark-field microscopy and by direct fluorescent antibody tests of lesion exudates or tissue. Serodiagnosis is normally based on the results of both nontreponemal antigen tests, such as the Venereal Disease Research Laboratory (VDRL) and rapid plasma reagin (RPR), and treponemal antigen tests, such as the fluorescent treponemal antibody absorption (FTA-ABS) assay and the microhemagglutination assay for T-pallidum (MHA-TP). Nontreponemal antibody titers correlate with disease activity, generally becoming positive during primary or secondary syphilis and dropping when the spirochetes are not active, such as during latent syphilis or after adequate antibiotic treatment. They are useful barometers for monitoring therapy for both systemic and ocular disease. The FTA-ABS test becomes positive during the secondary stage of syphilis and remains positive, with rare exceptions, throughout the patient's lifetime; as such, it is not useful in assessing a therapeutic response. Testing for HIV should be performed in all patients with syphilis, given the high frequency of coinfection.

False-positive test results for nontreponemal tests are seen in a variety of medical conditions, including systemic lupus erythematosus (SLE), leprosy, advanced age, intravenous drug abuse, bacterial endocarditis, tuberculosis, vaccinations, infectious mononucleosis, HIV, atypical pneumonia, malaria, pregnancy, rickettsial infections, and spirochetal infections (Lyme disease), besides syphilis. Likewise, false-positive treponemal test results may be seen in association with other spirochetal infections (leptospirosis), autoimmune disease (SLE, primary biliary cirrhosis, and rheumatoid arthritis), leprosy, malaria, and advanced age. Although nontreponemal tests are appropriate for screening large populations with a relatively lower risk for syphilis, specific treponemal tests, such as the FTA-ABS, have a higher predictive value in the setting of uveitis and should be used in conjunction with nontreponemal tests in diagnosing and treating ocular syphilis. Both the false-positive and false-negative rates of serologic testing may be greater in HIV-positive patients.

A lumbar puncture with examination of the cerebrospinal fluid (CSF) is warranted in every case of syphilitic uveitis. A positive CSF-VDRL is diagnostic for neurosyphilis, but it may be nonreactive in some cases of active central nervous system involvement. Although less specific, CSF-FTA-ABS is highly sensitive and may be useful in excluding neurosyphilis. Follow-up for patients with chorioretinitis and abnormal CSF requires spinal fluid examination every 6 months until the cell count, protein, and VDRL results return to normal. Finally, specific ELISA and PCR-based DNA amplification techniques are being used with increasing frequency in the serodiagnosis of syphilis. Given their high sensitivity and specificity, these techniques, particularly PCR analysis of intraocular and/or cerebrospinal fluids, may be valuable in confirming the diagnosis in atypical cases.

A confirmed case of congenital syphilis is one in which *T pallidum* is identified by dark-field microscopy, fluorescent antibody, or other specific stains in specimens from cutaneous lesions, placenta, or umbilical cord, or the autopsy material of an infected infant. As a result of the passive transfer of immunoglobulin (IgG) across the placenta, the VDRL and FTA-ABS tests are positive among infants born with congenital syphilis. For this reason, serodiagnosis of congenital syphilis is made using the IgM FTA-ABS test, because this antibody does not cross the placenta and its presence is indicative of the infection originating with the infant.

Treatment

Parenteral penicillin G is the preferred treatment for all stages of syphilis (Table 8-3). Although the formulation, dose, route of administration, and duration of therapy vary with the stage of the disease, patients with syphilitic uveitis should be considered as having a central nervous system disease, thus requiring neurologic dosing regimens regardless of immune status. The current CDC recommendation for the treatment of neurosyphilis is 18–24 million units (MU) of aqueous crystalline penicillin G per day, administered as 3–4 MU intravenously every 4 hours or as a continuous infusion for 10–14 days. Thereafter, patients may be supplemented with intramuscular benzathine pencillin G at a dose of 2.4 MU weekly for 3 weeks. Alternatively, neurosyphilis may be treated with 2.4 MU of intramuscular procaine penicillin daily plus probenecid 500 mg 4 times a day, each for 10–14 days.

The recommended treatment regimen for congenital syphilis for infants during the first months of life is crystalline penicillin G at 100,000–150,000 units/kg/day administered as 50,000 units/kg/day intravenously every 12 hours during the first 7 days of life and every 8 hours thereafter, for a total of 10 days. Alternatively, procaine penicillin G at 50,000 units/kg/dose intramuscularly per day in a single dose for 10 days may be given.

Table 8-3 Treatment of Syphilis

Stage of Disease	Primary Treatment Regimen	Alternative Treatment Regimen
Congenital syphilis	Crystalline penicillin G 100,000–150,000 MU*/kg/d given IV as 50,000 MU/kg/dose every 12 hours during the first 7 days of life and every 8 hours thereafter, for a total of 10 days	Procaine penicillin G 50,000 MU/kg/dose IM as a single dose × 10 days
Primary, secondary, or early latent disease	Benzathine penicillin G 2.4 MU IM as a single dose	Doxycycline 100 mg po bid × 2 weeks or tetracycline 500 mg po qid × 2 weeks
Late latent or latent syphilis of uncertain duration, tertiary disease in the absence of neurosyphilis	Benzathine penicillin G 2.4 MU IM, weekly × 3 doses	Doxycycline 100 mg po bid × 4 weeks or tetracycline 500 mg po qid × 4 weeks
Neurosyphilis	Aqueous penicillin G 18–24 MU per day given IV as 3–4 MU every 4 hours × 10–14 days	Procaine penicillin 2.4 MU IM daily × 10–14 days *and* probenecid 500 mg po qid × 10–14 days

*Million units

Adapted from Centers for Disease Control and Prevention. Sexually transmitted diseases treatment guidelines 2002. *MMWR.* 2002;51(RR06):1–80.

There are no proven alternatives to penicillin for the treatment of neurosyphilis, congenital infection or that arising during pregnancy or among patients coinfected with HIV; for that reason, patients with penicillin allergy require desensitization and then treatment with penicillin. Alternative treatments in penicillin-allergic patients who show no signs of neurosyphilis and who are HIV-negative include doxycyline 200 mg orally once daily or tetracycline 500 mg orally 4 times daily for 30 days. Ceftriaxone and chloramphenicol have been reported to be effective alternatives in penicillin-allergic, HIV coinfected patients with ocular syphilis.

Patients should be monitored for the development of the Jarisch-Herxheimer reaction, a hypersensitivity response of the host to treponemal antigens that are released in large numbers as spirochetes are killed during the first 24 hours of treatment. Patients present with constitutional symptoms but may also experience a concomitant increase in the severity of ocular inflammation that may require local and/or systemic corticosteroids. In the vast majority of cases, however, supportive care and observation are sufficient.

Topical, periocular, and/or systemic corticosteroids, under appropriate antibiotic cover, may be useful adjunctively in the treatment of the anterior and posterior segment inflammation associated with syphilitic uveitis. Finally, the sexual contacts of the patient must be identified and treated, as a high percentage of these individuals are at risk for developing and transmitting this disease.

Aldave AJ, King JA, Cunningham ET Jr. Ocular syphilis. *Curr Opin Ophthalmol.* 2001;12:433–441.

Barile GR, Flynn TE. Syphilis exposure in patients with uveitis. *Ophthalmology.* 1997;104:1605–1609.

Browning DJ. Posterior segment manifestations of active ocular syphilis, their response to a neurosyphilis regimen of penicillin therapy, and the influence of human immunodeficiency virus status on response. *Ophthalmology.* 2000;107:2015–2023.

Centers for Disease Control and Prevention. *Sexually Transmitted Diseases Surveillance 2003.* Atlanta, GA: U.S. Department of Health and Human Services; September 2004.

Centers for Disease Control and Prevention. Sexually transmitted diseases treatment guidelines 2002. *MMWR.* 2002;51(RR06):1–80.

Gass JD, Braunstein RA, Chenoweth RG. Acute syphilitic posterior placoid chorioretinitis. *Ophthalmology.* 1990;97:1288–1297.

Jumper JM, Machemer R, Gallemore RP, Jaffe GJ. Exudative retinal detachment and retinitis associated with acquired syphilitic uveitis. *Retina.* 2000;20:190–194.

Mendelsohn AD, Jampol LM. Syphilitic retinitis. A cause of necrotizing retinitis. *Retina.* 1984;4:221–224.

Tamesis RR, Foster CS. Ocular syphilis. *Ophthalmology.* 1990;97:1281–1287.

Villanueva AV, Sahouri MJ, Ormerod LD, Puklin JE, Reyes MP. Posterior uveitis in patients with positive serology for syphilis. *Clin Infect Dis.* 2000;30:479–485.

Lyme Disease

Lyme disease (LD) is the most common tickborne illness in the United States. It has protean systemic and ocular manifestations and is caused by the spirochete *Borrelia burgdorferi.* Animal reservoirs include deer, horses, cows, rodents, birds, cats, and dogs. The spirochete is transmitted to humans through the bite of infected ticks, *Ixodes scapularis* in the northeast, mid-Atlantic, and midwestern United States and *Ixodes pacificus* in the western United States. In 2002, the number of reported cases increased 40% from the previous year, yielding a national incidence of 8.2 cases per 100,000 population. The disease affects men (53%) slightly more often than women and has a bimodal distribution, with incidence peaks in children ages 5–14 years and in adults 50–59 years. There is a seasonal variation, with most cases occurring between May and August.

The clinical manifestations of LD have been divided into 3 stages; ocular findings vary within each stage. The most characteristic feature of *stage 1,* or local disease, is the appearance of a macular rash known as *erythema migrans* at the site of the tick bite within 2–28 days in 60%–80% of patients. As the lesion enlarges and becomes papular, the paracentral area may clear, forming a bull's eye, with the site of the bite marking the center (Figs 8-51, 8-52). Constitutional symptoms appear at this stage and include fever, malaise, fatigue, myalgias, and arthralgias.

Stage 2, or disseminated disease, occurs several weeks to 4 months following exposure. Spirochetes spread hematogenously to the skin, central nervous system, joints, heart, and eyes. A secondary rash known as *erythema chronicum* may be seen at sites remote from the site of tick inoculation. Left untreated, up to 80% of erythema migrans patients in the United States develop joint manifestations, most commonly a monoarthritis or oligoarthritis involving the large joints, typically the knee (Fig 8-53). Joint manifestations may be the only clinical manifestation of Lyme disease in children, in whom the differential diagnosis of juvenile rheumatoid/idiopathic arthritis (JRA/JIA)-associated iridocyclitis must be considered.

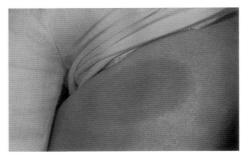

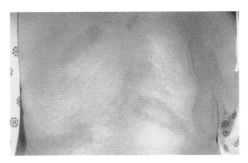

Figure 8-51 Erythema chronicum migrans, a single dense erythematous lesion. *(Courtesy of Alan B. MacDonald, MD.)*

Figure 8-52 Erythema chronicum migrans, multiple bull's-eye lesions. *(Courtesy of Alan B. MacDonald, MD.)*

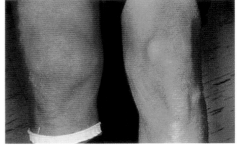

Figure 8-53 Lyme disease arthritis. *(Courtesy of Alan B. MacDonald, MD.)*

Neurologic involvement, which occurs in 30%–40% of patients, may present with meningitis, encephalitis, painful radiculitis, or unilateral or bilateral Bell's palsy. As many as 25% of new-onset CN VII palsies may be attributed to *B burgdorferi* infection in endemic areas.

The most frequent systemic manifestation of *stage 3*, or persistent disease, which occurs 5 months or more after the initial infection, is episodic arthritis that may become chronic. Chronic arthritis has been associated with the HLA-DR4 and HLA-DR2 haplotypes in North America; HLA-DR4 individuals have a poorer response to antibiotics. Acrodermatitis chronica atrophicans, a bluish-red lesion found on the extremities, along with fibrous bands and nodules, may occur in some patients, as well as chronic neurologic syndromes, including neuropsychiatric disease, radiculopathy, chronic fatigue, peripheral neuropathy, and memory loss.

The spectrum of ocular findings of LD is expanding and varies with the stage of the disease. The most common ocular manifestation of early stage 1 disease is a follicular conjunctivitis, which occurs in approximately 11% of patients; less commonly seen is episcleritis. See BCSC Section 8, *External Disease and Cornea,* for further discussion and the differential diagnosis.

Intraocular inflammatory disease is reported most often in stage 2 and, less frequently, in stage 3 disease and may manifest as anterior uveitis, intermediate uveitis, posterior uveitis, or panuveitis. Intermediate uveitis is one of the most common intraocular presentations. Vitritis may be severe and may be accompanied by a granulomatous anterior

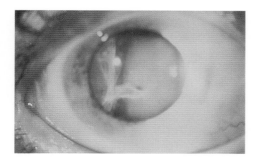

Figure 8-54 Dense anterior vitreous debris causing floaters and blurring in ocular Lyme disease. *(Courtesy of William W. Culbertson, MD.)*

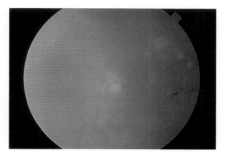

Figure 8-55 Grade III vitreous opacification in Lyme vitritis, as seen by indirect ophthalmoscopy, is reminiscent of severe pars planitis. *(Courtesy of John D. Sheppard, Jr, MD.)*

chamber reaction, papillitis, neuroretinitis, choroiditis, retinal vasculitis, and exudative retinal detachment (Figs 8-54, 8-55).

A distinct clinical entity of peripheral multifocal choroiditis has been described in association with LD; it is characterized by multiple small, round, punched-out lesions associated with vitritis, similar to those seen with sarcoidosis. Choroidal involvement may lead to pigment epithelial clumping resembling the inflammatory changes seen with syphilis or rubella. Retinal vasculitis, seen in association with peripheral multifocal choroiditis or vasculitic branch retinal vein occlusion, may be more common than previously known.

Neuro-ophthalmic manifestations include multiple cranial nerve involvement (second, third, fourth, fifth, sixth, and, most commonly, seventh cranial nerves) unilaterally or bilaterally, either sequentially or simultaneously. Optic nerve findings include optic neuritis, papilledema associated with meningitis, and papillitis most commonly seen with Lyme uveitis. Horner syndrome has also been reported.

Keratitis is the most common ocular manifestation of stage 3 disease; much less common is episcleritis. Both may present months to years after the onset of infection. Typically, infiltrates are bilateral, patchy, focal, and stromal, or they are subepithelial infiltrates with indistinct borders. However, infiltrates may also present as a peripheral keratitis with stromal edema and corneal neovascularization. The keratitis is thought to represent an immune phenomenon rather than an infectious process because it responds to topical corticosteroids alone.

The diagnosis of LD is based on the history, clinical presentation, and supportive serology. In the appropriate clinical context, the rash of erythema migrans is diagnostic of the disease. However, interpreting serologic data is problematic due to the lack of standardization of values by which a positive test is defined—the degree of cross-reactivity with other spirochetes—thus leading to frequent occurrences of false-positive and false-negative test results. The CDC recommends a 2-step protocol for the diagnosis of active disease or previous infection:

1. IFA or ELISA for IgM and IgG, followed by
2. Western immunoblot testing

PCR-based assays have been successfully used to amplify both genomic and plasmid *B burgdorferi* DNA from a variety of tissues, including ocular fluids, with the highest yields being obtained from the skin.

The current treatment recommendations for the various clinical manifestations of LD are listed in Table 8-4. For patients with ocular involvement, the route and duration of antibiotic treatment has not been established; however, as with syphilitic uveitis, intraocular inflammation associated with Lyme disease is best regarded as a manifestation of central nervous system involvement and warrants careful neurologic evaluation, including a lumbar puncture. Patients with severe posterior segment manifestations—and certainly those with confirmed central nervous system involvement—require intravenous antibiotic therapy with neurologic dosing regimens. Likewise, patients with less severe disease who respond incompletely or relapse when oral antibiotics are discontinued should probably be treated with intravenous regimens as outlined. New ketolide antibiotics such as telithromycin and cethromycin, which are both very effective against *Borrelia* and achieve high plasma and tissue concentrations following oral administration, hold promise as alternative treatments for LD.

Following the initiation of appropriate antibiotic therapy, anterior segment inflammation may be treated with topical corticosteroids and mydriatics. The use of systemic

Table 8-4 Treatment of Lyme Disease

		Drug	Adult Dosage	Pediatric Dosage
Early localized Lyme disease				
Erythema migrans		Doxycycline*	100 mg po bid × 10–21 d	≥8 yrs: 1–2 mg/kg bid
	or	Amoxicillin	500 mg po tid × 14–21 d	25–50 mg/kg/d divided tid
	or	Cefuroxime axetil	500 mg po bid × 14–21 d	30 mg/kg/d divided bid
Acute neurologic or cardiac disease				
Facial nerve palsy		Doxycycline*	100 mg po bid × 14–21 d	≥8 yrs: 1–2 mg/kg bid
	or	Amoxicillin	500 mg po tid × 14–21 d	25–50 mg/kg/d divided tid
Meningitis, radiculopathy or third-degree heart block		Ceftriaxone†	2 g/d IV once/d × 14–28 d	75–100 mg/kg once/d IV
Late disease				
Arthritis without neurologic disease		Doxycycline*	100 mg po bid × 28 d	≥8 yrs: 1–2 mg/kg bid
	or	Amoxicillin	500 mg po tid × 28 d	25–50 mg/kg/d divided tid
Recurrent arthritis, CNS or peripheral nervous system disease		Ceftriaxone†	2 g once/d IV × 14–28 d	50–100 mg/kg once/d IV

* Should not be used for children younger than 8 years old or for pregnant or lactating women
† Or cefotaxime 2 g IV q8h × 14–28 d for adults and 150–200 mg/kg/d in 3–4 doses for children

Adapted from Wormser GP, Nadelman RB, Dattwyler RJ, et al. Practice guidelines for the treatment of Lyme disease. The Infectious Diseases Society of America. *Clin Infect Dis.* 2000;31(Suppl 1):1–14.

corticosteroids has been described as part of the management of LD; however, the routine use of corticosteroids is controversial, as it has been associated with an increase in antibiotic treatment failures. As with syphilis, the Jarisch-Herxheimer reaction may complicate antibiotic therapy. Patients may become reinfected with *B burgdorferi* following successful antibiotic therapy, especially in the endemic areas, or they may experience a more severe or chronic course by virtue of coinfection with either babesiosis or human granulocytic erlichosis and require retreatment with antibiotics. Prevention strategies include avoiding tick-infested habitats, using insect repellents, wearing protective outer garments, removing ticks promptly, and reducing tick populations. A Lyme vaccine that was approved by the Food and Drug Administration (FDA) in 1998 was removed from the market in February 2002 and is no longer available.

Centers for Disease Control and Prevention (CDC). Lyme disease—United States 2001–2002. *MMWR Morb Mortal Wkly Rep.* 2004;53:365–369.

Hilton E, Smith C, Sood S. Ocular Lyme borreliosis diagnosed by polymerase chain reaction on vitreous fluid. *Ann Intern Med.* 1996;125:424–425.

Karma A, Seppala I, Mikkila H, Kaakkola S, Viljanen M, Tarkkanen A. Diagnosis and clinical characteristics of ocular Lyme borreliosis. *Am J Ophthalmol.* 1995;119:127–135.

Mikkila HO, Seppala IJ, Viljanen MK, Peltomaa MP, Karma A. The expanding clinical spectrum of ocular Lyme borreliosis. *Ophthalmology.* 2000;107:581–587.

Winterkorn JM. Lyme disease: neurologic and ophthalmic manifestations. *Surv Ophthalmol.* 1990;35:191–204.

Winward KE, Smith JL, Culbertson WW, Paris-Hamelin A. Ocular Lyme borreliosis. *Am J Ophthalmol.* 1989;180:651–657.

Wormser GP, Nadelman RB, Dattwyler RJ, et al. Practice guidelines for the treatment of Lyme disease. The Infectious Disease Society of America. *Clin Infect Dis.* 2000;31:1–14.

Leptospirosis

Leptospirosis, a zoonotic infection with a worldwide distribution, occurs most frequently in tropical and subtropical regions and is caused by the gram-negative spirochete *Leptospira interrogans*. The natural reservoirs for *Leptospira* are animals, including livestock, horses, dogs, and rodents, which excrete the organism in their urine. Humans contract the disease upon exposure to contaminated soil, water, or tissues or to infected animals; the organism gains systemic access through mucous membranes or abraded skin surfaces. The disease is not known to be spread from person to person, but maternal-fetal transmission may occur, albeit uncommonly. Occupational groups at risk include farmers, sewer workers, veterinarians, fish workers, dairy farmers, and military personnel, as well as individuals participating in water sports and activities such as swimming, wading, white water rafting, and even triathlon competitions. An estimated 100 to 200 cases are identified annually in the United States, with about half of these occurring in Hawaii.

There are over 200 pathologic strains belonging to the species *Leptospira interrogans*. Leptospirosis is frequently a biphasic disease with the initial, or leptospiremic phase, following an incubation period of 2–4 weeks, heralded by the abrupt onset of fever, chills, headache, myalgias, vomiting, and diarrhea. Circumcorneal conjunctival congestion commonly appears on the third to fourth day of the illness and is considered pathognomonic for severe systemic leptospirosis. The initial febrile attack varies in its severity, with 85%–90% of patients experiencing a self-limiting anicteric illness; 10%–15% develop severe septicemic leptospirosis or Weil disease. Weil disease is characterized by renal and hepatocellular dysfunction; it occurs 3–6 days after infection and carries a mortality rate of between 15% and 30% due to multiorgan failure. Leptospires may be isolated from the blood and cerebrospinal fluid 8–10 days after infection but are cleared rapidly from most host tissues as the patient progresses to the second, or immune, phase of the illness. The organism may persist for longer periods of time in immunologically privileged sites such as the brain and the eye. The clinical course of the immune phase is variable, the most important features being meningitis and leptospiruria. Other manifestations include the development of cranial nerve palsies, myelitis, and uveitis, all of which may appear many months after the acute stage of the illness.

The burden of ocular disease due to leptospirosis is undoubtedly underestimated because the disease itself is underdiagnosed and there is a prolonged interval between systemic and ocular disease. Circumcorneal conjunctival hyperemia is the earliest and most common sign of ocular leptospirosis, but the development of intraocular inflammation, either anterior or diffuse uveitis, in 10% and 44% of patients, respectively, is the more serious, potentially vision-threatening ocular complication.

The onset of predominantly anterior uveitis is marked by blurred vision, photophobia, and pain, but it may be insidious and mild and escape detection. The presentation of panuveitis, however, is often acute, severe, and relapsing, with 1 or both eyes being affected. A recent case series reported panuveitis to be distinctly more common than isolated anterior disease. The hallmarks include nongranulomatous anterior uveitis, with hypopyon in 12% of cases; moderate to dense vitritis with membranous veil-like opacities; optic disc edema; and retinal periphlebitis. Associated complications include glaucoma and rapid maturation of cataract, with the uncommon occurrence of spontaneous absorption of cataractous lens material. Macular edema, epiretinal membrane formation, and intermediate uveitis are uncommon.

The differential diagnosis includes uveitis associated with HLA-B27–associated seronegative spondyloarthropathies, idiopathic pars planitis, Adamantiades-Behçet disease, Eales disease, sarcoidosis, tuberculosis, and syphilis. Appropriate history and laboratory evaluation help distinguish syphilis, tuberculosis, and sarcoidosis from leptospiral uveitis. The high prevalence of bilaterality and vitreal inflammation, the infrequency of CME, and the absence of occlusive retinal vasculitis and peripheral retinal neovascularization differentiate this entity from HLA-B27–associated uveitis, idiopathic pars planitis, Adamantiades-Behçet disease, and Eales disease, respectively.

A definitive diagnosis requires isolation of the organism from bodily fluids, but this is seldom possible given that the acute phase of the disease, when leptospires may be isolated from the blood and cerebrospinal fluid, is very short, and that the process itself is very resource intensive. A presumptive diagnosis is made on the basis of serologic tests such as the microagglutination test (MAT) with seroconversion or on a fourfold or greater rise in paired serum samples in the appropriate clinical context. Although the MAT is considered the gold standard test, it is labor intensive and not widely available. Recently, rapid serologic assays such as ELISA and complement-fixation tests for the detection of IgM antibody against leptospiral antigens have been developed that are highly sensitive and specific. In addition, lipoprotein L2 and lipopolysaccharide (LPS) antigen for serodiagnosis of uveitis associated with leptospirosis have been identified, and PCR-based assays are under evaluation for rapid diagnostic evaluation. Leptospirosis may cause a positive RPR or FTA-ABS result.

Intravenous antibiotic therapy with 1.5 MU of penicillin G given every 6 hours for 1 week beginning within the first 4 days of the acute illness provides the greatest benefit for severe systemic leptospirosis. Oral doxycycline, 100 mg twice daily for 1 week, may be used for mild or moderate cases. It is not known whether systemic antibiotic treatment during the leptospiremic phase is protective with respect to long-term complications such as uveitis; however, because pathogenic leptospires may survive and multiply in the blood and anterior chamber for long periods of time, systemic antibody treatment should be considered for ocular disease that occurs even months after onset of the acute systemic disease. In addition, topical, periocular, or systemic corticosteroids, together with mydriatic/cycloplegic agents, are routinely used to suppress intraocular inflammation. The visual prognosis of leptospiral uveitis is quite favorable in spite of severe panuveal inflammation.

Martins MG, Matos KT, da Silva MV, de Abreu M. Ocular manifestations in the acute phase of leptospirosis. *Ocul Immunol Inflamm.* 1998;6:75–79.

Rathinam SR. Ocular manifestations of leptospirosis. *J Postgrad Med.* 2005;51:189–194.

Rathinam SR, Rathinam S, Selvaraj S, Dean D, Nozik RA, Namperumalsamy P. Uveitis associated with an epidemic outbreak of leptospirosis. *Am J Ophthalmol.* 1997;124:71–79.

Ocular Nocardiosis

Although ocular involvement with *Nocardia asteroides* is rare, ocular disease may be the presenting complaint in this potentially lethal but treatable systemic disease characterized by pneumonia and disseminated abscesses. Ocular involvement occurs by hematogenous spread of the bacteria. Choroidal abscess has been described in heart transplant recipients. The responsible organism is commonly found in soil, and initial infection occurs by ingestion or inhalation. Symptoms of ocular infection caused by *N asteroides* may vary from the mild pain and redness of iridocyclitis to the severe pain and decreased vision of panophthalmitis. Findings range from an isolated, unilateral chorioretinal mass with minimal vitritis to diffuse iridocyclitis with cell and flare, vitritis, and multiple choroidal abscesses with overlying retinal detachment.

Diagnosis can be established with a culture of the organism taken from tissue or fluid, by vitreous aspiration for Gram stain and culture, or occasionally by enucleation and microscopic identification of organisms. Treatment of systemic *N asteroides* infection is systemic sulfonamide for 6 weeks in immunologically competent patients and up to 1 year in immunomodulated patients.

Davitt B, Gehrs K, Bowers T. Endogenous *Nocardia* endophthalmitis. *Retina.* 1998;18:71–73.

Ng EW, Zimmer-Galler IE, Green WR. Endogenous *Nocardia asteroides* endophthalmitis. *Arch Ophthalmol.* 2002;120:210–213.

Tuberculosis

Tuberculosis was once considered the most common cause of uveitis; today ocular involvement due to tuberculosis (TB) is an uncommon event in the United States, affecting 1%–2% of patients. Worldwide, however, it remains the most important systemic infectious disease, with more than 8 million new cases and 3 million deaths reported annually. Nearly a third of the world's population is infected, and 95% of cases occurs in developing countries. In the United States, following many years of annual decline, the incidence of TB increased coincident with the AIDS epidemic and has reemerged as an important public health problem; nearly half the cases reported in 2001 involved foreign-born individuals. Although the frequency of ocular disease parallels the prevalence of TB in general, it is relatively uncommon both in endemic areas and among institutionalized populations with unequivocal systemic disease. In the United States, the incidence of uveitis attributable to TB at a large tertiary care facility was only 0.6%, whereas at major referral centers in India, it ranged from 0.6% to 10%, and in similar institutions in Japan and Saudi Arabia, it ranged from 7.9% to 10.5%, respectively.

Tuberculosis is caused by *Mycobacterium tuberculosis,* an acid-fast–staining, obligate aerobe, most commonly transmitted by aerosolized droplets. The organism has an affinity for highly oxygenated tissues, and tuberculous lesions are commonly found in the apices of the lungs as well as in the choroid, which has the highest blood flow rate in the body. Systemic infection may occur primarily, as a result of recent exposure, or secondarily, in the vast majority (90%) of patients, with reactivation of the disease due to compromised immune function. Hematogenous dissemination of TB, or miliary disease, likewise occurs most often in the setting of immunomodulation. High-risk groups include health care professionals, recent immigrants from endemic areas, the indigent, patients immunomodulated for whatever reason (chronic disease, HIV/AIDS, or medication), and the elderly.

Pulmonary TB develops in approximately 80% of patients, whereas extrapulmonary disease is seen in about 20%, with half of these patients exhibiting a normal chest radiograph and up to 20% having a negative purified protein derivative (PPD) skin test. Patients coinfected with HIV present more often with extrapulmonary disease, the frequency of which increases with deteriorating immune function. Only 10% of infected individuals develop symptomatic disease; half of these manifest within the first 1–2 years. The vast majority, however, remain infected but asymptomatic. The classic presentation of symptomatic disease—fever, night sweats, and weight loss—is seen with both pulmonary and extrapulmonary infection. This is important to keep in mind when conducting a review of systems for patients suspected of tuberculous uveitis because histopathologically proven intraocular TB has been shown to occur in patients with both asymptomatic disease and extrapulmonary disease.

The ocular manifestations of tuberculosis may be due to either active infection or an immunologic reaction to the organism. Primary ocular TB is defined as that in which the eye is the primary portal of entry, manifesting mainly as conjunctival, corneal, and scleral disease. Secondary ocular TB, of which uveitis is the most common manifestation, occurs by virtue of hematogenous dissemination of the organism or by contiguous spread from adjacent structures. External ocular and anterior segment findings include scleritis, phlyctenulosis, interstitial keratitis, corneal infiltrates, anterior chamber and iris nodules, and isolated granulomatous anterior uveitis; the last is exceedingly uncommon in the absence of posterior segment disease.

Tuberculous uveitis is classically a chronic granulomatous disease that may affect the anterior and/or posterior segments; it is replete with mutton-fat keratic precipitates, iris nodules, posterior synechiae, and secondary glaucoma, although a nongranulomatous uveitis may also occur. Patients typically experience a waxing and waning course, with long-term degradation of the blood–aqueous barrier, an accumulation of vitreous opacities, and CME (Figs 8-56, 8-57).

Disseminated choroiditis is the most common presentation and is characterized by deep, multiple, discrete, yellowish lesions between 0.5 and 3.0 mm in diameter, numbering from 5 to several hundred (Fig 8-58). These lesions, or tubercles, are located predominantly in the posterior pole and may be accompanied by disc edema, nerve fiber hemorrhages, and varying degrees of vitritis and granulomatous anterior uveitis. Alternatively, they may present as a focal, single, large elevated choroidal mass (tuberculoma) that varies in size from 4 mm to 14 mm and may be accompanied by neurosensory retinal detachment and macular star formation (Fig 8-59). Choroidal tubercles may be one of the earliest signs of disseminated disease and are more commonly observed among immunocompromised hosts. On fluorescein angiography, active choroidal lesions display early hyperfluorescence with late leakage and cicatricial lesions show early blocked fluorescence with late staining. Indocyanine green angiography reveals early- and late-stage hypofluorescence corresponding to the choroidal lesions, which are frequently more numerous than those seen on fluorescein angiography or even on clinical examination. Other manifestations of tuberculous infection of the choroid include multifocal choroiditis and a serpiginous-like choroiditis (Fig 8-60). In the setting of HIV/AIDS, tuberculous choroiditis may progress despite effective antituberculous therapy.

Retinal involvement in tuberculosis is usually secondary to extension of the choroidal disease or an immunologic response to mycobacteria. Eales disease is a peripheral retinal perivasculitis that presents in otherwise healthy young men aged 20–40 years with recurrent, unilateral retinal and vitreous hemorrhage and subsequent involvement of the fellow eye. A periphlebitis is most commonly observed, which may be accompanied by venous occlusion, peripheral nonperfusion, neovascularization, and the eventual development of tractional retinal detachment (Fig 8-61). The association between TB and retinal vasculitis is supported by the identification

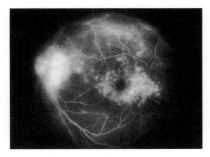

Figure 8-56 Chronic tuberculous uveitis with disc edema, vasculitis, periphlebitis, and CME. *(Courtesy of John D. Sheppard, Jr, MD.)*

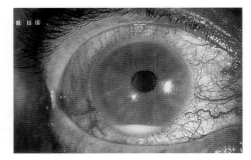

Figure 8-57 Acute tuberculous uveitis with hypopyon, posterior synechiae, vitritis, retinal vasculitis, and CME. *(Courtesy of John D. Sheppard, Jr, MD.)*

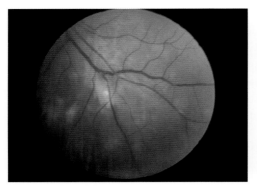

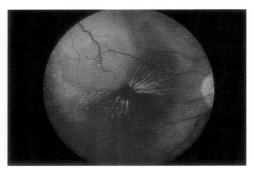

Figure 8-58 Multifocal, discrete, yellowish choroidal lesions in a patient with pulmonary tuberculosis. *(Reproduced with permission from Vitale AT, Foster CS. Uveitis affecting infants and children: infectious. In: Hartnett ME, Trese M, Capone A, Steidl SM, Keats B, eds. Pediatric Retina: Medical and Surgical Approaches. Philadelphia: Lippincott Williams & Wilkins; 2004:277, Fig 16-10; photograph courtesy of Albert T. Vitale, MD.)*

Figure 8-59 Choroidal tubercle with a macular star formation (miliary tuberculosis).

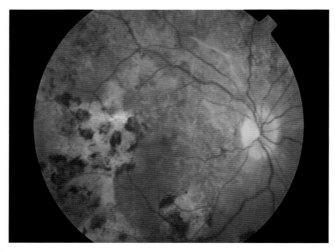

Figure 8-60 Tuberculous choroiditis masquerading as atypical serpiginous choroiditis. The patient showed progression and recurrence while on immunomodulatory agents; however, after antituberculous treatment, the patient showed improvement in vision and resolution of the vitritis without recurrences. *(Courtesy of Narsing A. Rao, MD.)*

by PCR-based assays of tuberculosis DNA from the aqueous, vitreous, and epiretinal membranes of patients with Eales disease. Other posterior segment findings of TB include subretinal abscess, choroidal neovascularization, optic neuritis, and acute panophthalmitis.

Definitive diagnosis of TB requires a finding of mycobacteria in bodily fluids or tissues. In many cases of ocular TB, this is not possible, and the diagnosis is instead presumptive, based on indirect evidence. A positive PPD is indicative of prior exposure to TB but

CHAPTER 9

Endophthalmitis

Endophthalmitis is a clinical diagnosis made when intraocular inflammation involving both the posterior and anterior chambers is attributable to bacterial or fungal infection. The retina or the choroid may be involved; occasionally there is concomitant infective scleritis or keratitis. *Infectious endophthalmitis,* confirmed by culture, is the focus of this chapter. *Sterile endophthalmitis* describes cases suspected of being infectious but with negative cultures. *Chronic postoperative inflammation* describes cases that are culture-negative and ultimately attributed to noninfectious stimuli such as retained lens material (lens-induced uveitis), malposition of the intraocular lens, or pro-inflammatory debris introduced into the eye during trauma or intraocular surgery.

Signs and Symptoms

Classic signs of endophthalmitis are decreased vision, conjunctival hyperemia, pain, lid swelling, and hypopyon. Hypopyon and pain were each absent in 25% of participants in the Endophthalmitis Vitrectomy Study (EVS), a national collaborative study. Conjunctival chemosis and corneal edema may be observed. There is a spectrum of clinical signs and symptoms from mild to severe that are generally more pronounced when the interval between surgery, or penetrating trauma, and onset of endophthalmitis is shorter. This is probably related to the virulence of the infecting organism or the infective load. Clinically worse eyes have a worse prognosis.

Types of Infectious Endophthalmitis

Infectious endophthalmitis can be classified according to how the infecting organism is introduced into the eye. *Exogenous endophthalmitis,* in which the organism enters the eye from the external environment, accounts for most cases, as in the following categories (Table 9-1):

- *postoperative endophthalmitis* after surgical incision (Fig 9-1)
- *posttraumatic endophthalmitis* after penetrating injury
- *bleb-associated endophthalmitis* after glaucoma surgery with a conjunctival filtering bleb

Table 9-1 Characteristics of Exogenous Endophthalmitis

Category	Incidence	Most Common Organisms	Onset After Surgery or Trauma	Symptoms	Common Clinical Findings
Acute postoperative (cataract surgery)	0.07%–0.12%				
Mild		Staphylococcus epidermidis Sterile	1–42 days	Photophobia, floaters	Slow progression, vision >20/400, ± hypopyon, mild vitritis, fundus visible
Severe		Staphylococcus aureus Streptococcus spp Gram-negative bacteria	1–4 days	Pain, decreased vision	Rapid progression, vision <20/400, ± hypopyon, marked vitritis, fundus not visible
Chronic postoperative	?	Propionibacterium acnes S epidermidis Fungus	6 weeks to 2 years	Photophobia, hazy vision	Sometimes appearing with granulomatous keratic precipitates, ± hypopyon, mild to moderate vitritis, capsular plaque
Posttraumatic	2.4%–8.0% (as high as 30.0% in rural settings)	S epidermidis Bacillus spp	1–5 days (fungi 1–4 weeks)	±Increasing pain, decreasing vision	Increasing inflammation, hypopyon, increasing vitritis
Associated with filtering bleb	0.2%–9.6%	Streptococcus spp Staphylococcus spp	Usually delayed	Red eye, discharge, pain, decreasing vision	Infected bleb, hypopyon, vitritis

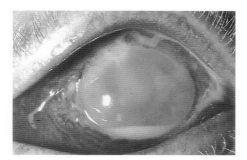

Figure 9-1 Exogenous postoperative endophthalmitis (bacterial).

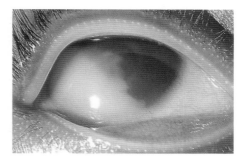

Figure 9-2 Endogenous endophthalmitis (meningococcal meningitis).

Postoperative Endophthalmitis

Exogenous infectious endophthalmitis can also occur after suture removal, late wound infection or wound leaks, microbial keratitis, or scleritis. *Endogenous endophthalmitis,* which is uncommon, occurs when infection hematogenously spreads to the eye (Fig 9-2).

A systematic review by Taban and colleagues of over 3 million published cataract surgeries indicated an increase in endophthalmitis during 2000–2003 to 0.265% vs an overall rate of 0.128% from 1963 to 2003. In the review, clear corneal incision was statistically associated with a higher risk of endophthalmitis. From 1992 to 2003, 0.189% of cases of clear corneal incision developed endophthalmitis vs 0.074% (relative risk, 2.55 [95% confidence interval, 1.75–3.71]) for scleral incision and 0.062% (relative risk, 3.06 [95% confidence interval, 2.48–3.76]) for limbal incision. A systematic review of over 90,000 penetrating keratoplasties revealed an incidence of endophthalmitis of 0.382%, a decline from 1992.

Pars plana vitrectomy has a low, 0.05%, rate of endophthalmitis. The cumulative incidence of bleb-related endophthalmitis after glaucoma filtering surgery has been reported to range from 0.2% to 9.6%. In one large series, the incidence of endophthalmitis due to glaucoma drainage devices was a low 1.7%; it was higher in children with these devices and when the device was exposed because of conjunctival erosion. High rates of endophthalmitis follow trauma. The incidence of posttraumatic endophthalmitis ranges between 2.4% and 8.0%. In rural settings or in cases with a retained intraocular foreign body, the incidence has been reported to be as high as 30%.

The spectrum of infecting organisms varies according to the etiology of the endophthalmitis.

In most cases of postoperative endophthalmitis, the causative organism is introduced into the eye at surgery; sutureless cataract wounds can also transmit organisms postoperatively. Studies of intraoperative contamination demonstrate positive bacterial cultures in a much higher percentage of cases than develop endophthalmitis. Because absolute sterility of the surgical site cannot be achieved, the eyelids and conjunctiva are the primary source of infection in postoperative endophthalmitis, and the organisms responsible are often normal ocular surface flora such as coagulase-negative *Staphylococcus* species. Strains isolated from the eyelids and from inside the eye were identical in two thirds of 105 comparisons made in the EVS. The ocular microbiology of the eyelids and conjunctiva is discussed in detail in BCSC Section 8, *External Disease and Cornea.*

Besides normal ocular flora, specific sources of contamination include

- secondary infection from other sites, such as the lacrimal system
- blepharitis
- contaminated eyedrops
- contaminated surgical instruments or irrigation fluids
- vital dyes or viscoelastics
- major breaches in sterile technique

Intraocular lenses can also introduce pathogens into the eye. Certain IOL materials, such as polypropylene (haptics), are associated with more positive bacterial cultures in aqueous humor at the conclusion of cataract surgery than other materials.

Aaberg TM Jr, Flynn HW Jr, Schiffman J, Newton J. Nosocomial acute-onset postoperative endophthalmitis survey: a 10-year review of incidence and outcomes. *Ophthalmology.* 1998;105:1004–1010.

Agrawal V, Gopinathan U, Singh S, Reddy M, Rao GN. Influence of intraocular lens haptic material on bacterial isolates from anterior chamber aspirate. *J Cataract Refract Surg.* 1997;23:588–592.

Al-Torbak AA, Al-Shahwan S, Al-Jadaan I, Al-Hommadi A, Edward DP. Endophthalmitis associated with the Ahmed glaucoma valve implant. *Br J Ophthalmol.* 2005;89:454–458.

Bannerman TL, Rhoden DL, McAllister SK, Miller JM, Wilson LA. The source of coagulase-negative staphylococci in the Endophthalmitis Vitrectomy Study. A comparison of eyelid and intraocular isolates using pulsed-field gel electrophoresis. *Arch Ophthalmol.* 1997;115:357–361.

Benz MS, Scott IU, Flynn HW Jr, Unonius N, Miller D. Endophthalmitis isolates and antibiotic sensitivities: a 6-year review of culture-proven cases. *Am J Ophthalmol.* 2004;137:38–42.

Essex RW, Yi Q, Charles PG, Allen PJ. Post-traumatic endophthalmitis. *Ophthalmology.* 2004;111:2015–2022.

Ozdal PC, Mansour M, Deschenes J. Ultrasound biomicroscopy of pseudophakic eyes with chronic postoperative inflammation. *J Cataract Refract Surg.* 2003;29:1185–1191.

Taban M, Behrens A, Newcomb RL, Nobe MY, McDonnell PJ. Incidence of acute endophthalmitis following penetrating keratoplasty: a systematic review. *Arch Ophthalmol.* 2005; 123:605–609.

Taban M, Behrens A, Newcomb RL, et al. Acute endophthalmitis following cataract surgery: a systematic review of the literature. *Arch Ophthalmol.* 2005;123:613–620.

Wisniewski SR, Capone A, Kelsey SF, Groer-Fitzgerald S, Lambert HM, Doft BH. Characteristics after cataract extraction or secondary lens implantation among patients screened for the Endophthalmitis Vitrectomy Study. *Ophthalmology.* 2000;107:1274–1282.

Acute-onset postoperative endophthalmitis

Acute-onset postoperative endophthalmitis can develop up to 6 weeks after intraocular surgery. When surgery is complicated, such as when posterior capsular rupture occurs during cataract surgery, the risk of contamination of the intraocular fluids increases.

Endophthalmitis may occur following any surgical procedure in which the intraocular space is entered or inadvertently violated:

- cataract surgery
- secondary IOL implantation
- glaucoma procedures
- penetrating keratoplasty
- keratorefractive surgery
- pterygium excision
- strabismus surgery
- scleral buckling surgery
- retinal/vitreous surgery
- anterior chamber paracentesis
- intravitreal administration of medication

For prognostic and therapeutic purposes, it is useful to distinguish between *mild* cases of acute endophthalmitis, with a slowly developing course, and *severe* cases, with a rapidly progressive course. The mild cases are less painful, involve a presenting visual acuity of 20/400 or better, and usually present 3–14 days postoperatively. *Staphylococus epidermidis* and other coagulase-negative *Staphylococcus* species are the organisms most commonly recovered in culture (Fig 9-3). In the EVS, approximately one third of clinically diagnosed acute postoperative endophthalmitis cases were culture-negative, regardless of whether the cultures were obtained by vitreous tap or by vitrectomy.

Severe acute-onset postoperative endophthalmitis usually presents within 1–4 days after surgery. Vision is usually worse than 20/400, and patients report pain. Marked vitritis is common, and the fundus details are not visible. In these cases, more virulent bacteria, including *Staphylococcus aureus; Streptococcus* species; and gram-negative organisms such as *Serratia marcescens* (Fig 9-4), *Proteus,* and *Pseudomonas* species, are often isolated. Despite prompt recognition and treatment of severe acute-onset postoperative endophthalmitis, significant damage may already have occurred at onset of symptoms, presumably based on the virulence of the infecting organism.

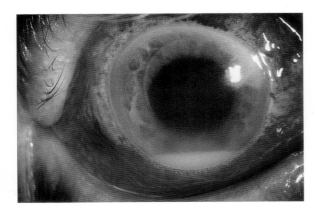

Figure 9-3 Mild acute postoperative endophthalmitis caused by *S epidermidis.*

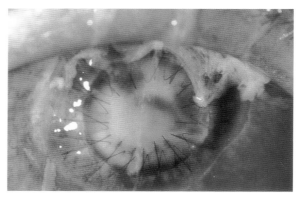

Figure 9-4 Severe acute postoperative endophthalmitis caused by *Serratia marcescens,* following penetrating keratoplasty.

Chronic, or delayed-onset, postoperative endophthalmitis

Chronic postoperative endophthalmitis is diagnosed 6 weeks to years after surgery, although signs and symptoms may have been gradually increasing since surgery. There is often good vision, minimal pain, and only mild vitritis. Development of hypopyon in an eye with chronic postoperative inflammation is often the clue that infection is present.

Infecting organisms in chronic postoperative endophthalmitis are usually slow growers of low virulence. Delayed-onset *Propionibacterium acnes* endophthalmitis often displays granulomatous keratic precipitates, a small hypopyon, vitritis, and a characteristic white plaque containing *P acnes* and residual lens material sequestered within the capsular bag (Fig 9-5). *S epidermidis* and fungi can also cause a chronic endophthalmitis. Candidal species are the most common fungal causes of chronic postoperative endophthalmitis.

Diagnosis of chronic postoperative endophthalmitis sometimes follows Nd:YAG laser capsulotomy. It is hypothesized that opening the capsule allows sequestered pathogens to enter the posterior and anterior chambers.

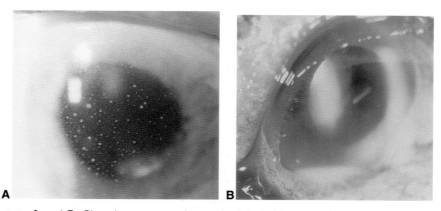

A   **B**

Figure 9-5 A and B, Chronic postoperative endophthalmitis caused by *P acnes*. Note granulomatous keratic precipitates and white plaque in the capsular bag. *(Photographs courtesy of David Meisler, MD.)*

Posttraumatic Endophthalmitis

Posttraumatic endophthalmitis can occur following any penetrating ocular injury; however, the incidence appears to be higher in rural settings and when intraocular foreign bodies are retained. The most common organisms found are *S epidermidis, Bacillus* species, *Streptococcus* species, *S aureus,* and various fungi. *Bacillus* species such as *B cereus,* which are recovered in 25%–50% of culture-positive cases, cause a particularly fulminant endophthalmitis. Delay in primary repair past 12 hours, rupture of the posterior capsule, and a dirty wound increased the odds of endophthalmitis in one Australian study of 250 patients with penetrating ocular injury. After primary repair, recognition of the signs of possible endophthalmitis may be obscured by coexisting ocular injuries and the expected inflammatory response that normally follows a severe injury, resulting in treatment delay. Endophthalmitis should be suspected whenever a patient exhibits signs of increasing pain, intraocular inflammation (retinal periphlebitis), or a hypopyon after repair of a penetrating injury. In one Indian study of 182 patients with posttraumatic endophthalmitis, visual prognosis was worse in patients with a retained intraocular foreign body.

Das T, Kunimoto DY, Sharma S, et al. Relationship between clinical presentation and visual outcome in postoperative and posttraumatic endophthalmitis in south central India. *Indian J Ophthalmol.* 2005;53:5–16.

Essex RW, Yi Q, Charles PG, Allen PJ. Post-traumatic endophthalmitis. *Ophthalmology.* 2004;111:2015–2022.

Foster RE, Martinez JA, Murray TG, Rubsamen PE, Flynn HW Jr, Forster RK. Useful visual outcomes after treatment of *Bacillus cereus* endophthalmitis. *Ophthalmology.* 1996;103:390–397.

Thompson JT, Parver LM, Enger CL, Mieler WF, Liggett PE. Infectious endophthalmitis after penetrating injuries with retained intraocular foreign bodies. National Eye Trauma System. *Ophthalmology.* 1993;100:1468–1474.

Endophthalmitis Associated With Filtering Blebs

Bacteria may enter the eye through either intact or leaking conjunctival filtering blebs. Preexisting diabetes, blebs created with antimetabolite therapy, and inferiorly placed blebs may increase the risk of bacterial infection. BCSC Section 10, *Glaucoma,* discusses filtering blebs and their complications in more detail. Infection may occur months to years after filtering surgery.

It is important to differentiate between low-grade bleb infection, or *blebitis,* and bleb-associated endophthalmitis. In blebitis, the organisms are usually of low virulence, the bleb appears thin and cystic, and there is no evidence of vitreous inflammation. These cases may be treated conservatively with good visual outcomes. However, the physician must be aware that bleb infection caused by more virulent organisms, such as *Streptococcus* species and *Haemophilus influenzae,* may progress rapidly to endophthalmitis with pain and loss of vision. Patients who have had previous, resolved blebitis are at increased risk for subsequent endophthalmitis.

In endophthalmitis, patients present with an infected bleb, marked intraocular inflammation with hypopyon, and vitritis. The most common infecting organisms are *Streptococcus* species and *S epidermidis*. Other infecting organisms include *Serratia* and *Enterococcus* species, *H influenzae,* and *Moraxella* species. The prognosis is usually poor, with profound visual loss. One nonrandomized study from Boston found poorer visual results in patients treated by tap and inject rather than by pars plana vitrectomy, and some clinicians feel that the results of the EVS are not generalizable to bleb-related endophthalmitis.

Busbee BG, Recchia FM, Kaiser R, Nagra P, Rosenblatt B, Pearlman RB. Bleb-associated endophthalmitis: clinical characteristics and visual outcomes. *Ophthalmology.* 2004;111: 1495–1503.

Greenfield DS. Dysfunctional glaucoma filtration blebs. *Focal Points: Clinical Modules for Ophthalmologists.* San Francisco: American Academy of Ophthalmology; 2002, module 4.

Lehmann OJ, Bunce C, Matheson MM, et al. Risk factors for development of post-trabeculectomy endophthalmitis. *Br J Ophthalmol.* 2000;84:1349–1353.

Mac I, Soltau JB. Glaucoma-filtering bleb infections. *Curr Opin Ophthalmol.* 2003;14:91–94.

Endogenous Endophthalmitis

Endogenous endophthalmitis results from the bloodborne spread of bacteria or fungi during generalized septicemia. The source may be remote and nonocular, such as an infected intravenous line or an infected organ, as in endocarditis, gastrointestinal disorders, pyelonephritis, meningitis, or osteomyelitis. Predisposed patients are chronically ill (eg, with diabetes or chronic renal failure) or immunosuppressed, use intravenous drugs, have indwelling catheters, or are in the immediate postoperative or postpartum period. Retinal lesions suggestive of disseminated bacterial or candidal infection in patients hospitalized in intensive care units can be explained in most cases as microangiopathy caused by systemic disease rather than endophthalmitis; such patients are often asymptomatic.

Accurate diagnosis of the agent causing endogenous endophthalmitis is crucial for proper antibiotic treatment of both ocular and systemic infections. Often, the cause may be presumed in light of existing positive cultures of blood or other suspected sites. If the agent is unknown, chest x-ray and fungal and bacterial blood and urine cultures should be obtained, as well as other indicated cultures and tests. In some patients, all extraocular cultures will be negative, with no signs of extraocular infection.

Endogenous bacterial endophthalmitis

Endogenous bacterial endophthalmitis is characterized by an acute onset with pain, decreased vision, hypopyon, and vitritis. Sometimes, both eyes are affected simultaneously. A wide variety of bacteria has been reported. The most common gram-positive organisms are *Streptococcus* species (endocarditis), *S aureus* (cutaneous infections), and *Bacillus* species (from intravenous drug use). The most common gram-negative organisms are *Neisseria meningitidis, H influenzae,* and enteric organisms such as *Escherichia coli* and *Klebsiella*. In Asia, endophthalmitis from *Klebsiella* species in liver abscesses is the most common type of endogenous endophthalmitis.

Endogenous fungal endophthalmitis

Endogenous fungal endophthalmitis develops slowly as focal or multifocal areas of chorioretinitis. Granulomatous or nongranulomatous inflammation is observed with keratic precipitates, hypopyon, and vitritis with cellular aggregates. The infection usually begins in the choroid, appearing as yellow-white lesions with indistinct borders, ranging in size from small cotton-wool spots to several disc diameters (Fig 9-6). It can subsequently break through into the vitreous, producing localized cellular and fungal aggregates overlying the original site(s).

Endogenous fungal endophthalmitis due to *Candida,* which is the most common cause (see Chapter 8, Figs 8-23, 8-24); *Aspergillus;* and *Coccidioides* can be considered a nonneoplastic masquerade syndrome because, in many patients, the condition can be mistaken for noninfectious uveitis and treated with corticosteroids alone. This usually worsens the clinical course of the disease, necessitating further investigation to establish the correct diagnosis. These conditions often require aggressive systemic and local therapy as well as surgical intervention.

Endogenous fungal endophthalmitis due to *Histoplasmosis capsulatum, Cryptococcus neoformans, Sporothrix schenckii,* and *Blastomyces dermatitidis* is less common than that due to *Candida* and *Aspergillus.*

Candida endophthalmitis Ocular inflammatory disease caused by *Candida albicans* (ocular candidiasis), although still uncommon, has increased notably as a result of the widespread use of immunosuppressive therapy, hyperalimentation, and intravenous drugs. Rarely, *Candida* retinitis is seen in AIDS patients following intravenous drug use (see Chapter 8, Figs 8-23, 8-24). Endogenous *Candida* endophthalmitis occurs in 10%–37% of patients with candidemia if they are not receiving antifungal therapy. Ocular involvement drops to 3% in patients who are receiving treatment. Classic 3-dimensional white lesions with vitreal extension were found in only 1% of candidemic patients in one study.

The organism spreads through metastasis to the choroid. Fungal replication results in secondary retinal and vitreous involvement. Symptoms of endogenous *Candida* endophthalmitis include decreased vision or floaters, depending on the location of the lesions. Mimicking toxoplasmic choroiditis, posterior pole lesions appear yellow-white with fluffy borders, ranging in size from small cotton-wool spots to several disc diameters wide. Peripheral lesions may resemble pars planitis.

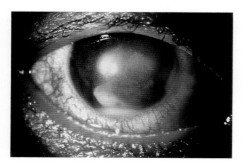

Figure 9-6 Fungal endophthalmitis.

Diagnosis of endogenous *Candida* endophthalmitis can be confirmed by positive blood cultures obtained during candidemia. Recent advances in polymerase chain reaction (PCR) assays allow detection of *C albicans* DNA in intraocular fluid. This method can be used in research settings to evaluate vitreous specimens obtained from pars plana vitrectomy in suspected cases. The physician should be alert to the possible diagnosis of candidiasis in hospitalized patients with indwelling intravenous catheters or those receiving hyperalimentation or systemic therapy with antibiotics, steroids, and antimetabolites. Symptomatic or newly diagnosed, untreated cases of candidemia should prompt examination for ocular involvement. These patients should undergo 2 dilated fundus examinations 1–2 weeks apart to detect ocular disease.

Treatment of endogenous *Candida* endophthalmitis includes intravenous, periocular, and intraocular administration of antifungal agents such as amphotericin B and ketoconazole. However, new antifungals have recently been developed that may be more effective against some of the most common ocular fungal pathogens. Voriconazole, a new triazole antifungal, can achieve therapeutic vitreous levels with oral administration and is effective against nearly all types of fungal pathogens. In addition, intravitreal injection of voriconazole (100 µg/0.1 mL) appears to be safe and effective in recent uncontrolled, small case series. Another new antifungal, caspofungin, the first approved echinocandin class of cell wall inhibitors, is also active against *Candida* and *Aspergillus*. It is administered intravenously once daily. Also in the echinocandin class is mycofungin, which is currently under investigation in phase 3 clinical trials. Oral voriconazole, flucytosine, fluconazole, or rifampin may be administered in addition to intravenous amphotericin B or caspofungin.

If the infectious process breaks through the retina into the vitreous cavity, intravitreal antifungal agents and vitrectomy should be considered. Prompt treatment of peripherally located lesions promotes a favorable prognosis. However, even early treatment of central lesions seldom salvages useful vision because of macular damage. Consultation with an infectious disease specialist is helpful.

Rao NA, Hidayat AA. Endogenous mycotic endophthalmitis: variations in clinical and histopathologic changes in candidiasis compared with aspergillosis. *Am J Ophthalmol.* 2001; 132:244–251.

***Aspergillus* endophthalmitis** Endogenous *Aspergillus* endophthalmitis is a rare disorder associated with disseminated aspergillosis among patients with severe chronic pulmonary diseases, severe immunocompromise, or intravenous drug abuse. It is particularly common among patients following orthotopic liver transplantation. Rarely, *Aspergillus* endophthalmitis may occur in immunocompetent patients with no apparent predisposing factors.

Aspergillus species are found in soils and decaying vegetation. The spores of these ubiquitous saprophytic spore-forming molds become airborne and seed the lungs and paranasal sinuses of humans. Human exposure is very common, but infection is rare and depends on the virulence of the fungal pathogen and immunocompetence of the host. Ocular disease occurs via hematogenous dissemination of *Aspergillus* to the choroid.

Endogenous *Aspergillus* endophthalmitis results in rapid onset of pain and visual loss. A confluent yellowish infiltrate is often seen in the macula beginning in the choroid and subretinal space. A "hypopyon" can develop in the subretinal or subhyaloidal space (see Chapter 8, Fig 8-25A). Retinal hemorrhages, retinal vascular occlusions, and full-thickness retinal necrosis may occur. The infection can spread to produce a dense vitritis and variable degrees of cells, flare, and hypopyon in the anterior chamber. The macular lesions form a central atrophic scar when healed.

The diagnosis of endogenous *Aspergillus* endophthalmitis is based on clinical findings combined with pars plana vitreous biopsy and cultures and Gram and Giemsa stains. Coexisting systemic aspergillosis can be a strong clue, especially among high-risk patients.

The differential diagnosis of endogenous *Aspergillus* endophthalmitis includes *Candida* endophthalmitis, cytomegalovirus retinitis, *Toxoplasma* retinochoroiditis, coccidioidomycotic choroiditis/endophthalmitis, and bacterial endophthalmitis.

Aspergillus endophthalmitis lesions are histologically angiocentric. Mixed acute (polymorphonuclear leukocytes) and chronic (lymphocytes and plasma cells) inflammatory cells infiltrate the infected areas of the choroid and retina. Hemorrhage is present in all retinal layers. Granulomas contain rare giant cells. Fungal hyphae may be seen spreading on the surface of Bruch's membrane without penetrating it. Polymorphonuclear leukocytes are present in the vitreous. Fungal hyphae are often surrounded by macrophages and lymphocytes, which form small vitreous abscesses (see Fig 8-25B). In *Candida* endophthalmitis, the vitreous is the prominent focus of infection, but in *Aspergillus* endophthalmitis, the principal foci are retinal and choroidal vessels and the subretinal/sub-RPE space.

Endogenous *Aspergillus* endophthalmitis usually requires aggressive treatment with diagnostic and therapeutic pars plana vitrectomy combined with intravitreal injection of amphotericin B or voriconazole; intravitreal corticosteroids may be used in conjunction with these. Because most patients with this condition have disseminated aspergillosis, systemic treatment with oral voriconazole, intravenous amphotericin B, or caspofungin is often required. Other systemic antifungals, such as itraconazole, miconazole, fluconazole, and ketoconazole, may also be used. Systemic aspergillosis is best managed by an infectious disease specialist.

Despite aggressive treatment, the visual prognosis is poor because of frequent macular involvement. Final visual acuity is usually less than 20/200.

Breit SM, Hariprasad SM, Mieler WF, Shah GK, Mills MD, Grand MG. Management of endogenous fungal endophthalmitis with voriconazole and caspofungin. *Am J Ophthalmol.* 2005;139:135–140.

Brooks RG. Prospective study of *Candida* endophthalmitis in hospitalized patients with candidemia. *Arch Intern Med.* 1989;149:2226–2228.

Chen YJ, Kuo HK, Wu PC, et al. A 10-year comparison of endogenous endophthalmitis outcomes: an east Asian experience with *Klebsiella pneumoniae* infection. *Retina.* 2004;24:383–390.

Crump JR, Elner SG, Elner VM, Kauffman CA. Cryptococcal endophthalmitis: case report and review. *Clin Infect Dis.* 1992;14:1069–1073.

Donahue SP, Greven CM, Zuravleff JJ, et al. Intraocular candidiasis in patients with candidemia. Clinical implications derived from a prospective multicenter study. *Ophthalmology.* 1994;101:1302–1309.

Essman TF, Flynn HW Jr, Smiddy WE, et al. Treatment outcomes in a 10-year study of endogenous fungal endophthalmitis. *Ophthalmic Surg Lasers.* 1997;28:185–194.

Gonzales CA, Scott IU, Chaudhry NA, et al. Endogenous endophthalmitis caused by *Histoplasma capsulatum* var. capsulatum: a case report and literature review. *Ophthalmology.* 2000;107:725–729.

Hidalgo JA, Alangaden GJ, Eliott D, et al. Fungal endophthalmitis diagnosis by detection of *Candida albicans* DNA in intraocular fluid by use of species-specific polymerase chain reaction assay. *J Infect Dis.* 2000;181:1198–1201.

Hunt KE, Glasgow BJ. *Aspergillus* endophthalmitis: an unrecognized endemic disease in orthotopic liver transplantation. *Ophthalmology.* 1996;103:757–767.

Menezes AV, Sigesmund DA, Demajo WA, Devenyi RG. Mortality of hospitalized patients with *Candida* endophthalmitis. *Arch Intern Med.* 1994;154:2093–2097.

Okada AA, Johnson RP, Liles WC, D'Amico DJ, Baker AS. Endogenous bacterial endophthalmitis: report of a ten-year retrospective study. *Ophthalmology.* 1994;101:832–838.

Rodriguez-Adrian LJ, King RT, Tamayo-Derat LG, Miller JW, Garcia CA, Rex JH. Retinal lesions as clues to disseminated bacterial and candidal infections: frequency, natural history, and etiology. *Medicine (Baltimore).* 2003;82:187–202.

Safneck JR, Hogg GR, Napier LB. Endophthalmitis due to *Blastomyces dermatitidis.* Case report and review of the literature. *Ophthalmology.* 1990;97:212–216.

Scherer WJ, Lee K. Implications of early systemic therapy on the incidence of endogenous fungal endophthalmitis. *Ophthalmology.* 1997;104:1593–1598.

Weishaar PD, Flynn HW Jr, Murray TG, et al. Endogenous *Aspergillus* endophthalmitis: clinical features and treatment outcomes. *Ophthalmology.* 1998;105:57–65.

Witherspoon CD, Kuhn F, Owens SD, White MF, Kimble JA. Endophthalmitis due to *Sporothrix schenckii* after penetrating ocular injury. *Ann Ophthalmol.* 1990;22:385–388.

Prophylaxis

No study has established a standard of care for prophylaxis of postoperative endophthalmitis. Rather, an accumulation of data has led to some common practices, some of which remain controversial.

For cataract surgery, current literature strongly supports the use of preoperative povidone-iodine antisepsis. Preparation of the eyelids and conjunctiva with a 5% povidone-iodine solution just before surgery substantially reduces the bacterial load of the external structures and is superior to 1% povidone-iodine.

Preoperative eyelid and conjunctival treatment with appropriate topical antibiotics may benefit patients who are at high risk for infection, such as those who have severe chronic blepharitis, lacrimal drainage abnormalities, cicatricial conjunctivitis, or a prosthesis in the other eye or who are diabetic or immunosuppressed. Preventive measures include preoperative, topically applied broad-spectrum antibiotics, which can decrease the number of eyelid and conjunctival bacteria compared to no treatment. Isolation of the eyelids and lashes from the surgical field with careful draping is also important.

Recent evidence indicates that repeated preoperative doses of topical fourth-generation quinolones achieves bactericidal levels in the anterior chamber for many bacteria at the time of surgery; however, it has not been proven that this reduces the risk of endophthalmitis. A large German survey indicated that intraocular antibiotics or periocular antibiotics given at the time of surgery led to a reduced risk of endophthalmitis. This benefit, however, may apply only to bacteria introduced through the anterior chamber. Topically administered moxifloxacin or gatifloxacin failed to achieve the 90% minimum inhibitory concentration in vitreous humor for common bacteria associated with endophthalmitis. Orally administered moxifloxacin does reach inhibitory concentrations in aqueous and vitreous but is not used as a routine prophylaxis for postoperative endophthalmitis.

The use of intraocular antibiotics, either as an injection into the anterior chamber or in irrigation fluids, has also been advocated. Subconjunctival antibiotics may be given at the end of intraocular surgery. The effectiveness of these methods in preventing endophthalmitis is uncertain. The efficacy of systemic administration of antibiotics in preventing endophthalmitis is also uncertain. Intravitreal antibiotics administered during repair of penetrating ocular trauma reduced the incidence of endophthalmitis in one randomized series of 70 patients.

In general, the true effectiveness of any of these prophylactic strategies in the actual prevention of endophthalmitis is unknown. Moreover, routine antibiotic prophylaxis has raised concerns regarding costs, the risk of toxicity, and the emergence of resistant organisms.

Ciulla TA, Starr MB, Masket S. Bacterial endophthalmitis prophylaxis for cataract surgery: an evidence-based update. *Ophthalmology.* 2002;109:13–24.

Costello P, Bakri SJ, Beer PM, et al. Vitreous penetration of topical moxifloxacin and gatifloxacin in humans. *Retina.* 2006;26:191–195.

Ferguson AW, Scott JA, McGavigan J, et al. Comparison of 5% povidone-iodine solution against 1% povidone-iodine solution in preoperative cataract surgery antisepsis: a prospective randomised double blind study. *Br J Ophthalmol.* 2003;87:163–167.

Hariprasad SM, Shah GK, Mieler WF, et al. Vitreous and aqueous penetration of orally administered moxifloxacin in humans. *Arch Ophthalmol.* 2006;124:178–182.

Kampougeris G, Antoniadou A, Kavouklis E, Chryssouli Z, Giamarellou H. Penetration of moxifloxacin into the human aqueous humour after oral administration. *Br J Ophthalmol.* 2005;89:628–631.

Katz HR, Masket S, Lane SS, et al. Absorption of topical moxifloxacin ophthalmic solution into human aqueous humor. *Cornea.* 2005;24:955–958.

Kim DH, Stark WJ, O'Brien TP, Dick JD. Aqueous penetration and biological activity of moxifloxacin 0.5% ophthalmic solution and gatifloxacin 0.3% solution in cataract surgery patients. *Ophthalmology.* 2005;112:1992–1996. Epub 2005 Sep 23.

Krummenauer F, Kurz S, Dick HB. Epidemiological and health economical evaluation of intraoperative antibiosis as a protective agent against endophthalmitis after cataract surgery. *Eur J Med Res.* 2005;10:71–75.

Narang S, Gupta V, Gupta A, Dogra MR, Pandav SS, Das S. Role of prophylactic intravitreal antibiotics in open globe injuries. *Indian J Ophthalmol.* 2003;51:39–44.

Sobaci G, Tuncer K, Tas A, Ozyurt M, Bayer A, Kutlu U. The effect of intraoperative antibiotics in irrigating solutions on aqueous humor contamination and endophthalmitis after phacoemulsification surgery. *Eur J Ophthalmol.* 2003;13:773–778.

Diagnosis

Differential Diagnosis

Infectious endophthalmitis caused by bacteria and fungi is often difficult to distinguish from other types of intraocular inflammation. Excessive inflammation without endophthalmitis is often encountered postoperatively in the setting of complicated surgery, preexisting uveitis and keratitis, diabetes, glaucoma therapy, and previous surgery. A vitreous and anterior chamber cellular reaction and a pseudohypopyon may be simulated by red blood cells, pigment, or debris. Retained lens material or other substances may cause sterile postoperative inflammation. Toxic anterior segment syndrome (TASS) should also be included in the differential diagnosis; TASS is attributed to the introduction of unknown toxic substances during surgery by instruments, fluids, or the intraocular lens. Keratitis and postsurgical incision infections are often accompanied by a hypopyon without intraocular infection. It is important to avoid introducing an external infection (as in the case of bacterial keratitis) into the eye by performing an unnecessary paracentesis. Tumor cells from a lymphoma may accumulate in the vitreous, or retinoblastoma cells may accumulate in the anterior chamber, simulating intraocular inflammation. Intraocular biopsy of retinoblastoma is contraindicated.

The most helpful distinguishing characteristic of true infectious endophthalmitis is that the vitritis is progressive and out of proportion to other anterior segment findings. When in doubt, the clinician should manage the condition as an infectious process.

Obtaining Intraocular Specimens

Identification of an infective pathogen establishes diagnosis. Whenever possible, aqueous and vitreous specimens should be obtained for culture and microscopic study before antibiotic therapy is initiated. Obtaining vitreous specimens is important because vitreous cultures are often positive, even when aqueous cultures in the same case are negative; the reverse may also be true.

Aqueous is obtained by passing a small-gauge needle through the limbus into the anterior chamber and withdrawing a 0.1-mL sample. Vitreous may be obtained by a vitreous tap using a needle or by a biopsy with an automated vitrector. For the tap, a 25- or 23-gauge 1-inch needle is passed through the pars plana 3.5 mm posterior to the limbus into the anterior vitreous cavity. If possible, the needle tip is visualized through the pupil to be in the proper position, and 0.2 mL of undiluted vitreous is withdrawn. If resistance to aspiration is encountered during the needle tap, mechanized vitreous biopsy can be performed.

Vitreous biopsy with a cutting instrument is presumed to create less traction on the retina and vitreous than a needle tap; however, microbiologic yields and complications were equivalent when needle tap and mechanized biopsy were compared in the EVS.

Dilute vitreous collected in the machine cassette during pars plana vitrectomy can be filtered or injected into blood culture bottles for culture. Yields from dilute vitreous were inferior to those from undiluted vitreous in the EVS.

Cultures and Laboratory Evaluation of Intraocular Specimens

Undiluted aqueous and vitreous specimens should promptly be inoculated directly onto culture media. Drops of the sample should be placed onto blood agar, Sabouraud's agar, chocolate agar, thioglycollate broth, or similar media and properly incubated. One drop each of the aqueous and vitreous specimens should be placed on clean slides for Gram and Giemsa stains for bacteria and fungi. Organisms visible after staining are predictive of positive cultures; negative stains are not predictive of negative cultures.

> Barza M, Pavan PR, Doft BH, et al. Evaluation of microbiological diagnostic techniques in postoperative endophthalmitis in the Endophthalmitis Vitrectomy Study. *Arch Ophthalmol.* 1997;115:1142–1150.
>
> Han DP, Wisniewski SR, Kelsey SF, Doft BH, Barza M, Pavan PR. Microbiologic yields and complication rates of vitreous needle aspiration versus mechanized vitreous biopsy in the Endophthalmitis Vitrectomy Study. *Retina.* 1999;19:98–102.

Treatment

Management should be tailored to the course, severity, and extent of inflammation.

Surgical Management of Acute Postoperative Endophthalmitis

For postoperative endophthalmitis following cataract surgery with IOL or secondary IOL implantation, the EVS established that outcomes of needle tap for culture and injection of intravitreal antibiotics were equivalent to those after pars plana vitrectomy and injection of intravitreal antibiotics for all eyes with at least hand-motions vision at presentation. The EVS did not address the role of vitrectomy for other categories of endophthalmitis (ie, posttraumatic, filtering bleb–associated, endogenous, and chronic postoperative cases). The potential benefits of vitrectomy include removing the vitreous scaffold, reducing bacterial load, and removing toxic bacterial and inflammatory products.

Medical Management of Acute Postoperative Endophthalmitis

Antibacterial treatment of endophthalmitis should provide broad-spectrum coverage for both gram-positive and gram-negative organisms when the organism is not known (Table 9-2). Vancomycin provides the best gram-positive coverage. Aminoglycosides, including gentamicin and amikacin, are usually effective treatment for gram-negative infection and may also be synergistic with vancomycin against certain gram-positive organisms. Ceftazidime can be substituted for an aminoglycoside to reduce the risk of macular ischemia. However, coverage for gram-negative bacilli is less complete with ceftazidime.

Antibiotics may be administered by topical, subconjunctival, intraocular (usually intravitreal), and intravenous routes. The EVS employed intravitreal (vancomycin/amikacin), subconjunctival (vancomycin/ceftazidime), and topical (vancomycin/amikacin) antibiotics to treat acute postoperative endophthalmitis. The use of systemic antibiotics remains controversial. Although systemic treatment with intravenous vancomycin and ceftazidime was found to be of no benefit in the EVS, oral fluoroquinolones penetrate

Table 9-2 Medications Used in Exogenous Endophthalmitis

	Topical	Subconjunctival	Route and Dose	Systemic
			Intravitreal	
Antibiotic				
Gentamicin	9 mg/mL	20 mg/0.5 mL	0.1 mg/0.1 mL	1 mg/kg IV q8hr
Vancomycin	50 mg/mL	25 mg/0.5 mL	1 mg/0.1 mL	1 g IV q12hr
Amikacin	—	—	0.4 mg/0.1 mL	—
Clindamycin	—	—	1 mg/0.1 mL	—
Chloramphenicol	—	—	1 mg/0.1 mL	—
Ceftazidime	—	50 mg/0.5 mL	2–2.25 mg/0.1 mL	1–2 g IV q8hr
Levoquin	—	—	—	400 mg PO daily
Antifungal				
Amphotericin B	—	—	5 µg/0.1 mL	Up to 1 mg/kg IV daily
Voriconazole	—	—	0.05–0.1 mg/0.1 mL	200 mg PO bid
Ketoconazole	—	—	—	400 mg PO daily
Fluconazole	—	—	—	200 mg PO daily
Itraconazole	—	—	—	100–200 mg PO daily
Corticosteroid Preparations				
Prednisolone acetate 1% drops	Every 1–2 hours	—	—	—
Dexamethasone 0.1% drops	Every 1–2 hours	—	—	—
Dexamethasone injection 4 mg/mL	—	0.5 mL (2 mg)	0.1 mL (0.4 mg)	—
Prednisone tablets	—	—	—	0.5–1 mg/kg/day PO

well into the eye and have a broad spectrum of activity except for anaerobic organisms, *Streptococcus* species, and gram-positive bacteria with emerging resistance to quinolones. Their use may therefore warrant further study. The efficacy of intravenous antibiotics for the other categories of endophthalmitis just mentioned has not been established through the use of randomized controlled trials. Subconjunctival and topical antibiotics may provide little extra benefit after treatment with intravitreal antibiotics. Intravitreal dexamethasone injection can accompany intravitreal antibiotic treatment. In one randomized study, this combination reduced early inflammation with no effect on final visual acuity.

Other Considerations for Treatment of Endophthalmitis

Milder cases of infectious endophthalmitis, as for acute postoperative endophthalmitis from any cause, are generally managed by aspiration for culture and injection of intraocular antibiotics, without vitrectomy, followed by topical antibiotics and steroids. In contrast, the treatment of more severe endophthalmitis includes pars plana vitrectomy with vitreous and aqueous cultures; intravitreal, subconjunctival, and topical antibiotics; and topical and periocular corticosteroids.

Chronic postoperative endophthalmitis therapy depends on the organism isolated. *S epidermidis* responds to intraocular vancomycin injection alone. In *P acnes* endophthalmitis, capsulectomy to remove visible deposits of bacteria, pars plana vitrectomy, and injection of intravitreal vancomycin have been successful, although removal of the intraocular lens is sometimes required to sterilize the eye.

Exogenous fungal endophthalmitis is treated by pars plana vitrectomy and intravitreal injection of amphotericin B or voriconazole. Topical, subconjunctival, and systemic antibiotics are given concomitantly, but their additional therapeutic value is unknown.

Treatment of endogenous bacterial and fungal endophthalmitis usually includes systemic antibiotic administration to treat not only the intraocular infection but also the systemic source of the pathogen. Treatment of endogenous bacterial endophthalmitis also usually includes intravitreal antibiotics. Systemic treatment of *Candida* chorioretinitis includes 5-flucytosine or oral fluconazole or, in more severe cases, IV amphotericin B. Intravenous amphotericin is nephrotoxic, and serum creatinine levels should be closely monitored during the course of treatment. When intravitreal involvement is present, intravitreal amphotericin B is usually used in combination with vitrectomy.

Blebitis usually responds to topical and subconjunctival antibiotic therapy. Infection in filtering blebs, however, may progress rapidly to endophthalmitis with pain and loss of vision. Vitreous inflammation dictates prompt intervention with vitreous cultures followed by intravitreal antibiotic injection, similar to the treatment of acute-onset postoperative cases.

Outcomes of Treatment

Visual loss in endophthalmitis results from the damage caused both by the toxins and proteases produced by the infectious organism and by the host's inflammatory response to the infection. The posterior and anterior segment structures may be directly injured, which may lead to tractional or rhegmatogenous retinal detachments, ciliary body damage, hypotony, and phthisis bulbi.

In the EVS, visual outcomes correlated best with presenting visual acuity but also correlated with the type of infecting organism. Vision of 20/100 or better was found with 84% of cases of coagulase-negative staphylococci, 50% of *S aureus*, 30% of streptococci, 14% of enterococci, and 56% of gram-negative organisms.

The EVS reported the following findings:

- *At 3 months:* 41% of patients achieved 20/40 or better visual acuity; 69% had 20/100 or better acuity
- *At 9–12 months:* 53% of patients achieved visual acuity of 20/40 or better; 74% achieved 20/100 or better; 15% had worse than 5/200 vision
- *At the final follow-up visit:* 5% of patients had no light perception

Chronic endophthalmitis usually carries a favorable visual prognosis, with one study showing visual acuity of 20/40 or better in 80% of cases. The incidence for achieving 20/400 or better visual acuity in endophthalmitis associated with infected filtering blebs was 47% in one study. Only 10% of patients who develop bacterial endophthalmitis after trauma obtain a visual acuity of 20/400 or better.

Aaberg TM Jr, Flynn HW Jr, Murray TG. Intraocular ceftazidime as an alternative to the aminoglycosides in the treatment of endophthalmitis. *Arch Ophthalmol.* 1994;112:18–19.

Breit SM, Hariprasad SM, Mieler WF, Shah GK, Mills MD, Grand MG. Management of endogenous fungal endophthalmitis with voriconazole and caspofungin. *Am J Ophthalmol.* 2005;139:135–140.

Campochiaro PA, Lim JI. Aminoglycoside toxicity in the treatment of endophthalmitis. The Aminoglycoside Toxicity Study Group. *Arch Ophthalmol.* 1994;112:48–53.

Das T, Jalali S, Gothwal VK, Sharma S, Naduvilath TJ. Intravitreal dexamethasone in exogenous bacterial endophthalmitis: results of a prospective randomised study. *Br J Ophthalmol.* 1999;83:1050–1055.

Han DP, Wisniewski SR, Wilson LA, et al. Spectrum and susceptibilities of microbiologic isolates in the Endophthalmitis Vitrectomy Study. *Am J Ophthalmol.* 1996;122:1–17. Erratum in: *Am J Ophthalmol.* 1996;122:920.

Microbiologic factors and visual outcome in the Endophthalmitis Vitrectomy Study. *Am J Ophthalmol.* 1996;122:830–846.

Results of the Endophthalmitis Vitrectomy Study. A randomized trial of immediate vitrectomy and of intravenous antibiotics for the treatment of postoperative bacterial endophthalmitis. Endophthalmitis Vitrectomy Study Group. *Arch Ophthalmol.* 1995;113:1479–1496.

Smiddy WE, Smiddy RJ, Ba'Arath B, et al. Subconjunctival antibiotics in the treatment of endophthalmitis managed without vitrectomy. *Retina.* 2005;25:751–758.

CHAPTER 10

Masquerade Syndromes

Masquerade syndromes are classically defined as those conditions that include, as part of their clinical findings, the presence of intraocular cells but are not due to immune-mediated uveitis entities. These may be divided into nonneoplastic conditions and neoplastic conditions. They account for nearly 5% of all uveitis patients at a tertiary referral center.

> Rothova A, Ooijman F, Kerkhoff F, Van der Lelij A, Lokhorst HM. Uveitis masquerade syndromes. *Ophthalmology.* 2001;108:386–399.

Nonneoplastic Masquerade Syndromes

The nonneoplastic masquerade syndromes classically include retinitis pigmentosa (RP), ocular ischemic syndrome, and chronic peripheral rhegmatogenous retinal detachment.

Retinitis Pigmentosa

Patients with RP often have variable numbers of vitreous cells. In addition, to confuse matters further, patients with RP can also develop cystoid macular edema (CME). Classically, CME is seen angiographically as leakage from the retinal pigment epithelium. Unlike the case with most uveitic entities, patients with RP uniformly complain of nyctalopia. Retinitis pigmentosa is usually a bilateral disease, and patients usually have a positive family history. In addition, fundus examination demonstrates waxy disc pallor, attenuation of arterioles, and a bone-spiculing pattern of pigmentary changes in the midperiphery. The electroretinogram of patients with RP often appears severely depressed or extinguished, even early in the course of the disease process. These criteria can be used to differentiate RP from true uveitis. Refer to BCSC Section 6, *Pediatric Ophthalmology and Strabismus,* and Section 12, *Retina and Vitreous,* for additional information.

Ocular Ischemic Syndrome

Ocular ischemic syndrome is defined by a generalized hypoperfusion of the entire eye and sometimes the orbit, usually due to carotid artery obstruction. Patients with ocular ischemic syndrome present with decreased vision and mild ocular pain. Examination may demonstrate corneal edema, a variable number of anterior chamber cells, and moderate flare. The flare often is greater and out of proportion to the number of cells in the anterior chamber. Rubeosis may be present on the iris, and neovascularization may be present in the angle on gonioscopy. A cataract may be more prominent on the side of the ocular ischemia. The vitreous is usually clear. Dilated fundus examination may show mild disc edema associated with dilated tortuous retinal venules, narrowed arterioles, and scattered blot intraretinal hemorrhages of medium to large size in the midperiphery and far periphery of the retina. Neovascularization may be present in the disc or elsewhere in the retina.

Fluorescein angiography shows delayed arteriolar filling, diffuse leakage in the posterior pole as well as from the optic disc, and signs of capillary nonperfusion in the posterior pole of the midperiphery. Retinal vascular staining may be present in the absence of any physical vascular sheathing on examination.

Patients with ocular ischemic syndrome should undergo carotid Doppler studies to determine whether there is ipsilateral carotid stenosis of greater than 75%, which often supports the diagnosis.

Treatment involves carotid endarterectomy of the ipsilateral site, if indicated, and a local ocular treatment with both topical corticosteroid agents and cycloplegics, as well as panretinal photocoagulation treatment, especially if rubeosis or retinal neovascularization is present. The 5-year mortality rate of patients with ocular ischemic syndrome is 40%. The visual prognosis is guarded, and many patients transiently improve with treatment but eventually worsen.

Differentiating ocular ischemia from true uveitis can be difficult. However, a combination of ischemic signs in the iris and in the posterior pole, along with the age of the patient, usually over 65 years, and ipsilateral carotid stenosis, can be very useful in differentiating ocular ischemic syndrome from uveitis.

Sivalingam A, Brown GC, Magargal LE. The ocular ischemic syndrome. III. Visual prognosis and the effect of treatment. *Int Ophthalmol.* 1991;15:15–20.

Sivalingam A, Brown GC, Magargal LE, Menduke H. The ocular ischemic syndrome. II. Mortality and systemic morbidity. *Int Ophthalmol.* 1989;13:187–191.

Chronic Peripheral Rhegmatogenous Retinal Detachment

Chronic peripheral rhegmatogenous retinal detachment can be associated with anterior segment cell and flare and vitreous inflammatory and pigment cells. Patients often have good vision that can sometimes deteriorate due to CME. The key to the diagnosis of peripheral retinal detachment is a dilated fundus examination with scleral depression. Peripheral pigment demarcation lines, subretinal fluid, retinal breaks, subretinal fibrosis, and peripheral retinal cysts may be present. In some cases, the anterior segment cells may represent not true inflammation but rather the presence of photoreceptor outer segments that have been liberated from the subretinal space. In such situations, IOP can be elevated. These photoreceptor outer segments are phagocytosed by the endothelial cells in the trabecular meshwork, resulting in secondary open-angle glaucoma. This condition is called *Schwartz syndrome.*

Matsuo N, Takabatake M, Ueno H, Nakayama T, Matsuo T. Photoreceptor outer segments in the aqueous humor in rhegmatogenous retinal detachment. *Am J Ophthalmol.* 1986;101:673–679.

Schwartz A. Chronic open-angle glaucoma secondary to rhegmatogenous retinal detachment. *Am J Ophthalmol.* 1973;75:205–211.

Intraocular Foreign Body

Retained intraocular foreign bodies may produce chronic anterior and posterior segment inflammation due to mechanical, chemical, toxic, or inflammatory irritation of uveal tissues (particularly the ciliary body). A careful history; clinical examination; and ancillary testing, including gonioscopy, ultrasonography, and computed tomography of the eye and orbits to rule out intraocular foreign bodies, are essential in any case of uveitis that is unexplained and resistant to standard treatment. If this condition is suspected and recognized quickly, identification and removal of the foreign body often results in a cure. If the diagnosis is delayed, ocular complications such as proliferative vitreoretinopathy and endophthalmitis result in a poorer visual prognosis.

Pigment Dispersion Syndrome

Pigment dispersion syndrome is characterized by pigment granules floating in the anterior chamber that have been released from the iris and/or ciliary body. These free-floating pigment granules may be confused with cells such as occur in anterior uveitis. Unlike with true anterior uveitis, however, ciliary injection and posterior synechiae are absent in pigment dispersion syndrome. The pigment granules are in turn deposited on the corneal endothelium (Krukenberg spindle), trabecular meshwork (Sampaolesi line), posterior surface of the lens, zonules, and anterior vitreous. Midperipheral iris transillumination defects are often present. The disease occurs in young Caucasian men with myopia. The cause of the disease is thought to be a mechanical denudation of the ciliary and iris pigment epithelium from an abnormally posteriorly bowed midperipheral iris, seen on gonioscopy. The released pigment granules are phagocytosed by the trabecular endothelium or intraocular macrophages, which can clog the trabecular outflow and result in IOP elevation and glaucoma. Treatment consists of prophylactic argon laser iridoplasty to change the concavity of the midperipheral iris and medical and surgical management of glaucoma. Corticosteroids should be avoided because their use may lead to worsening of the glaucoma.

> Yao L, Foster CS. Nonmalignant, noninfectious masquerade syndromes. In: Foster CS, Vitale AT, eds. *Diagnosis and Treatment of Uveitis.* Philadelphia: Saunders; 2002:537–572.

Other Syndromes

Certain infectious uveitic entities may also be mistaken for immunologic uveitis. Thus, nonneoplastic masquerade syndromes can also include bacterial uveitis due to *Nocardia* spp and *Tropheryma whippelii* (Whipple disease), and fungal endophthalmitis due to *Candida* spp, *Aspergillus* spp, *or Coccidioides immitis.* These entities are discussed in Chapter 8, Infectious Uveitis, and Chapter 9, Endophthalmitis.

Neoplastic Masquerade Syndromes

Neoplastic masquerade syndromes may account for 2%–3% of all patients seen in tertiary uveitis referral clinics. The vast majority of these are patients with intraocular involvement from primary CNS lymphoma.

Primary Central Nervous System Lymphoma

Nearly all (98%) primary CNS lymphomas (PCNSLs) are non-Hodgkin B-lymphocyte lymphomas. Approximately 2% are T-lymphocyte lymphomas. Although PCNSL mainly affects patients in their fifth to seventh decade of life, it also occurs, in rare instances, in children and adolescents. (It is not necessarily just a disease of "the elderly.") The incidence of PCNSL appears to be increasing and is projected to occur in 1 out of every 100,000 immunocompetent patients.

Clinical features and findings

Approximately 25% of patients with PCNSL have ocular involvement. Approximately 15% may have ocular involvement alone. Fifteen percent may have ocular and visceral involvement. Approximately 60% have ocular and CNS involvement, and 4% have ocular, CNS, and visceral involvement. Sites of ocular involvement include the vitreous, retina, sub-RPE, and any combination thereof. The most common complaints of presenting patients are decreased vision and floaters.

Examination reveals spillover anterior chamber cells and a variable degree of vitritis, often severe. Retinal examination shows characteristic retinal lesions. These often appear as creamy yellow subretinal infiltrates with overlying retinal pigment epithelial detachments (Fig 10-1). They can look like discrete white lesions from acute retinal necrosis, toxoplasmosis, frosted branch angiitis, or retinal arteriolar obstruction with coexisting multifocal chorioretinal scars and retinal vasculitis. The lesions vary in thickness from about 1 mm to 2 mm.

Many of these patients are mistakenly treated with systemic corticosteroids. This can improve the vitreous cellular infiltration, but the effect is not long lasting and the uveitis often becomes resistant to corticosteroid therapy. In these situations, immunomodulatory agents are then added, which also reduce vitreous cells temporarily. However, this therapy too eventually meets with failure. Subsequently, a vitrectomy is often performed, but the vitrectomy specimens are nondiagnostic because of the previous intensive treatment. Diagnosis is much easier to make when retinal lesions are present because the lesions have a characteristic appearance (see Fig 10-1).

Central nervous system signs may vary. Behavioral changes appear to be the single most frequent symptom reported, often when patients are admitted for hospitalization. These behavioral changes occur because of the periventricular location of many of the CNS lesions in PCNSL. Other neurologic signs include hemiparesis, cerebellar signs,

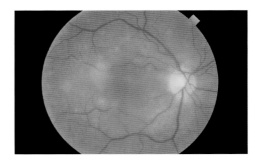

Figure 10-1 Primary CNS lymphoma. Fundus photograph of multifocal, subretinal pigment epithelial lesions. *(Courtesy of E. Mitchel Opremcak, MD.)*

epileptic seizures, and cranial nerve palsies. Cerebrospinal fluid seeding of lymphoma cells occurs in 42% of patients with PCNSL. A new syndrome can also occur in which glaucoma, uveitis, and neurologic symptoms *(GUN syndrome)* are all associated together in PCNSL.

Ancillary tests

Ultrasonography shows choroidal thickening, vitreous debris, elevated chorioretinal lesions, and serous retinal detachment. Fluorescein angiography shows hypofluorescent areas due to blockage from a sub-RPE tumor mass or from RPE clumping. Hyperfluorescent window defects may also be present due to RPE atrophy from spontaneously resolved RPE infiltration. An unusual leopard spot pattern of alternating hyper- and hypofluorescence may also be noted.

MRI studies of the brain show isointense lesions on T1 and iso- to hyperintense lesions on T2. Computed tomography shows multiple diffuse periventricular lesions when no contrast is present. If intravenous contrast is used, these periventricular lesions may enhance.

Results of cerebrospinal fluid analysis are positive in one third of patients with PCNSL and show lymphoma cells.

Diagnostic testing

Tissue diagnosis is the most effective and accurate method of determining whether a patient has PCNSL. If lymphoma cells are found in the cerebrospinal fluid from a lumbar puncture, or if MRI demonstrates characteristic intracranial lesions, pars plana vitreous biopsy may not be necessary. However, the presence of vitreous cells of unidentifiable cause, especially in a patient over age 65, necessitates a vitreous biopsy. Usually this is performed via a pars plana vitrectomy. Ideally, 1 mL of undiluted vitreous sample should be obtained in a syringe that contains 3 mL of tissue culture medium to maximize cellular viability. In addition, a retinal biopsy, an aspirate of sub-RPE material, or both may also be obtained during vitrectomy. This approach may improve diagnostic yield when previous vitreous biopsies have been negative. The vitreous specimen should be fixed in an equal volume of 95% alcohol immediately after its removal from the eye. Samples stored in balanced salt solution will undergo cellular degradation and loss of detail. Proper diagnosis requires an expert cytopathologist with experience in interpreting lymphomas. Despite these measures, diagnostic yield from vitrectomy specimens is rarely more than 65% positive. Repeat biopsies of the vitreous may be performed if the clinical picture warrants.

Cytokine analysis in vitreous samples can be helpful in confirming the diagnosis of intraocular lymphoma when histopathologic evaluation is equivocal. Interleukin-10 (IL-10) is elevated in the vitreous of patients with lymphoma because it is preferentially produced by malignant B lymphocytes. In contrast, high levels of IL-6 are found in the vitreous of patients with inflammatory uveitis. Thus, the relative ratio of IL-10 to IL-6 is often elevated in intraocular lymphoma and supports the diagnosis.

Histopathology

Cytologic specimens obtained from the vitreous or subretinal space often show pleomorphic cells with hyperchromatic nuclei and an elevated nuclear/cytoplasmic ratio (Fig 10-2). The cytoplasm is very scant, and multiple irregular nucleoli may be seen. Necrotic cellular

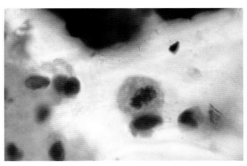

Figure 10-2 Vitreous aspirate showing mitotic figure and cellular atypia in large cell lymphoma. *(Courtesy of E. Mitchel Opremcak, MD.)*

debris is present in the background. Equivocal vitreous biopsies may require immunophenotypic or genetic testing. Immunophenotyping is used to establish clonality of B lymphocytes by demonstrating the presence of abnormal immunoglobulin κ or λ light chain predominance and specific B-lymphocyte markers (CD19, CD20, and CD22). This is performed by flow cytometry and immunohistochemistry. Monoclonal populations of cells are likely to be present in cases of PCNSL. Molecular diagnosis using genetic techniques relies on the fact that cancers such as PCNSL are clonal growths. As a result, gene translocations or oncogene translocations or gene rearrangements are often repeated in all of the cells in a given PCNSL. Polymerase chain reaction (PCR) techniques are invaluable in the detection of these oncogene translocations or gene rearrangements.

Abnormal lymphocytes may be isolated manually or by laser capture, and PCR-based assays may be performed to detect IgH, bcl-2 (a protein family that regulates apoptosis), or T-lymphocyte receptor gamma gene rearrangements. This improves diagnostic yield of paucicellular samples.

If diagnosis by vitreous aspiration or subretinal aspiration cannot be performed, either internal or external chorioretinal biopsy techniques may be used to aid in the diagnosis of PCNSL. This is discussed in Chapter 6, Clinical Approach to Uveitis, in detail.

Treatment

Without treatment and supportive care, the prognosis of PCNSL is dismal. Median survival is 2–3 months with supportive care alone. With surgical removal of the CNS lesions, the patient does not fare much better; with surgery alone, median survival is in the range of 1–5 months. However, even with disease isolated to the eye, prophylactic CNS treatment is warranted because approximately 56% of patients with ocular involvement eventually develop CNS involvement with PCNSL. Currently, a combination of chemotherapy and coned-down radiotherapy is advocated.

Investigators from the Memorial Sloan-Kettering Cancer Center have reported some success using high-dose methotrexate delivered intravenously, along with intrathecal administration via the Ommaya reservoir, in combination with radiation therapy and intravenous cytarabine. In addition, local ocular treatment with repeated biweekly or weekly intravitreal methotrexate injections of 400 μg can also be used in conjunction with systemic treatment. The role of this treatment alone in isolated ocular disease has been studied; the treatment may be effective in controlling local disease. The regimen's effect on median survival compared to that of systemic treatment is not known. Based on the available information, chemotherapy alone is indicated for patients 60 years and older because of potential CNS toxicity from radiation; for patients younger than 60, combination radiation therapy and chemotherapy is preferred. The effect of whole-brain radiation on reducing quality of life is an important consideration among therapeutic options.

Prognosis

Despite the availability of multiple treatment modalities and regimens, the long-term prognosis for PCNSL remains poor. The longest median survival in various reports approaches 40 months with treatment. Factors that can influence outcome include age; neurologic functional classification level; single versus multiple lesions in the CNS; and superficial cerebral, cerebellar hemispheric lesions versus deep nuclei/periventricular lesions.

Baehring JM, Androudi S, Longtine JJ, Betensky RA, et al. Analysis of clonal immunoglobulin heavy chain rearrangements in ocular lymphoma. *Cancer.* 2005;104:591–597.

Chan CC. Molecular pathology of primary intraocular lymphoma. *Trans Am Ophthalmol Soc.* 2003;101:275–292.

Chan CC, Wallace DJ. Intraocular lymphoma: update on diagnosis and management. *Cancer Control.* 2004;11:285–295.

Chan CC, Whitcup SM, Solomon D, Nussenblatt RB. Interleukin-10 in the vitreous of patients with primary intraocular lymphoma. *Am J Ophthalmol.* 1995;120:671–673.

Davis JL. Diagnosis of intraocular lymphoma. *Ocul Immunol Inflamm.* 2004;12:7–16.

Davis JL, Miller DM, Ruiz P. Diagnostic testing of vitrectomy specimens. *Am J Ophthalmol.* 2005;140:822–829.

Read RW, Zamir E, Rao NA. Neoplastic masquerade syndromes. *Surv Ophthalmol.* 2002;47:81–124.

Rothova A, Ooijman F, Kerkhoff F, Van der Lelij A, Lokhorst HM. Uveitis masquerade syndromes. *Ophthalmology.* 2001;108:386–399.

Valluri S, Moorthy RS, Khan A, Rao NA. Combination treatment of intraocular lymphoma. *Retina.* 1995;15:125–129.

Whitcup SM, de Smet MD, Rubin BI, et al. Intraocular lymphoma. Clinical and histopathologic diagnosis. *Ophthalmology.* 1993;100:1399–1406.

Zaldivar RA, Martin DF, Holden JT, Grossniklaus HE. Primary intraocular lymphoma: clinical, cytologic, and flow cytometric analysis. *Ophthalmology.* 2004;111:1762–1767.

Neoplastic Masquerade Syndromes Secondary to Systemic Lymphoma

Systemic lymphomas hematogenously spread to the choroid, to the subretinal space, into the vitreous, and occasionally into the anterior chamber. These entities often present with vitritis and creamy subretinal infiltrates of variable size, number, and extent. Retinal vasculitis, necrotizing retinitis, and diffuse choroiditis or uveal masses may also be present. All T-lymphocyte lymphomas (including mycosis fungoides, HTLV-1 lymphoma, systemic B-lymphocyte lymphoma, and anaplastic large cell lymphoma), Hodgkin disease, and primary intravascular lymphoma can present in this fashion. Reports of these entities are rare and scattered throughout the literature.

Neoplastic Masquerade Syndromes Secondary to Leukemia

Patients with leukemia may have retinal findings, including intraretinal hemorrhages, cotton-wool spots, white-centered hemorrhages, microaneurysms, and peripheral neo-vascularization. Rarely, leukemic cells may invade the vitreous cavity. If the choroid is involved, exudative retinal detachment may be present and is angiographically similar to Vogt-Koyanagi-Harada disease. Leukemia may also present with a hypopyon/hyphema, iris heterochromia, or a pseudohypopyon, which can be gray-yellow.

> Kincaid MC, Green WR. Ocular and orbital involvement in leukemia. *Surv Ophthalmol.* 1983;27:211–232.

Neoplastic Masquerade Syndromes Secondary to Uveal Lymphoid Proliferations

The uveal tract may also be a site for lymphoid proliferations that can mimic chronic uve-itis. These proliferations can range from benign reactive uveal lymphoid proliferations to frank lymphomas that may or may not be associated with systemic lymphomas. Patients with these conditions clinically may present with gradual painless unilateral or bilateral vision loss. Early stages show multifocal creamy choroidal lesions that may mimic inflam-matory entities, including sarcoid uveitis or birdshot choroidopathy. Cystoid macular edema may be present. Anterior uveitis with acute symptoms of pain, redness, and pho-tophobia may also be present. Glaucoma and elevated IOP are common. Angle structures may be infiltrated by lymphocytes, resulting in elevation of IOP.

Clinical appearances may seem malignant even though the processes may be benign histopathologically. These intraocular processes may extend to the epibulbar area and may manifest as fleshy episcleral or conjunctival masses that may be salmon pink in color. Unlike subconjunctival lymphomas, they are not mobile and are attached firmly to the sclera. These conditions should be differentiated from posterior scleritis as well as from uveal effusion syndrome. Needle aspiration biopsy and biopsy of extrascleral portions of the tumors can help in diagnosis. Biopsy specimens demonstrate mature lymphocytes and plasma cells that are quite different from those seen with PCNSL. Therapy with cortico-steroids, radiation, or both has been used with variable results. Systemic and periocular corticosteroid therapy can result in rapid regression of the lesions, as can external-beam radiation.

> Jakobiec FA, Sacks E, Kronish JW, Weiss T, Smith M. Multifocal static creamy choroidal infil-trates. An early sign of lymphoid neoplasia. *Ophthalmology.* 1987;94:397–406.

Nonlymphoid Malignancies

Uveal melanoma

Approximately 5% of patients with uveal melanoma may present with ocular inflammation, including episcleritis, anterior or posterior uveitis, endophthalmitis, or panophthalmitis. Most of the tumors that present in this fashion are epithelioid cell or mixed cell choroidal melanoma. Ultrasonography can be very useful in diagnosing atypical cases because of the characteristic low internal reflectivity of these lesions. The management of uveal melano-mas is discussed in BCSC Section 4, *Ophthalmic Pathology and Intraocular Tumors.*

> Fraser DJ Jr, Font RL. Ocular inflammation and hemorrhage as initial manifestations of uveal malignant melanoma. Incidence and prognosis. *Arch Ophthalmol.* 1979;97:1311–1314.

Retinoblastoma

Approximately 1%–3% of retinoblastomas may present with inflammation. Patients are usually between 4 and 6 years of age at presentation. Most cases that present with inflammation are due to the relatively rare variant of diffuse infiltrating retinoblastoma. These cases can be diagnostically confusing because of the limited visibility of the fundus and the lack of calcification on radiography or ultrasonography. Patients may have conjunctival chemosis, pseudohypopyon, and vitritis. The pseudohypopyon typically shifts with changes in head position. The pseudohypopyon of retinoblastoma is usually white. Diagnostic aspiration of the aqueous humor may be required, but there is a significant risk of tumor spread through the needle tract. Histopathologic examination shows round cells with hyperchromatic nuclei and scanty cytoplasm.

Bhatnagar R, Vine AK. Diffuse infiltrating retinoblastoma. *Ophthalmology.* 1991;98:1657–1661.

Juvenile xanthogranuloma

Juvenile xanthogranuloma is a histiocytic process affecting mainly the skin and eyes, and, in rare instances, viscera. Patients usually present before the age of 1 with characteristic skin lesions that are reddish yellow. Histopathologic investigation shows large histiocytes with foamy cytoplasm and Touton giant cells containing fat. Ocular lesions can involve the iris, from which spontaneous hyphema may occur. Iris biopsy shows fewer foamy histiocytes and fewer Touton giant cells than a skin biopsy. Other ocular structures may be involved, but this is rare. If the skin of the eyelids is involved, the globe is usually spared. Intraocular lesions may respond to topical, periocular, or systemic corticosteroid therapy. Resistant cases may require local resection, radiation, or immunomodulatory therapy.

Zamir E, Wang RC, Krishnakumar S, Aiello Leverant A, Dugel PU, Rao NA. Juvenile xanthogranuloma masquerading as pediatric chronic uveitis: a clinicopathologic study. *Surv Ophthalmol.* 2001;46:164–171.

Metastatic Tumors

The most common intraocular malignancies in adults are metastatic tumors. The most common primaries include lung and breast cancer. Choroidal metastasis may be marked by vitritis, serous retinal detachment, and, occasionally, CME. These lesions are often bilateral and multifocal. Vitritis may be very mild.

Anterior uveal metastasis may present with cells in the aqueous humor, iris nodules, rubeosis iridis, and elevated IOP. Anterior chamber paracentesis may help in the diagnosis.

Retinal metastases are extremely rare. The most common primary cancers metastatic to the retina include cutaneous melanoma (the most common), followed by lung cancer, gastrointestinal cancer, and breast cancer. Metastatic tumors to the retina can present with vitreous cells. Metastatic melanoma often produces brown spherules in the retina, whereas other metastatic cancers are white to yellow and result in perivascular sheathing, simulating a retinal vasculitis or necrotizing retinitis. Vitreous biopsy and aspiration may be diagnostic if vitreous cells are present.

Bilateral Diffuse Uveal Melanocytic Proliferation

Bilateral diffuse uveal melanocytic tumors have been associated with systemic malignancy. Such tumors can be associated with rapid vision loss; cataracts; multiple pigmented and nonpigmented, placoid iris and choroidal nodules; and serous retinal detachments. This condition can mimic Vogt-Koyanagi-Harada disease. Histopathologic investigation shows diffuse infiltration of the uveal tract by benign nevoid or spindle-shaped cells. Necrosis within the tumors may be present, and scleral involvement is common. The cause of this entity is unknown. Treatment should be directed at finding and treating the underlying primary lesion.

Barr CC, Zimmerman LE, Curtin VT, Font RL. Bilateral diffuse melanocytic uveal tumors associated with systemic malignant neoplasms. A recently recognized syndrome. *Arch Ophthalmol.* 1982;100:249–255.

CHAPTER 11

Complications of Uveitis

Calcific Band-Shaped Keratopathy

Patients with chronic uveitis lasting many years, especially those with childhood-onset uveitis, may develop calcium deposits in the epithelial basement membrane and Bowman's layer. Calcium deposits are usually found in the interpalpebral zone, often extending into the visual axis. This calcific band-shaped keratopathy may become visually significant in some cases and require removal. The procedure is done in the operating room by first gently removing the central corneal epithelium with a #15 Bard-Parker blade, leaving the limbal stem cells intact. Then 0.35% sodium EDTA is placed in a plastic or steel well, 7–8 mm in diameter, that is then placed over the cornea. The well containing EDTA is left in place for 5 minutes and then removed. The cornea is irrigated with balanced salt solution, and loose flakes of calcium are gently lifted off the cornea. The process may be repeated several times until all the desired calcium is removed. A soft bandage contact lens is then placed, along with topical antibiotics and cycloplegics, and the eye is patched overnight. The bandage contact lens, topical antibiotics, and cycloplegics are continued. Visual improvement can be significant. Late recurrences may require repeat EDTA scrubs.

Cataracts

Any eye with chronic or recurrent uveitis may develop cataract due to both the inflammation itself and the corticosteroids used to treat it. Cataract surgery should be considered whenever functional benefit is likely. Cataract surgery in uveitic eyes is generally more complex and more likely to lead to postoperative complications when improperly managed. The key to a successful visual outcome in these cases is careful long-term control of pre- and postoperative inflammation. The absence of inflammation for 3 or more months before surgery is a prerequisite for any elective intraocular surgery in uveitic eyes. The control of perioperative inflammation is as important as the technical feat of performing successful complex cataract extraction in uveitic eyes. See also BCSC Section 11, *Lens and Cataract,* for more information on many of the issues covered in this discussion.

Careful preoperative evaluation is necessary to ascertain how much the cataract is actually contributing to visual dysfunction, because visual loss in uveitis may stem from a variety of other ocular problems, such as macular edema or vitritis. Sometimes a cataract precludes an adequate view of the posterior segment of the eye, and surgery can be justified to permit examination, diagnosis, and treatment of posterior segment abnormalities.

Studies have shown that phacoemulsification with posterior chamber (in-the-bag) intraocular lens (IOL) implantation effectively improves vision and is well tolerated in many eyes with uveitis, even over long periods. For example, excellent surgical and visual results have been reported for eyes with Fuchs heterochromic iridocyclitis. Cataract surgery in other types of uveitis—including idiopathic uveitis, pars planitis, and uveitis associated with sarcoidosis, herpes simplex virus, herpes zoster, syphilis, toxoplasmosis, and spondyloarthropathies—can be more problematic, although such surgery may also yield very good results.

Juvenile Rheumatoid Arthritis/Juvenile Idiopathic Arthritis–associated Uveitis

Pars plana lensectomy/vitrectomy is advocated for cataracts that occur in patients with juvenile rheumatoid arthritis/juvenile idiopathic arthritis (JRA/JIA)–associated uveitis. Although acceptable results have also been reported with combined phacoemulsification and vitrectomy, phacoemulsification with IOL implantation in the capsular bag is increasingly being performed in children with JRA/JIA-associated iridocyclitis with good results as long as there is meticulous control of pre- and postoperative intraocular inflammation and long-term follow-up. These eyes must be quiet, without cells, for 3 months or longer before cataract surgery can even be considered. Frequent (hourly) preoperative corticosteroids are given for 1–2 weeks. Synechiolysis with viscoelastic or iridodialysis spatula is performed, if necessary, followed by capsulorrhexis, standard phacoemulsification, and in-the-bag IOL implantation (with a hydrophobic acrylic or heparin-coated polymethylmethacrylate [PMMA] lens). Meticulous cortical cleanup and placement of both haptics in the capsular bag are essential. Topical corticosteroids are slowly tapered over 3–5 months based on the level of intraocular inflammation. If IOLs are not well tolerated and recalcitrant intraocular inflammation develops, they should be removed. The threshold for IOL removal in these cases should be low. Long-term postoperative complications include increasing rate of posterior capsular opacity, glaucoma, and cystoid macular edema (CME). Longer preoperative duration of immunosuppressive therapy (with no intraocular inflammation for more than 3 months); tight control of perioperative inflammation, with liberal use of topical corticosteroids for 3–5 months postoperatively; and continuation of aggressive perioperative immunosuppressive therapy also appear to reduce the risk of these complications and improve visual outcomes.

Other Uveitis Entities

Phacoemulsification may be more challenging in uveitic eyes than in noninflamed eyes, and intraocular inflammation should be well controlled before surgery is performed. It is imperative to eliminate anterior chamber cells and to have the eye quiet, without inflammatory flare-ups for at least 3 months prior to cataract surgery. Approximately 1–2 weeks before surgery, oral corticosteroids (0.5–1.0 mg/kg per day) and hourly topical corticosteroids should be administered. These may be tapered over 3–5 months after surgery, depending on the postoperative inflammatory response.

Phacoemulsification using a clear corneal approach is preferred. This is particularly true in cases of scleritis that may be prone to postoperative scleral necrosis. Extensive posterior synechiae and pupillary miosis may require mechanical or viscoelastic pupil stretching, sphincterotomies, or the use of flexible iris retractors. Pupillary membranes should be removed if possible. Continuous curvilinear capsulorrhexis is preferred, as it appears to reduce posterior synechiae formation, reduces the risk of posterior capsular tear, and facilitates placing IOL haptics in the capsular bag. A fibrotic anterior capsule may be more difficult to open with a capsulorrhexis. The zonules may be inherently weak, which may make phacoemulsification and lens implantation challenging or impossible. In such cases there may be few alternatives. It may be preferable in these cases to perform pars plana lensectomy and vitrectomy and, because of the lack of capsular support or zonular dehiscence, avoid placing an IOL. This scenario is fortunately rare.

Nucleus extraction is performed using phacoemulsification, the preferred technique. Cortical cleanup should be meticulous. A hydrophobic acrylic posterior chamber IOL is preferred. The IOL may be placed in the capsular bag using a "shooter" through the small, clear corneal incision; or, the corneal incision is enlarged to admit a forceps containing a folded IOL to be inserted into the capsular bag.

The use of surface-modified IOLs has also been advocated to minimize deposit formation on the optics. Heparin-surface-modified IOLs have been shown to have fewer surface deposits than PMMA lenses for up to 1 year after cataract extraction. Among patients with uveitis, the frequency of postoperative posterior synechiae formation and CME appears similar with both PMMA and heparin-surface-modified lenses. Modern hydrophobic acrylic posterior chamber lenses appear to have good capsular and uveal compatibility and can be safely used as long as the implant is placed in the capsular bag. These acrylic lenses have the advantage of being foldable and requiring very small corneal incisions for placement. Foldable silicone lenses should be avoided in uveitic eyes, because they may be associated with greater postoperative inflammation and because future vitreoretinal surgery may be necessary. If posterior segment pathology is present, silicone IOLs should be avoided because silicone oil would need to be used as a vitreous substitute. Ciliary sulcus and anterior chamber placement of IOLs must be avoided at all costs. Removal of IOLs, even after strict adherence to inflammatory control guidelines, may be unavoidable in 5%–10% of patients with uveitis due to lens intolerance or dislocation.

After IOL insertion, viscoelastic must be removed. Periocular or intravitreal corticosteroids may be administered after surgery. Preoperative immunomodulation is continued after surgery and supplemented with liberal use of topical corticosteroids, which are slowly tapered.

Combined Phacoemulsification and Pars Plana Vitrectomy

Phacoemulsification can also be done in conjunction with pars plana vitrectomy if clinical or ultrasonographic examination suggests the presence of substantial vision-limiting vitreous debris or macular pathology such as epiretinal membranes. This scenario may occur in certain intermediate uveitis, posterior uveitis, and panuveitis syndromes. Nucleus removal and cortical cleanup are performed first. The aphakic capsular bag is kept intact. Then, a standard 3-port pars plana vitrectomy is performed. The posterior hyaloid should be separated from the retina, and the vitreous gel is shaved to the edge of the vitreous base with scleral depression. The IOL is then placed in the capsular bag after the vitrectomy surgery. Intravitreal triamcinolone acetonide (Kenalog) 4 mg can be given at the conclusion of the surgery to help control postoperative fibrin formation and inflammation. Perioperative corticosteroids (eg, topical, subconjunctival, and oral), other immunomodulators, or both should be administered to help control postoperative intraocular inflammation.

Postoperative complications commonly occur in uveitic eyes. Their rates of occurrence may be reduced with effective perioperative inflammatory control using immunomodulators and corticosteroids. Visual compromise following phacoemulsification with posterior chamber lens implantation in patients with uveitis is usually attributed to posterior segment abnormalities, most commonly CME. The postoperative course may also be complicated by the recurrence or exacerbation of uveitis. The incidence of posterior capsule opacification is higher in uveitic eyes, leading to earlier use of Nd:YAG laser capsulotomy. In some uveitic conditions, such as pars planitis, inflammatory debris may accumulate and membranes may form on the surface of the IOL, necessitating frequent Nd:YAG laser procedures. On occasion, posterior chamber IOLs have been removed from these eyes. Frequent follow-up, a high index of suspicion, and aggressive immunomodulatory treatment can optimize short- and long-term visual results in these patients.

Alio JL, Chipont E, BenEzra D, et al. Comparative performance of intraocular lenses in eyes with cataract and uveitis. International Ocular Inflammation Society Study Group of Uveitic Cataract Surgery. *J Cataract Refract Surg.* 2002;28:2096–2108.

Androudi S, Ahmed M, Fiore T, Brazitikos P, Foster CS. Combined pars plana vitrectomy and phacoemulsification to restore visual acuity in patients with chronic uveitis. *J Cataract Refract Surg.* 2005;31:472–478.

Estafanous MF, Lowder CY, Meisler DM, Chauhan R. Phacoemulsification cataract extraction and posterior chamber lens implantation in patients with uveitis. *Am J Ophthalmol.* 2001;131:620–625.

Flynn HW Jr, Davis JL, Culbertson WW. Pars plana lensectomy and vitrectomy for complicated cataracts in juvenile rheumatoid arthritis. *Ophthalmology.* 1988;95:1114–1119.

Foster CS. Cataract surgery in the patient with uveitis. *Focal Points: Clinical Modules for Ophthalmologists.* San Francisco: American Academy of Ophthalmology; 1994, module 4.

Foster CS, Barrett F. Cataract development and cataract surgery in patients with juvenile rheumatoid arthritis–associated iridocyclitis. *Ophthalmology.* 1993;100:809–817.

Kaufman AH, Foster CS. Cataract extraction in patients with pars planitis. *Ophthalmology.* 1993;100:1210–1217.

Krishna R, Meisler DM, Lowder CY, Estafanous M, Foster RE. Long-term follow-up of extracapsular cataract extraction and posterior chamber intraocular lens implantation in patients with uveitis. *Ophthalmology.* 1998;105:1765–1769.

Lam LA, Lowder CY, Baerveldt G, Smith SD, Traboulsi EI. Surgical management of cataracts in children with juvenile rheumatoid arthritis-associated uveitis. *Am J Ophthalmol.* 2003;135:772–778.

Probst LE, Holland EJ. Intraocular lens implantation in patients with juvenile rheumatoid arthritis. *Am J Ophthalmol.* 1996;122:161–170.

Trocme SD, Li H. Effect of heparin-surface-modified intraocular lenses on postoperative inflammation after phacoemulsification: a randomized trial in a United States patient population. Heparin-Surface-Modified Lens Study Group. *Ophthalmology.* 2000;107:1031–1037.

Glaucoma

Uveitic ocular hypertension is common and must be differentiated from uveitic glaucoma, a well-recognized complication of uveitis. Uveitic ocular hypertension refers to IOP 10 mm Hg or greater above baseline without evidence of glaucomatous optic nerve damage. Uveitic glaucoma is defined as elevated IOP resulting in progressive neuroretinal rim loss and/or development of typical, perimetric, glaucomatous field defects.

Elevated IOP in uveitic eyes may be acute, chronic, or recurrent. In eyes with long-term ciliary body inflammation, the IOP may fluctuate between abnormally high and low values. Numerous morphologic, cellular, and biochemical alterations occur in the uveitic eye that cause uveitic glaucoma and ocular hypertension (Table 11-1). Successful management of uveitic glaucoma and ocular hypertension requires the identification and treatment of each of these contributing factors.

Elevation of IOP to levels above 24 mm Hg seems to substantially increase the risk of glaucoma. However, most practitioners tend to treat IOPs greater than 30 mm Hg even without evidence of glaucomatous optic nerve damage. Assessment of patients with uveitis and elevated IOP should, in addition to slit-lamp and dilated fundus examination, include gonioscopy, disc photos and OCT evaluation of the optic nerve head, and serial automated visual fields.

Table 11-1 Pathogenesis of Uveitic Glaucoma

    I. Cellular and biochemical alterations of aqueous in uveitis
       A. Inflammatory cells
       B. Protein
       C. Prostaglandins
       D. Inflammatory mediators (cytokines) and toxic agents (oxygen-free radicals)
    II. Morphologic changes in anterior chamber angle
       A. Closed angle
          1. Primary angle-closure glaucoma
          2. Secondary angle-closure glaucoma
             a. Posterior synechiae and pupillary block
             b. Peripheral anterior synechiae (PAS)
                i. PAS secondary to inflammation
                ii. PAS secondary to iris neovascularization
                iii. PAS secondary to prolonged iris bombé
             c. Forward rotation of ciliary body (due to inflammation)
       B. Open angle
          1. Primary open-angle glaucoma
          2. Secondary open-angle glaucoma
             a. Aqueous misdirection
             b. Mechanical blockage of trabecular meshwork
                i. Serum components (proteins)
                ii. Precipitates (cells, cellular debris)
             c. Trabeculitis (trabecular dysfunction)
             d. Damage to trabeculum and endothelium from chronic inflammation
             e. Corticosteroid-induced glaucoma
       C. Combined-mechanism glaucoma

Uveitic Ocular Hypertension

Early in the course of uveitis, ocular hypertension is treated with intensive corticosteroids. Clinicians should resist the tendency to back off on corticosteroids because of the unsubstantiated fear of corticosteroid-induced ocular hypertension. Corticosteroid-induced ocular hypertension rarely occurs before 3 weeks after initiation of corticosteroid therapy. Early IOP elevations with active inflammation are almost always due to inflammation that requires aggressive treatment. When the inflammation becomes quiet but IOP is still 30 mm Hg or higher, topical corticosteroids may be slowly tapered and aqueous suppressants may be added.

Uveitic Glaucoma

Uveitic ocular hypertension that results in neuroretinal rim loss and typical glaucomatous visual field defects is defined as *uveitic glaucoma*. Because many cellular, biochemical, and morphologic variables contribute to the development of uveitic glaucoma, many classification methods are possible. However, glaucoma associated with uveitis is best classified by morphologic changes in angle structure; thus, uveitic glaucoma may be divided into secondary angle-closure and secondary open-angle glaucoma. These entities may be further subdivided into acute and chronic types. Most cases of chronic uveitic glaucoma, however, result from a combination of mechanisms. In addition, corticosteroid-induced ocular hypertension and glaucoma are yet other components that must be addressed in these cases of chronic uveitic glaucoma. Gonioscopic evaluation of the peripheral angle, optic nerve evaluation with disc photos and OCT, and automated visual fields are essential in the management of all uveitic glaucoma patients, especially those with chronic inflammation. See also BCSC Section 10, *Glaucoma*.

Secondary angle-closure glaucoma

Acute Acute secondary angle-closure glaucoma may occur when choroidal inflammation results in forward rotation of the ciliary body and lens iris diaphragm. This can be the presenting sign of Vogt-Koyanagi-Harada (VKH) syndrome or sympathetic ophthalmia. Patients present with pain, elevated IOP, no posterior synechiae, and severe inflammation. Ultrasound biomicroscopy (UBM) or ultrasound evaluation showing choroidal thickening and anterior rotation of the ciliary body is diagnostic. Treatment with aggressive corticosteroid therapy and aqueous suppressants is required. As the inflammation subsides, the chamber deepens and the IOP normalizes. Peripheral iridotomy or iridectomy is not useful in these acute cases because the underlying cause is severe choroidal inflammation.

Subacute Chronic anterior segment inflammation may result in the formation of circumferential posterior synechiae, pupillary block, and iris bombé, resulting in subacute secondary peripheral angle closure. This condition occasionally occurs in patients with chronic granulomatous iridocyclitis associated with sarcoidosis or VKH disease and in those with recurrent nongranulomatous iridocyclitis, as is seen with ankylosing spondylitis. In patients with light-colored (blue, green, hazel) irides, peripheral iridotomy with the Nd:YAG or argon laser results in resolution of the bombé and angle closure if performed before permanent peripheral synechiae form. Iridotomies should be multiple and as large as possible. Considerable inflammation can be anticipated following laser iridotomy procedures in these eyes, making them prone to close. Intensive topical corticosteroid and cycloplegic therapy is given following the procedure. In patients with brown irides or if laser iridotomy is not successful in patients with blue, green, or hazel irides, surgical iridectomy is the procedure of choice. The procedure may be supplemented with goniosynechiolysis if peripheral anterior synechiae have started to develop. It is important that the iridectomy specimen be submitted for histopathologic, immunohistochemical, and possibly microbiologic studies to help determine or confirm the etiology of the uveitis. This step is often overlooked in uveitic eyes.

Chronic Chronic intraocular inflammation may result in insidious peripheral anterior synechiae (PAS) and chronic secondary angle-closure glaucoma. These eyes often have superimposed chronic secondary open-angle glaucoma and corticosteroid-induced glaucoma. Topical aqueous suppressants may be inadequate to prevent progression of optic nerve head damage. These eyes may require goniosynechiolysis and trabeculectomy with mitomycin C or glaucoma tube shunt placement.

Secondary open-angle glaucoma

Acute Inflammatory open-angle glaucoma occurs when the trabecular meshwork is inflamed or blocked by inflammatory cells and debris, as commonly occurs with infectious causes of uveitis, such as *Toxoplasma* retinitis, acute retinal necrosis, and herpes simplex and varicella-zoster iridocyclitis. This type of glaucoma usually responds to topical cycloplegics, corticosteroids, and specific treatment of the infectious agent.

Chronic Chronic outflow obstruction in anterior chamber inflammation may be caused by PAS, as well as by direct damage to the trabecular meshwork. Common examples of these mechanisms are chronic iridocyclitis associated with JRA/JIA, sarcoidosis, and Fuchs heterochromic iridocyclitis. Initial treatment is with topical and oral glaucoma medications such as carbonic anhydrase inhibitors, β-blockers, and α-agonists. However, parasympathomimetic medications should be avoided. The β-blocker metipranolol (OptiPranolol) has been associated with granulomatous intraocular inflammation. The prostaglandin analogs latanoprost, travoprost, and bimatoprost should also be avoided as they may also provoke inflammation, especially in eyes with a history of anterior uveitis. There have also been case reports of iriodocyclitis induced by these 3 agents in eyes without a history of intraocular inflammation. Serial automated perimetry, serial OCT evaluation of optic nerve head and nerve fiber layer thickness, and serial stereoscopic optic disc photos must all be carefully evaluated every 6 months to assess treatment success. Medical management is often inadequate in uveitic glaucoma. Failure of medical management may be defined as out-of-control IOP, and/or progressive optic disc cupping and OCT-defined nerve fiber layer loss, and/or progressive visual field loss.

When medical management fails, glaucoma filtering surgery is indicated. Standard trabeculectomy has a greater risk of failure in these eyes. Results may be improved by using mitomycin C with intensive topical corticosteroids. However, intense and recurrent postoperative inflammation can often lead to filtering surgery failure in uveitic eyes. In Adamantiades-Behçet disease, trabeculectomy with mitomycin C can result in successful control of IOP with no medicines in 83% of patients at the end of the first year after surgery and in 62% of patients 5 years after surgery. Surgical complications include cataract formation, bleb leakage (early and late) that could lead to endophthalmitis, and choroidal effusions. Because peripheral iridotomy is performed with trabeculectomy, the excised trabecular block and iris should be submitted for pathologic evaluation, as discussed earlier.

Alternatives to classical trabeculectomy are numerous and have been used with some success in uveitic glaucoma. Nonpenetrating deep sclerectomy with or without a drainage implant has been effective in controlling IOP in 90% of uveitic eyes for 1 year after surgery. Among pediatric uveitis patients, goniotomy has up to a 75% chance of reducing IOP to 21 mm Hg or less after 2 surgeries. This procedure may be complicated by transient hyphema and worsening of the preexisting cataract. Trabeculodialysis, a modified goniotomy, and laser sclerostomy have also been suggested for treatment of uveitic glaucomas, but these procedures have a high rate of failure due to postoperative and recurrent inflammation. Viscocanalostomy has shown higher success rates in a limited number of studies.

Many eyes, especially if pseudophakic or aphakic, require aqueous drainage devices such as Molteno, Ahmed valve, and Baerveldt implants. These tube shunts may be tunneled into the anterior chamber or placed directly into the vitreous cavity in eyes that have undergone previous vitrectomy. In addition, the unidirectional valve design of the Ahmed valve implant can prevent postoperative hypotony. These implants are more likely than trabeculectomy to successfully control IOP long term, with a 70%–75% reduction of IOP from preoperative levels and with most patients achieving target IOPs with 1 or no topical antiglaucoma medications. Complications of tube shunt surgery can include shallow anterior chamber, hypotony, suprachoroidal hemorrhage, and blockage of the tube by blood, fibrin, or iris. Long-term complications include tube erosion through the conjunctiva, valve migration, corneal decompensation, tube–cornea touch, and retinal detachment. Unlike trabeculectomy, these tube shunts have proven to be robust and continue to function despite chronic, recurrent inflammation; they provide excellent long-term IOP control in eyes with uveitic glaucoma.

Cyclodestructive procedures may worsen ocular inflammation and lead to hypotony and phthisis bulbi. Diode cyclophotocoagulation and other cyclodestructive procedures are best avoided in uveitic eyes. Also, laser trabeculoplasty should be avoided in eyes with active intraocular inflammation or iris neovascularization.

As with all surgeries in uveitic patients, tight and meticulous control of perioperative inflammation using immunomodulators and corticosteroids not only improves the success of glaucoma surgery but also improves visual acuity outcomes by limiting sight-threatening complications such as CME and hypotony.

Corticosteroid-induced ocular hypertension and glaucoma

Early in the course of all uveitis entities, priority should be given first and foremost to the control of intraocular inflammation, even if the IOP is high. As the inflammation subsides and is brought under control, IOP will spontaneously decrease, if elevated on presentation. Clinicians must resist the temptation to reduce corticosteroid dosing and frequency prematurely.

However, progressive elevation of IOP after the inflammation is brought under control over the first 3–4 weeks may represent a corticosteroid-induced ocular hypertension. Topical, periocular, and oral corticosteroid therapy for uveitis may all produce a corticosteroid-induced elevation in IOP, which may be difficult to distinguish from other causes of glaucoma in uveitis. This IOP rise may be avoided with a less potent topical corticosteroid preparation, a less frequent administration schedule, or both. Fluorometholone, loteprednol, or rimexolone may be less likely to cause a corticosteroid-induced IOP elevation but may also be less effective in controlling intraocular inflammation than other topical ocular corticosteroid preparations. If these measures do not reduce IOP and further optic nerve head damage, medical and possibly surgical treatment of the glaucoma may be required. This corticosteroid complication may be prevented by earlier institution of corticosteroid-sparing immunomodulatory therapy in the treatment of chronic, recurrent intraocular inflammation.

Combined-mechanism uveitic glaucoma

Multiple mechanisms may be responsible in many cases of uveitic glaucoma. Treatment should be aimed at controlling the inflammation and IOP through a multimodal approach of both medical and surgical therapy aimed at each of the responsible mechanisms.

Auer C, Mermoud A, Herbort CP. Deep sclerectomy for the management of uncontrolled uveitic glaucoma: preliminary data. *Klin Monatsbl Augenheilkd.* 2004;221:339–342.

Ceballos EM, Parrish RK 2nd, Schiffman JC. Outcome of Baerveldt glaucoma drainage implants for the treatment of uveitic glaucoma. *Ophthalmology.* 2002;109:2256–2260.

Freedman SF, Rodriguez-Rosa RE, Rojas MC, Enyedi LB. Goniotomy for glaucoma secondary to chronic childhood uveitis. *Am J Ophthalmol.* 2002;133:617–621.

Ho CL, Wong EY, Walton DS. Goniosurgery for glaucoma complicating chronic childhood uveitis. *Arch Ophthalmol.* 2004;122:838–844.

Kafkala C, Hynes A, Choi J, Topalkara A, Foster CS. Ahmed valve implantation for uncontrolled pediatric uveitic glaucoma. *J AAPOS.* 2005;9:336–340.

Kumarasamy M, Desai SP. Anterior uveitis is associated with travaprost. *BMJ.* 2004;329:205.

Miserocchi E, Carassa RG, Bettin P, Brancato R. Viscocanalostomy in patients with glaucoma secondary to uveitis: preliminary report. *J Cataract Refract Surg.* 2004;30:566–570.

Molteno AC, Sayawat N, Herbison P. Otago glaucoma surgery outcome study: long-term results of uveitis with secondary glaucoma drained by Molteno implants. *Ophthalmology.* 2001;108:605–613.

Moorthy RS, Mermoud A, Baerveldt G, Minckler DS, Lee PP, Rao NA. Glaucoma associated with uveitis. *Surv Ophthalmol.* 1997;41:361–394.

Packer M, Fine IH, Hoffman RS. Bilateral nongranulomatous anterior uveitis associated with bimatoprost. *J Cataract Refract Surg.* 2003;29:2242–2243.

Patel NP, Patel KH, Moster MR, Spaeth GL. Metipranolol-associated nongranulomatous anterior uveitis. *Am J Ophthalmol.* 1997;123:843–844.

Patitsas CJ, Rockwood EJ, Meisler DM, Lowder CY. Glaucoma filtering surgery with postoperative 5-fluorouracil in patients with intraocular inflammatory disease. *Ophthalmology.* 1992;99:594–599.

Schlote T, Derse M, Zierhut M. Transscleral diode laser cyclophotocoagulation for the treatment of refractory glaucoma secondary to inflammatory eye diseases. *Br J Ophthalmol.* 2000;84:999–1003.

Towler HM, McCluskey P, Shaer B, Lightman S. Long-term follow-up of trabeculectomy with intraoperative 5-fluorouracil for uveitis-related glaucoma. *Ophthalmology.* 2000;107:1822–1828.

Watanabe TM, Hodes BL. Bilateral anterior uveitis associated with a brand of metipranolol. *Arch Ophthalmol.* 1997;115:421–422.

Yalvac IS, Sungur G, Turhan E, Eksioglu U, Duman S. Trabeculectomy with mitomycin-C in uveitic glaucoma associated with Behçet disease. *J Glaucoma.* 2004;13:450–453.

Hypotony

Hypotony in uveitis is usually caused by decreased aqueous production from the ciliary body and may follow intraocular surgery in patients with uveitis. Acute inflammation of the ciliary body may cause temporary hyposecretion, whereas chronic ciliary body damage with atrophic or absent ciliary processes results in permanent hypotony. Serous choroidal detachment often accompanies hypotony and complicates management.

Hypotony early in the course of uveitis usually responds to intensive corticosteroid and cycloplegic therapy, although prolonged choroidal effusions may require surgical drainage. Chronic hypotony in long-standing uveitis with preservation of the ciliary process on UBM may respond to topical ibopamine, a nonselective dopaminergic drug with activity on DA1 and DA2 receptors and also on α_1-, α_2-, β_1-, and β_2-adrenergic receptors. Unlike more selective dopaminergic drugs that reduce IOP, ibopamine increases aqueous production by three- to fourfold by stimulating the DA1 receptor. Ibopamine 2% drops, currently available only from Italy, can raise IOP for 8 hours by more than 2 mm Hg when administered twice daily. In eyes with ciliary body traction from cyclitic membranes with absence of ciliary processes, pars plana vitrectomy and membranectomy may restore normal pressure. In select cases, vitrectomy and intraocular silicone oil may help maintain ocular anatomy and IOP. In some of these cases, visual improvement after surgery can be significant.

de Smet MD, Gunning F, Feenstra R. The surgical management of chronic hypotony due to uveitis. *Eye.* 2005;19:60–64.

Ugahary LC, Ganteris E, Veckeneer M, et al. Topical ibopamine in the treatment of chronic ocular hypotony attributable to vitreoretinal surgery, uveitis, or penetrating trauma. *Am J Ophthalmol.* 2006;141:571–573.

Virno M, De Gregorio F, Pannarale L, Arrico L. Topical ibopamine and corticosteroids in the treatment of post-surgery ocular hypotony. *Int Ophthalmol.* 1996;20:147–150.

Cystoid Macular Edema

Cystoid macular edema is a common cause of visual loss in eyes with uveitis. It most commonly occurs in pars planitis, birdshot retinochoroiditis, and retinal vasculitis but can occur in any chronic uveitis. CME is usually caused by active intraocular inflammation and less commonly caused by mechanical vitreomacular traction; the two can easily be differentiated by OCT. CME can also be quantitatively evaluated and followed by serial OCTs. The severity of CME can correspond to the level of inflammatory disease activity, but it is often slow to respond and clear and often remains even after visible, active inflammation has resolved.

Treatment of CME must first be directed toward control of intraocular inflammation with corticosteroids and immunomodulatory therapy. Therapy that reduces intraocular inflammation in general often reduces CME. Topical, periocular, intraocular, and oral corticosteroids are used to control the inflammation. When periocular therapy is used specifically to treat CME, a superotemporal posterior sub-Tenon's injection of 20–40 mg of triamcinolone acetonide (Kenalog) is preferred (see Chapter 6). Theoretically, this technique delivers juxtascleral corticosteroid closest to the macula. The injections may be administered as a series of 3 or 4, repeated monthly. If, after 3 or 4 posterior sub-Tenon's triamcinolone injections, CME still persists, then 2–4 mg of intravitreal triamcinolone may be considered (see Chapter 6). Intravitreal triamcinolone can be highly effective in reducing CME, particularly in nonvitrectomized eyes, but its effect is time-limited; the drug is eliminated more quickly from the vitreous cavity of vitrectomized eyes, reducing its efficacy. Maximum visual improvement and reduction of CME after intravitreal triamcinolone injection occurs within 4 weeks. Eyes with a longer duration of CME and worse vision on presentation with uveitic CME tend to have the least amount of visual improvement after treatment with intravitreal triamcinolone. Corticosteroid-induced IOP elevation may occur in up to 40% of patients, especially in those younger than 40 years. Most of the data on intravitreal triamcinolone is from small, retrospective, uncontrolled studies. This treatment modality is actively being investigated.

Other agents have been used to treat uveitic CME but with limited success. Topical ketorolac can be beneficial in treating pseudophakic CME. Its effectiveness in the treatment of uveitic CME has not been established. Oral acetazolamide, 500 mg once or twice daily, has also been effective in reducing uveitic CME, particularly in patients whose inflammation is well controlled. Recently, the somatostatin analog ocreotide has shown some promise in reducing uveitic CME in a patient with intermediate uveitis.

Surgical therapy for uveitic CME is still controversial. Pars plana vitrectomy for uveitic CME in the presence of hyaloidal traction on the macula (as seen on OCT imaging) may be visually and anatomically beneficial. In the absence of vitreomacular traction, however, the efficacy of pars plana vitrectomy in treating CME is not well understood. In a recent review of 39 studies of eyes with uveitis that underwent pars plana vitrectomy, the median reported percentage of patients per study with CME was 36% preoperatively and 18% postoperatively. Thus, there is some suggestion that vitrectomy may be beneficial in managing recalcitrant uveitic CME. The role of vitrectomy for the treatment of uveitic CME requires further investigation. See BCSC Section 12, *Retina and Vitreous*.

Androudi S, Letko E, Meniconi M, Papadaki T, Ahmed M, Foster CS. Safety and efficacy of intravitreal triamcinolone acetonide for uveitic macular edema. *Ocul Immunol Inflamm.* 2005;13:205–212.

Angunawela RI, Heatley CJ, Williamson TH, et al. Intravitreal triamcinalone acetonide for refractory uveitic cystoid macular oedema: long-term management and outcome. *Acta Ophthalmol Scand.* 2005;83:595–599.

Becker M, Davis J. Vitrectomy in the treatment of uveitis. *Am J Ophthalmol.* 2005;140:1096–1105.

Farber MD, Lam S, Tessler HH, Jennings TJ, Cross A, Rusin MM. Reduction of macular oedema by acetazolamide in patients with chronic iridocyclitis: a randomised prospective crossover study. *Br J Ophthalmol.* 1994;78:4–7.

Jennings T, Rusin MM, Tessler HH, Cunha-Vaz JG. Posterior sub-Tenon's injections of corticosteroids in uveitis patients with cystoid macular edema. *Jpn J Ophthalmol.* 1988;32:385–391.

Kok H, Lau C, Maycock N, McCluskey P, Lightman S. Outcome of intravitreal triamcinolone in uveitis. *Ophthalmology.* 2005;112:1916–1921.

Papadaki T, Zacharopoulos I, Iaccheri B, Fiore T, Foster CS. Somatostatin for uveitic cystoid macular edema (CME). *Ocul Immunol Inflamm.* 2005;13:469–470.

Schilling H, Heiligenhaus A, Laube T, Bornfeld N, Jurklies B. Long-term effect of acetazolamide treatment of patients with uveitic chronic cystoid macular edema is limited by persisting inflammation. *Retina.* 2005;25:182–188.

Vitreous Opacification and Vitritis

Permanent vitreous opacification affecting vision occasionally occurs in uveitis, particularly in eyes with toxoplasma retinitis and pars planitis. In fact, in a review of 39 recent studies of eyes with chronic uveitis that had undergone pars plana vitrectomy, visual acuity improved in 68%. In other cases of vitritis, the diagnosis is uncertain. Pars plana vitrectomy may be therapeutic or diagnostic in eyes with vitritis. This procedure can be used both to debride vitreous and to obtain a vitreous sample that may be studied by culture, stains, and cytology to determine the cause of the vitritis. In a recent retrospective review of diagnostic testing of vitrectomy specimens, the positive predictive values of cytologic evaluation of vitreous for lymphoma and bacterial and fungal cultures for infection were 100%. Carefully planned testing of the samples obtained from diagnostic vitrectomy is an effective method of supporting the suspected clinical diagnosis of atypical chorioretinitis, chronic ocular infections, and primary intraocular lymphoma. It may alter the clinical management of 10% or more of patients with unusual posterior segment uveitides.

A standard 3-port pars plana vitrectomy is the preferred technique, with a few minor variations. Core vitrectomy is performed with the hand-held cutter and a syringe attached to a stopcock that interrupts the aspiration line of the cutter handpiece. This syringe is used to manually aspirate and collect 0.5–1.0 cc of undiluted vitreous prior to opening the irrigation line. The core vitrectomy is then completed in the usual manner; the posterior hyaloid should be separated from the retina if this has not already occurred naturally. The vitreous gel should then be dissected to the edge of the vitreous base with careful scleral depression under direct visualization. Membrane peeling may be performed in cases when epiretinal membranes are present. The peripheral retina should be checked for tears, dialyses, or detachments. At the conclusion of the procedure, the cassette containing the diluted vitreous may be used for cultures and additional testing if needed.

Becker M, Davis J. Vitrectomy in the treatment of uveitis. *Am J Ophthalmol.* 2005;140:1096–1105.

Davis JL, Miller DM, Ruiz P. Diagnostic testing of vitrectomy specimens. *Am J Ophthalmol.* 2005;140:822–829.

Manku H, McCluskey P. Diagnostic vitreous biopsy in patients with uveitis: a useful investigation? *Clin Experiment Ophthalmol.* 2005;33:604–610.

Retinal Detachment

Rhegmatogenous retinal detachment (RRD) occurs in 3% of patients with uveitis. The high prevalence of RRD means that uveitis itself may be an independent risk factor for the condition. Panuveitis and infectious uveitis are the entities most frequently associated with RRD. Pars planitis and posterior uveitis can also be associated with rhegmatogenous or tractional retinal detachments. Uveitis is often still active in eyes that present with RRD. Because these are surgical emergencies, there is not adequate time available for preoperative control of intraocular inflammation. Up to 30% of patients with uveitis and RRD may have proliferative vitreoretinopathy (PVR) at presentation; this percentage is significantly higher than that in primary RRD in patients without uveitis. Repair is often complicated by preexisting PVR, vitreous organization, and poor visualization. Scleral buckling with cryoretinopexy is still useful in cases of retinal detachment associated with pars planitis. Acute retinal necrosis and cytomegalovirus retinitis frequently lead to retinal detachments that are difficult to repair because of multiple, large posterior retinal breaks. Pars plana vitrectomy and endolaser treatment with internal silicone oil tamponade are required to repair the detachment and remove epiretinal membranes. When PVR is present, combined scleral buckling and pars plana vitrectomy is often required to reattach the retina. The retinal reattachment rate after 1 surgery in uveitic eyes with RRD is 60%. Final vision was less than 20/200 in 70% of eyes in one study, and 10% of these had no light perception. Thus, the prognosis in eyes with uveitis and RRD is particularly poor compared to that in nonuveitic eyes with RRD. In some conditions, such as acute retinal necrosis syndrome, prophylactic barrier laser photocoagulation around areas of necrotic retina may prevent retinal detachment.

Freeman WR, Friedberg DN, Berry C, et al. Risk factors for development of rhegmatogenous retinal detachment in patients with cytomegalovirus retinitis. *Am J Ophthalmol.* 1993;116:713–720.

Kerkhoff FT, Lamberts QJ, van den Biesen PR, Rothova A. Rhegmatogenous retinal detachment and uveitis. *Ophthalmology.* 2003;110:427–431.

Kuppermann BD, Flores-Aguilar M, Quiceno JI, et al. A masked prospective evaluation of outcome parameters for cytomegalovirus-related retinal detachment surgery in patients with acquired immune deficiency syndrome. *Ophthalmology.* 1994;101:46–55.

Nussenblatt RB, Whitcup SM, Palestine AG. *Uveitis: Fundamentals and Clinical Practice.* 3rd ed. St Louis: Mosby; 2004.

Sternberg P Jr, Han DP, Yeo JH, et al. Photocoagulation to prevent retinal detachment in acute retinal necrosis. *Ophthalmology.* 1988;95:1389–1393.

Retinal and Choroidal Neovascularization

Retinal neovascularization may develop in any chronic uveitic condition but is particularly common in pars planitis, sarcoid panuveitis, and retinal vasculitis of various causes, including Eales disease. Retinal neovascularization occurs from chronic inflammation or capillary nonperfusion. Treatment is directed toward the underlying etiology. Treatment options include reduction of inflammation with corticosteroids and/or immunomodulatory agents or scatter laser photocoagulation in the ischemic areas and associated watershed zones. The presence of retinal neovascularization does not always require panretinal photocoagulation. Some cases of sarcoid panuveitis, for example, may present with neovascularization of the disc that resolves completely with immunomodulatory and corticosteroid therapy alone.

Choroidal neovascularization (CNV) can develop in posterior uveitis and panuveitis. It can commonly occur in ocular histoplasmosis syndrome, punctate inner choroidopathy, idiopathic multifocal choroiditis, and serpiginous choroiditis. CNV can also occur in VKH syndrome and other panuveitis entities. In such cases, CNV results from a disruption of Bruch's membrane from choroidal inflammation and the presence of inflammatory cytokines that promote angiogenesis. The prevalence of CNV varies among different entities. It can occur in up to 10% of patients with VKH disease. Patients present with metamorphopsia and rapid-onset scotoma. Diagnosis is based on clinical and angiographic findings. Treatment should be directed toward reducing inflammation as well as on anatomical ablation of the CNV. Focal laser photocoagulation of peripapillary, extrafoveal, and juxtafoveal CNV may be performed. The treatment of subfoveal CNV is more difficult. Corticosteroids (systemic, periocular, and intraocular) and immunomodulators alone may be used in an attempt to promote involution of CNV. Immunomodulators may be combined with vascular endothelial growth factor (VEGF) inhibitors such as pegaptanib, bevacizumab, and ranibizumab or may be used in conjunction with ocular photodynamic therapy. If these agents alone do not work, pars plana vitrectomy and subfoveal CNV extraction may be considered. See Ocular Histoplasmosis Syndrome in Chapter 8, Infectious Uveitis, for discussion of the results of photodynamic therapy for subfoveal CNV in the Verteporfin in Ocular Histoplasmosis study.

Kuo IC, Cunningham ET. Ocular neovascularization in patients with uveitis. *Int Ophthalmol Clin.* 2000;40:111–126.

Moorthy RS, Chong LP, Smith RE, Rao NA. Subretinal neovascular membranes in Vogt-Koyanagi-Harada syndrome. *Am J Ophthalmol.* 1993;116:164–170.

O'Toole LL, Tufail A, Pavesio C. Management of choroidal neovascularization in uveitis. *Int Ophthalmol Clin.* 2005;45:157–177.

Sanislo SR, Lowder CY, Kaiser PK, et al. Corticosteroid therapy for optic disc neovascularization secondary to chronic uveitis. *Am J Ophthalmol.* 2000;130:724–731.

CHAPTER 12

Ocular Involvement in AIDS

Acquired immunodeficiency syndrome (AIDS) is the first pandemic since influenza in the first half of the 20th century. First described in 1981 in Los Angeles, AIDS is now thought to have originated in central Africa, perhaps in the 1950s, then spread to the Caribbean, the United States, Europe, and other parts of the world. This syndrome is caused by a retrovirus, human lymphotropic virus type III, commonly known as *human immuno-deficiency virus (HIV)*.

By 2005, an estimated 40.3 million people were living with AIDS (see http://www.unaids.org/en/). In that same year, 3 million people died of AIDS and 5 million were newly infected. The steepest increases in cases occurred in central and east Asia and eastern Europe. In the United States, cases continue to increase by about 40,000 per year and are approaching a cumulative 1 million cases. The spread of HIV is of particular concern in countries with large populations and much poverty. Sub-Saharan Africa has 10% of the world's population and 60% (25.8 million) of the people living with AIDS; 3.2 million of its people became newly infected in 2005. India has 10 million of its 1 billion people living with AIDS, but it is considered highly vulnerable to further spread of the disease; the government provides free antiretroviral treatment. Overall, the proportion of new cases involving homosexual and bisexual men is dropping, whereas the proportion of new HIV infections in intravenous drug users, women, minorities, and children is rising. At the end of 2005, 2.3 million children under the age of 15 were living with AIDS.

During the first decade of the HIV epidemic, mass education programs tried to change high-risk sexual behavior in the United States and other parts of the industrialized world. Today, HIV-infected persons with access to medical care live longer, with improved quality of life, due to antiretroviral drugs and other treatments that reduce morbidity and mortality from opportunistic infections.

> Cunningham ET Jr, Belfort R Jr. *HIV/AIDS and the Eye: A Global Perspective.* Ophthalmology Monograph 15. San Francisco: American Academy of Ophthalmology; 2002.

Virology of HIV

HIV is a lentivirus that is a member of the retrovirus family of RNA viruses. Currently, 2 lentiviruses are known to infect humans:

1. HIV-1, the more prevalent, is seen worldwide.
2. HIV-2 is identified primarily in western Africa.

The HIV-2 virus shares roughly 40% homology in nucleotide sequence with HIV-1 and about 75% homology with simian immunodeficiency virus.

HIV-1 and HIV-2 viruses are each approximately 100 nm in diameter. The virion has a cylindrical nucleocapsid that contains the single-stranded RNA and viral enzymes, including proteinase, integrase, and reverse transcriptase. Surrounding the capsid is a lipid envelope, which is derived from the infected host cell. This envelope contains virus-encoded glycoproteins. The viral genome contains 3 structural genes: *gag, pol,* and *env.* HIV-1 and HIV-2 are genetically similar in the *gag* and *pol* regions; the *env* regions, however, are different, resulting in differences in the envelope glycoproteins of these viruses. Such heterogeneity leads to specific immune responses and necessitates different HIV-1 and HIV-2 immunoassays or Western blot procedures for serologic diagnosis. In addition to the 3 structural genes, HIV contains 6 regulatory genes: *tat, rev, nef, vif, vpr,* and *vpu.* Two of these regulatory genes *(tat* and *rev)* are essential for virus replication. HIV isolates show marked heterogeneity in the *env* and the *nef* genes, with the following results:

- differing tissue and cell tropisms
- variations in pathogenesis
- disparate responses to therapy
- potential challenges in developing a broadly cross-reactive protective vaccine

This viral heterogeneity exists from continent to continent, from one infected individual to another, and even within the same infected host. Causes of the heterogeneity may include spontaneous mutation of the virus, the frequent error rate of the reverse transcriptase enzyme, and, possibly, antiviral therapy. See also BCSC Section 2, *Fundamentals and Principles of Ophthalmology,* Part III, Genetics.

Pathogenesis

Initial events in HIV infection include attachment of the virus to a distinct group of T lymphocytes and monocytes/macrophages that display a membrane antigen complex known as *CD4.* However, other molecules on these cells may also play a role in the attachment of HIV, particularly chemokine receptors such as CCR5 and CXCR4. After attachment, the lipid membrane of the virus fuses with the target cell, allowing entry of the viral core into host cell cytoplasm. This viral core is subsequently uncoated and transcribed by reverse transcriptase enzyme, resulting in a complementary strand of DNA. The action of cellular enzymes transforms this DNA into the typical double-stranded form that subsequently enters the cell nucleus.

Once inside the nucleus, the proviral DNA integrates into the genome of the host cell by means of a viral endonuclease. This host cell can be either latently or actively infected. If latently infected, no viral RNA is produced, and a productive infection may not develop. If actively infected, however, the cell may produce mature virions by transcription of proviral DNA. This transcription also generates messenger RNA (mRNA). In the cytoplasm, mRNA is translated into HIV-specific structural proteins that are integrated with the viral core particles.

Table 12-2 Antiretroviral Agents

Nucleoside/nucleotide reverse transcriptase inhibitors (NRTIs)	Nonnucleoside reverse transcriptase inhibitors (NNRTIs)
Zidovudine (ZDV, AZT; Retrovir)	Nevirapine (NVP; Viramune)
Didanosine (ddl; Videx)	Delavirdine (DLV; Rescriptor)
Zalcitabine (ddC; Hivid)	Efavirenz (EFV; Sustiva)
Stavudine (d4T; Zerit)	**Protense inhibitors (PIs)**
Lamivudine (3TC; Epivir)	Amprenavir/fosamprenavir (APV; Agenerase/ FPV; Lexiva)
Abacavir (ABC; Ziagen)	Atazanavir (ATZ; Reyataz)
Emtricitabine (FTC; Emtriva)	Indinavir (IDV; Crixivan)
Tenofovir (TDF; Viread)	Nelfinavir (NFV; Viracept)
Combined NRTIs	Ritonavir (RTV; Norvir)
ABC + 3TC (Epzicom)	Saquinavir (SQV; Invirase, Fortovase)
ABC + AZT + 3TC (Trivizir)	Lopinavir + ritonavir (LPV; Kaletra)
AZT + 3TC (Combivir)	Tipranavir (TPV; Aptivus)
TDF + FTC (Truvada)	**Fusion or entry inhibitors**
	Enfuvirtide (ENF; Fuzeon)

200 and 350. Highly active antiretroviral therapy for initial treatment consists of 2 NRTIs, 1 NNRTI, and 1 PI. Three-NRTI regimens can be considered in special circumstances. A typical starting regimen might consist of zidovudine and lamivudine (NRTIs), efavirenz (NNRTI), and lopinavir + ritonavir (PI).

Yeni PG, Hammer SM, Hirsch MS, et al. Treatment for adult HIV infection: 2004 recommendations of the International AIDS Society-USA Panel. *JAMA.* 2004;292:251–265.

When the CD4$^+$ T-lymphocyte count falls below 200 cells/mm^3, prophylaxis against *Pneumocystis* pneumonia is begun with trimethoprim/sulfamethoxazole (TMP/SMX). Among pulmonary diseases, tuberculosis must also be considered. Tuberculosis is 500 times more common in HIV-infected persons than in the general population; multidrug, directly observed therapy is recommended for its treatment. Purified protein derivative (PPD) testing may be unreliable, and minor reactions of 5 mm should be considered positive. Multidrug-resistant tuberculosis occurs in the HIV-infected population. HIV-infected patients with low CD4$^+$ T-lymphocyte counts also require prophylaxis against recurrent opportunistic infections such as cerebral toxoplasmosis, cryptococcosis, *Mycobacterium avium–intracellulare* complex (MAI), oroesophageal or vulvovaginal candidiasis, and histoplasmosis. Rifabutin is commonly used for prophylaxis against MAI, and fluconazole is used for mycotic infections. All HIV-infected patients should be tested for syphilis.

Ophthalmic Complications

Ocular manifestations have been reported in up to 70% of people infected with HIV and may be the first sign of disseminated systemic infection. The ophthalmologist thus has the opportunity to make not only a sight-saving but indeed a life-prolonging diagnosis in some patients with AIDS. These ocular manifestations include

- HIV-related microangiopathy of the retina
- various opportunistic viral, bacterial, and fungal infections
- Kaposi sarcoma
- lymphomas involving the retina (primary intraocular lymphoma), adnexal structures, and orbit
- squamous cell carcinoma of the conjunctiva

Reports also suggest that HIV itself may cause anterior uveitis or an inflammatory reaction in the vitreous that is not responsive to corticosteroids but improves with antiretroviral therapy.

Cunningham ET Jr. Uveitis in HIV positive patients. *Br J Ophthalmol.* 2000;84:233–235.

HIV retinopathy is the most common ocular finding in patients with AIDS, occurring in about 50%–70% of cases. It is characterized by retinal hemorrhages, microaneurysms, and cotton-wool spots (Fig 12-1). HIV has been isolated from the human retina, and its antigen has been detected in retinal endothelial cells by immunohistochemistry. It is thought that such HIV endothelial infection and/or rheologic abnormalities such as increased leukocyte activation and rigidity may play a role in the development of cotton-wool spots and other vascular alterations.

Goldenberg DT, Holland GN, Cumberland WG, et al. An assessment of polymorphonuclear leukocyte rigidity in HIV-infected individuals after immune recovery. *Invest Ophthalmol Vis Sci.* 2002;43:1857–1861.

Other infectious agents that can affect the eye in patients with AIDS include CMV, herpes zoster virus, *Toxoplasmosis gondii, Mycobacterium tuberculosis,* MAI, *Cryptococcus neoformans, Pneumocystis carinii, Histoplasma capsulatum, Candida* spp, molluscum contagiosum, Microsporida, and others. These agents can infect the ocular adnexa, anterior segment, or posterior segment. Visual morbidity, however, occurs primarily with posterior segment involvement, particularly retinitis caused by CMV, herpes zoster virus, or *T gondii.*

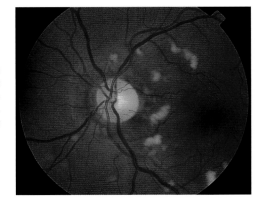

Figure 12-1 HIV retinopathy with numerous cotton-wool spots. *(Reprinted with permission from Cunningham ET Jr, Belfort R Jr. HIV/AIDS and the Eye: A Global Perspective. Ophthalmology Monograph 15. San Francisco: American Academy of Ophthalmology; 2002:55.)*

Cytomegalovirus retinitis

Disseminated CMV infection was the most common opportunistic infection in AIDS before HAART, and retinal infection was its most clinically important manifestation, occurring in 15%–40% of patients with AIDS. CMV retinitis remains the most common ocular opportunistic infection in patients with AIDS and is occasionally the first AIDS-defining infection for an individual. CMV retinitis most commonly occurs in people whose CD4$^+$ T-lymphocyte counts are below 50 cells/mm^3. (See also Chapter 8, Infectious Uveitis.)

CMV is a double-stranded DNA virus that belongs to the Herpesviridae family, which also includes the herpes simplex, varicella-zoster, and Epstein-Barr viruses. Transmission of CMV probably occurs with close or intimate contact with infected individuals who are shedding virus in their urine, saliva, or other secretions. CMV infection in otherwise healthy adults and children is usually asymptomatic but occasionally is associated with a mononucleosis-like syndrome. In contrast to the generally benign course of CMV infection in healthy persons, CMV is a major cause of morbidity and mortality in immunocompromised patients. The high prevalence of anti-CMV antibodies in the general population is evidence of widespread exposure to this virus. In the 1980s, the median survival time following diagnosis of CMV retinitis was 6 weeks in patients receiving no treatment. Survival time increased in patients who responded to ganciclovir treatment. Progressively longer survival times have resulted from improved treatment of HIV infection and other opportunistic infections and neoplasms. However, the presence of CMV retinitis or a detectable CMV viral load in the blood is associated with an increased risk of death, even in the HAART era.

CMV retinitis is characterized by yellow-white retinal lesions that often follow a vascular distribution because the virus initially infects the endothelium of the blood vessels. Posterior involvement usually follows a fulminant pattern, with marked retinal opacification, hard exudates, and intraretinal hemorrhages (Fig 12-2). In the periphery, the retinitis has a more granular pattern, with less opacification and hemorrhage. Because of severe immunosuppression in patients with AIDS, the amount of overlying vitreous inflammation is usually minimal. Expansion of lesions usually occurs along all borders. Because viral replication is somewhat slow, there is usually some central healing. Vessels are occluded within lesions. Very early CMV retinitis lesions may resemble cotton-wool spots; a lesion size over 750 μm is suggestive of CMV retinitis.

Diagnosis The diagnosis of CMV retinitis is based on its characteristic clinical appearance. Serologic investigation and viral culture are of limited value, because many persons show evidence of previous exposure to CMV on serologic testing. Equivocal cases of active retinitis can usually be diagnosed by PCR to amplify CMV DNA in aqueous humor. Urine cultures are somewhat more reliable than blood cultures in detecting systemic infection. However, a quantitative CMV PCR for blood can also be used to assess systemic infection.

Treatment In the United States, 5 medications are currently approved for treatment of CMV retinitis:

1. oral or intravenous ganciclovir
2. oral valganciclovir

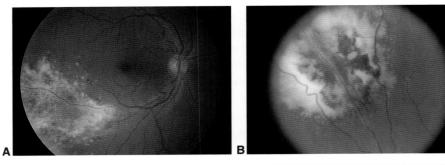

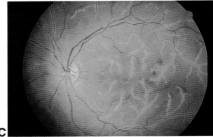

Figure 12-2 Types of cytomegalovirus retinitis. **A,** Granular CMV retinitis. **B,** Fulminant, or hemorrhagic, CMV retinitis. **C,** Perivascular CMV retinitis mimicking frosted-branch retinitis. *(A–C reprinted with permission from Cunningham ET Jr, Belfort R Jr. HIV/AIDS and the Eye: A Global Perspective. Ophthalmology Monograph 15. San Francisco: American Academy of Ophthalmology; 2002:57. Part C photograph courtesy of J. Michael Lahey, MD.)*

3. intravenous foscarnet
4. ganciclovir via intraocular device
5. intravenous cidofovir

Intravenous *ganciclovir* was the first therapy developed for the treatment of CMV retinitis. The initial, high-dose induction therapy (5 mg/kg twice daily for 2 weeks) is aimed at controlling the infection and is followed by long-term maintenance therapy (5 mg/kg once daily 7 days a week). The primary side effect of ganciclovir is myelosuppression. Concomitant use of granulocyte-macrophage colony-stimulating factor can reduce or reverse neutropenia, the most serious component of myelosuppression, and may allow continuation of ganciclovir therapy. Neutropenia is usually reversible but may also necessitate interruption of the drug therapy. Thrombocytopenia has been reported to occur in 5%–10% of patients treated with ganciclovir. When CMV retinitis is diagnosed, patients may already be undergoing treatment with zidovudine (ZDV). Because ZDV also has toxic effects on the bone marrow, the dosage is usually decreased when the drug is used concomitantly with ganciclovir.

Ganciclovir is also available for oral administration, and this route of administration can be used as a maintenance therapy for patients with CMV retinitis who respond well to intravenous induction therapy with this agent. Drug toxicity is lower in patients maintained on oral administration. However, median time to progression of retinitis on oral ganciclovir (29 days) is less than with intravenous maintenance therapy (49 days). Moreover, the risk of CMV in the fellow eye is greater in patients receiving oral ganciclovir compared to those on intravenous maintenance.

Valganciclovir, a pro-drug of ganciclovir, achieves blood levels comparable to those of intravenous ganciclovir during both induction and maintenance therapy. Induction therapy is 900 mg twice daily for 21 days, followed by 900 mg once daily as maintenance therapy. The systemic side effects and toxicities are similar to those of intravenous ganciclovir, but the oral agent is much more convenient for the patient and eliminates complications associated with placement of an indwelling catheter or repeated IV administration. Treatment with oral valganciclovir is preferred by most specialists and patients.

Foscarnet is administered intravenously and, like ganciclovir, requires an initial 2-week, high-dose induction therapy (90 mg/kg every 12 hours for 2 weeks), followed by long-term maintenance therapy (90–120 mg/kg daily). Although foscarnet does not have a toxic effect on the bone marrow and can be used concurrently with full-dose ZDV therapy, it is toxic to the kidneys. Renal dysfunction and metabolic abnormalities of calcium and magnesium have been reported in up to 30% of patients who are receiving foscarnet, and seizures have been reported in approximately 10%.

Off-label intravitreal ganciclovir or foscarnet can be considered for patients who have shown retinitis progression despite high-dose systemic therapy with ganciclovir, foscarnet, or both, or those who cannot tolerate systemic therapy. Under topical anesthesia, an intravitreal injection of 200 μg to 2.0 mg in 0.1 mL of ganciclovir is given once a week as maintenance therapy. Foscarnet, 2.4 mg in 0.1 mL, can be given instead of ganciclovir. Induction therapy is given twice a week for 2–3 weeks. Initial success rates are very high, with almost all patients showing early resolution of retinitis. The risks associated with repeated intravitreal injections include cataract formation, vitreous hemorrhage, retinal detachment, and infectious endophthalmitis. Perhaps the most serious drawback of the intravitreal route of administration is that it does not provide the benefits of systemic anti-CMV treatment to the other eye and to extraocular sites of CMV infection.

A second proven method of intravitreal administration of ganciclovir is through an intravitreal device, which is surgically implanted and delivers the drug in effective concentrations over 6–8 months. Intraocular concentrations are 4 times higher than that achieved by intravenous ganciclovir. Surgery to place the implant has a low risk of serious complications. Concomitant use of oral valganciclovir provides optimal benefits in reducing second eye involvement or systemic CMV disease.

Cidofovir is administered intravenously with efficacy similar to that of intravenous ganciclovir. Cidofovir has a prolonged intracellular half-life and is administered at a dose of 5 mg/kg once a week for 2 weeks for induction therapy and 5 mg/kg every 2 weeks for maintenance therapy. During the administration of this agent, the patient requires IV hydration and probenecid to avoid severe renal toxicity. Up to 50% of patients may develop hypotony, anterior uveitis, or both while on cidofovir.

When assessing response to treatment, the most important clinical characteristic to evaluate is the size of the lesion. Careful attention to the border of the lesion, not the central area, is essential. The clinical appearance of the lesion can be compared against earlier clinical photographs to detect enlargement or stabilization of its size. The second most important clinical parameter is the degree of activity of the lesion, which is determined by the presence of retinal whitening and hemorrhage at the border of the lesion. Lesions in recurrent disease usually demonstrate fluffy white areas of active retinitis at the border of the original CMV lesion. In some cases of recurrence, lesions may enlarge despite minimal signs of retinal whitening or hemorrhage. As with the primary disease, it is the border of the lesion that reflects disease activity. In chronic stages of the disease, large atrophic holes may develop that can lead to retinal detachment.

Healing of lesions with resolution of retinal whitening and no further progression is expected within 4–6 weeks of starting therapy. Without HAART, active retinitis recurs in 50% of patients within the next 6–8 weeks of maintenance therapy and in virtually all patients who discontinue anti-CMV therapy. Rates of progression are lower in patients who are taking HAART, even if they do not have high CD4 counts; use of HAART also reduces the risk of second eye involvement. Most investigators think that, given enough time, all patients eventually suffer a relapse, although they generally respond to a second course of induction (reinduction) therapy. If a patient experiences recurrence while receiving ganciclovir, foscarnet, or cidofovir, the following choices must be considered:

- reinduction with the current medication
- new induction using the second or third medication
- concomitant use of 2 medications

Concomitant use of ganciclovir and foscarnet is synergistic against CMV and beneficial in preventing progression if the disease fails to respond to either agent administered alone. In some cases, for example, viral resistance develops that may limit the usefulness of 1 of the agents. Although blood CMV viral load does not predict resistance, if CMV cannot be detected by PCR in the blood, such resistance is unlikely to be present. A switch to a more effective means of administration, such as intravitreal, may be appropriate, rather than a switch to a different medication entirely, as higher intraocular levels can be achieved with intravitreal injection.

In patients on HAART, the CD4 cell count may increase sufficiently to allow a decrease or discontinuation of anti-CMV therapy. Such patients need to be monitored closely every 6–12 months, however, for 2 reasons: CMV retinitis may recur even with CD4 counts over 100 cells/mm^3, and partial viral resistance, intolerance, or both occur in a sizable proportion of patients on HAART. More frequent follow-up may be warranted if CD4 counts drop.

Immune recovery uveitis Patients with preexisting CMV retinitis who improve their immune status with HAART are susceptible to anterior or intermediate uveitis and cystoid macular edema. The inflammation occurs only in eyes infected with CMV and seems to be proportional to the surface area of retina involved. Widely disparate estimates of the prevalence of immune recovery have appeared in the literature.

A large cohort study with prospective data collection recorded *immune recovery uveitis (IRU)* in 9.6% of 374 patients. Immune recovery was defined as an increase in the CD4$^+$ T-lymphocyte count of at least 50 cells to at least 100 cells/mm^3. Immune recovery uveitis was associated with a CMV retinitis surface area of greater than 25%. The odds ratio of IRU was 10.6 greater in patients who had ever used cidofovir.

Eyes with IRU were much more likely to have macular edema or epiretinal membrane. The macular edema seen in IRU can be resistant to treatment with sub-Tenon's injections of depot corticosteroids, although such injections do not seem to cause reactivation of CMV infection. Intravitreal injections of corticosteroids must be avoided. Immune recovery uveitis has been associated with moderate vision loss in eyes in which it occurs but is not associated with active replication of CMV or with the continuance or discontinuation of anti-CMV medication.

Retinal detachment An additional complication of CMV retinitis is retinal detachment, which occurs in up to 50% of patients. It may occur either when the retinitis is active or when it is quiescent during successful treatment. In the HAART era, the rate of retinal detachment has been reduced among patients with CD4[+] T-lymphocyte counts greater than 50 cells/mm^3 to 0.50 per patient-year. Involvement of all 3 retinal zones, lower CD4[+] T-lymphocyte count, and more extensive retinitis are risk factors for developing retinal detachment. The repair of retinal detachments in patients with CMV retinitis requires special techniques because of extensive retinal necrosis and multiple, often posterior, hole formation. Most investigators agree that these detachments are not amenable to repair by scleral buckling alone; a common procedure is pars plana vitrectomy with long-term silicone oil tamponade. Anatomical reattachment can be achieved in 90% of these patients. Functional success, however, depends on the condition of the macula and the extent of affected retina.

Dunn JP, Van Natta M, Foster G, et al. Complications of ganciclovir implant surgery in patients with cytomegalovirus retinitis: the Ganciclovir Cidofovir Cytomegalovirus Retinitis Trial. *Retina.* 2004;24:41–50.

El-Bradey MH, Cheng L, Song MK, Torriani FJ, Freeman WR. Long-term results of treatment of macular complications in eyes with immune recovery uveitis using a graded treatment approach. *Retina.* 2004;24:376–382.

Goldberg DE, Wang H, Azen SP, Freeman WR. Long term visual outcome of patients with cytomegalovirus retinitis treated with highly active antiretroviral therapy. *Br J Ophthalmol.* 2003;87:853–855.

Jabs DA, Holbrook JT, Van Natta ML, et al. Risk factors for mortality in patients with AIDS in the era of highly active antiretroviral therapy. *Ophthalmology.* 2005;112:771–779.

Jabs DA, Martin BK, Forman MS, Ricks MO, Cytomegalovirus Retinitis and Viral Resistance Research Group. Cytomegalovirus (CMV) blood DNA load, CMV retinitis progression, and occurrence of resistant CMV in patients with CMV retinitis. *J Infect Dis.* 2005;192:640–649.

Jabs DA, Van Natta ML, Thorne JE, et al. Course of cytomegalovirus retinitis in the era of highly active antiretroviral therapy: 1. Retinitis progression. *Ophthalmology.* 2004;111:2224–2231.

Jabs DA, Van Natta ML, Thorne JE, et al. Course of cytomegalovirus retinitis in the era of highly active antiretroviral therapy: 2. Second eye involvement and retinal detachment. *Ophthalmology.* 2004;111:2232–2239.

Kempen JH, Jabs DA, Wilson LA, Dunn JP, West SK. Incidence of cytomegalovirus (CMV) retinitis in second eyes of patients with the acquired immune deficiency syndrome and unilateral CMV retinitis. *Am J Ophthalmol.* 2005;139:1028–1034.

Kempen JH, Min YI, Freeman WR, et al. Risk of immune recovery uveitis in patients with AIDS and cytomegalovirus retinitis. *Ophthalmology.* 2006;113:684–694.

Kuo IC, Kempen JH, Dunn JP, Vogelsang G, Jabs DA. Clinical characteristics and outcomes of cytomegalovirus retinitis in persons without human immunodeficiency virus infection. *Am J Ophthalmol.* 2004;138:338–346.

Schrier RD, Song MK, Smith IL, et al. Intraocular viral and immune pathogenesis of immune recovery uveitis in patients with healed cytomegalovirus retinitis. *Retina.* 2006;26:165–169.

Song MK, Azen SP, Buley A, et al. Effect of anti-cytomegalovirus therapy on the incidence of immune recovery uveitis in AIDS patients with healed cytomegalovirus retinitis. *Am J Ophthalmol.* 2003;136:696–702.

Necrotizing herpetic retinitis

Patients with AIDS may develop aggressive forms of necrotizing herpetic retinitis, which appear to manifest as a spectrum of disease; the severity of these forms is directly proportional to the level of immunologic compromise. Hence, patients with HIV infection with profound reductions in CD4[+] T-lymphocyte counts may develop more severe forms of necrotizing herpetic retinitis.

A rare infection in HIV-infected patients, progressive outer retinal necrosis (PORN), a variant of necrotizing herpetic retinitis, may be caused by the varicella-zoster virus or herpes simplex virus (Fig 12-3). It may occur in the absence of, at the same time as, or subsequent to a cutaneous zoster infection. (See also Chapter 8, Infectious Uveitis.)

In its early stages, PORN may be difficult to differentiate from peripheral CMV retinitis. However, PORN's characteristic rapid progression and relative absence of vitreous inflammation usually allow this entity to be distinguished from CMV retinitis and from the acute retinal necrosis syndrome (ARN). PORN is associated with a high incidence of retinal detachment, and bilateral involvement is common. Intravitreal ganciclovir or foscarnet or both seem to provide better control of infection than intravenous acyclovir. Intravenous ganciclovir and/or foscarnet also seem to be more effective than intravenous acyclovir, the use of which is associated with a high rate of bilateral blindness.

Herpes zoster ophthalmicus may increase the risk of developing necrotizing herpetic retinitis in the same eye in patients with HIV infection.

Engstrom RE Jr, Holland GN, Margolis TP, et al. The progressive outer retinal necrosis syndrome. A variant of necrotizing herpetic retinopathy in patients with AIDS. *Ophthalmology.* 1994;101:1488–1502.

Scott IU, Luu KM, Davis JL. Intravitreal antivirals in the management of patients with acquired immunodeficiency syndrome with progressive outer retinal necrosis. *Arch Ophthalmol.* 2002;120:1219–1222.

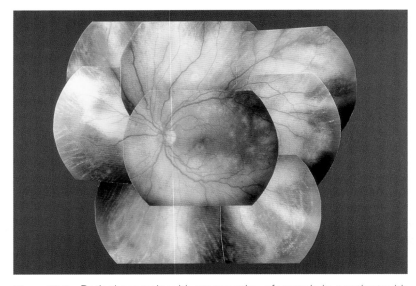

Figure 12-3 Retinal necrosis with preservation of vessels in a patient with progressive outer retinal necrosis. *(Courtesy of Narsing A. Rao, MD.)*

Toxoplasma *retinochoroiditis*

A number of reports of toxoplasmosis in patients with AIDS have revealed important clinical differences from toxoplasmosis in immunocompetent patients. In general, the size of the retinochoroidal lesions is larger in patients with AIDS, with up to one third of lesions greater than 5 disc diameters. Bilateral disease is seen in 18%–38% of these cases. Solitary, multifocal, and miliary patterns of retinitis have been observed (Fig 12-4). A vitreous inflammatory reaction usually appears overlying the area of active retinochoroiditis, but the degree of vitreous reaction may be less than that observed in immunocompetent patients. (See also Chapter 8, Infectious Uveitis.)

The diagnosis of ocular toxoplasmosis may also be more difficult in patients with AIDS. In immunocompetent patients, this diagnosis is frequently helped by the presence of old retinochoroidal scars; in patients with AIDS, however, such preexisting scars are rarely seen (present in only 4%–6% of patients with ocular toxoplasmosis). Because the clinical manifestations in this latter population are so varied and may be more severe than those seen in immunocompetent patients, ocular toxoplasmosis in patients with AIDS may be difficult to distinguish from ARN, necrotizing herpetic retinitis, or syphilitic retinitis.

The histologic features of ocular specimens from patients with AIDS reflect the immunologic abnormalities of the host. In general, the inflammatory reaction in the choroid, retina, and vitreous is less prominent than in patients with an intact immune system. Trophozoites and cysts can be observed in greater numbers within areas of retinitis, and *T gondii* organisms can occasionally be seen invading the choroid, which is not the case in immunocompetent patients.

Ocular toxoplasmosis in immunocompetent patients is usually the result of reactivation of a congenital infection. In contrast, newly acquired infection or dissemination from a nonocular site of infection is the most likely cause among patients with AIDS. These conclusions are drawn from the observations that preexisting retinochoroidal scars are rarely present and *Toxoplasma*-specific IgM titers are found in 6%–12% of patients.

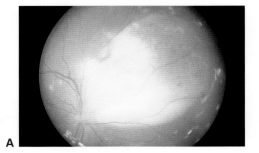 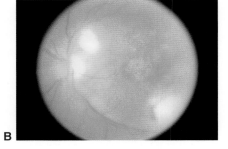

Figure 12-4 **A,** A large area of macular toxoplasmic retinochoroiditis in an HIV-infected patient. **B,** Multifocal toxoplasmic retinochoroiditis in another HIV-infected patient. *(Courtesy of Emmett T. Cunningham, Jr, MD.)*

The prompt diagnosis of ocular toxoplasmosis is especially important in patients with immunosuppression because the condition inevitably progresses if left untreated, in contrast to the self-limited disease of immunocompetent patients. In addition, ocular toxoplasmosis in immunocompromised patients may be associated with cerebral or disseminated toxoplasmosis, an important cause of morbidity and mortality in patients with AIDS. HIV-infected patients with active ocular toxoplasmosis should therefore undergo MRI of the brain to rule out CNS involvement.

Antitoxoplasmic therapy with various combinations of pyrimethamine, sulfadiazine, and clindamycin is required. Corticosteroids should be used with caution and only in the presence of appropriate antimicrobial cover because of the risk of further immunosuppression in this population. In selecting the therapeutic regimen, the physician should consider the possibility of coexisting cerebral or disseminated toxoplasmosis and the toxic effects of pyrimethamine and sulfadiazine on the bone marrow. Continued maintenance therapy may be necessary for patients with poor immune status that is not improving.

Moshfeghi DM, Dodds EM, Couto CA, et al. Diagnostic approaches to severe, atypical toxoplasmosis mimicking acute retinal necrosis. *Ophthalmology.* 2004;111:716–725.

Syphilitic chorioretinitis

The clinical presentations of ocular syphilitic chorioretinitis include uveitis, optic neuritis, and nonnecrotizing retinitis. Patients may also experience dermatologic and CNS manifestations. A classic manifestation of syphilis in patients with AIDS is unilateral or bilateral pale yellow placoid, retinal lesions that preferentially involve the macula *(syphilitic posterior placoid chorioretinitis)*. Exudative retinal detachment can also be seen. Some HIV-positive patients with syphilis may present with dense vitritis without clinical evidence of chorioretinitis. In these patients, vitritis can be the first manifestation of syphilis. (See also Chapter 8, Infectious Uveitis.)

The course of syphilis may be more aggressive in patients with AIDS. These patients require treatment with 12–24 million units of intravenous penicillin G administered daily for 10–14 days, followed by 2.4 million units of intramuscular benzathine penicillin G administered weekly for 3 weeks. Monitoring of the quantitative rapid plasma reagin (RPR) test is recommended, as symptomatic disease can recur.

Browning DJ. Posterior segment manifestations of active ocular syphilis, their response to a neurosyphilis regimen of penicillin therapy, and the influence of human immunodeficiency virus status on response. *Ophthalmology.* 2000;107:2015–2023.

Pneumocystis carinii *choroiditis*

Patients with AIDS are at much greater risk for *P carinii* pneumonia, an infection that can be the opportunistic disease initially seen in these patients. In rare instances, this infection can disseminate, and patients with such disseminated infection may present with choroidal infiltrates containing the responsible microorganisms.

Fundus changes characteristic of *P carinii* choroiditis consist of slightly elevated, plaquelike, yellow-white lesions located in the choroid with minimal vitritis (Figs 12-5, 12-6, 12-7). On fluorescein angiography, these lesions tend to be hypofluorescent in the early phase and hyperfluorescent in the later phases. If disseminated *P carinii* is suspected, an extensive examination is required, including

- chest radiography
- arterial blood gas analysis
- liver function testing
- abdominal CT

Treatment of *P carinii* choroiditis is a 3-week regimen of intravenous trimethoprim (20 mg/kg per day) and sulfamethoxazole (100 mg/kg per day) or pentamidine (4 mg/kg per day). Within 3–12 weeks, most of the yellow-white lesions disappear, leaving mild overlying pigmentary changes. Vision is usually not affected.

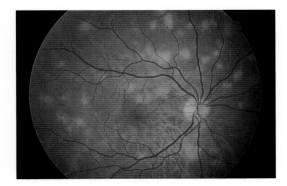

Figure 12-5 *Pneumocystis carinii* choroiditis. The fellow eye revealed similar findings. *(Reprinted with permission from Cunningham ET Jr, Belfort R Jr. HIV/AIDS and the Eye: A Global Perspective. Ophthalmology Monograph 15. San Francisco: American Academy of Ophthalmology; 2002:67.)*

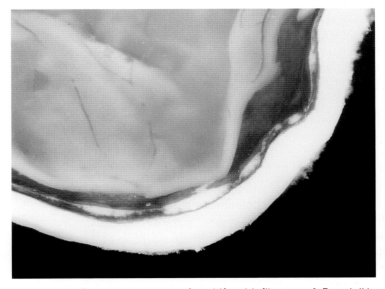

Figure 12-6 Gross appearance of multifocal infiltrates of *P carinii* in the choroid.

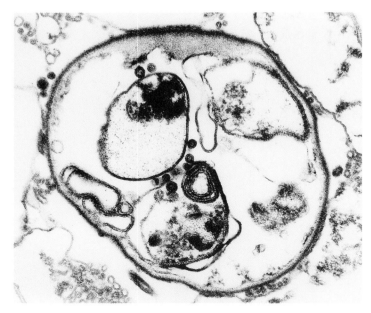

Figure 12-7   Electron micrograph showing a cyst of *P carinii*.

Cryptococcus neoformans *choroiditis*

The dissemination of *C neoformans* in patients with AIDS may result in a multifocal cho-roiditis similar to *P carinii* choroiditis. Some patients with *C neoformans* choroiditis show choroidal lesions before they develop clinical evidence of dissemination. More typically, *C neoformans* involves the cerebrospinal fluid and there is secondary optic nerve edema from increased intracranial pressure that can slowly lead to optic atrophy. Direct invasion of the optic nerve by organisms is also possible and can lead to more rapid vision loss.

> Kestelyn P, Taelman H, Bogaerts J, et al. Ophthalmic manifestations of infections with *Crypto-coccus neoformans* in patients with the acquired immunodeficiency syndrome. *Am J Oph-thalmol*. 1993;116:721–727.

Multifocal choroiditis and systemic dissemination

Multifocal choroidal lesions from a variety of infectious agents, including those just dis-cussed, are seen in about 5%–10% of patients with AIDS. Most of these lesions are caused by *C neoformans, P carinii, M tuberculosis,* or atypical mycobacteria. Although multifocal choroiditis caused by any 1 of these infectious organisms is seen in many patients with AIDS, occasionally 2 or more in combination can be responsible.

Because it is so often the site of opportunistic disseminated infections, the choroid is a critical structure that needs to be carefully examined in patients with AIDS. Although nonspecific, multifocal choroiditis is alarming and should prompt an exhaustive workup for disseminated infection. Because multifocal choroiditis frequently represents dissemi-nated infection, the ophthalmologist may have a life-prolonging role in the diagnosis and treatment of these patients.

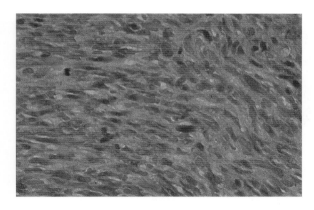

Figure 12-8 Histopathologically, Kaposi sarcoma is made up of large spindle cells forming slitlike spaces. These spaces contain erythrocytes.

External Eye Manifestations

Other ophthalmic manifestations of AIDS include Kaposi sarcoma; molluscum contagiosum; herpes zoster ophthalmicus; and keratitis caused by various viruses, protozoa, conjunctival infections, and microvascular abnormalities. All of these conditions affect mainly the anterior segment of the globe and the ocular adnexa. These conditions are also discussed in BCSC Section 8, *External Disease and Cornea.*

Ocular adnexal Kaposi sarcoma

Since the initial description of Kaposi sarcoma in 1872, 2 more-aggressive variants of this tumor have been described. An endemic variety was described in 1959 in Africa; it is especially prevalent in Kenya and Nigeria, where it accounts for nearly 20% of all malignancies. The second variant, *epidemic Kaposi sarcoma,* was first noted in renal transplant recipients and currently occurs in 30% of all patients with AIDS. AIDS-associated Kaposi sarcoma is particularly aggressive, disseminating to visceral organs (gastrointestinal tract, lung, and liver) in 20%–50% of patients. Prior to 1981, fewer than 25 patients with ocular adnexal Kaposi sarcoma had been reported, but in the pre-HAART era, the condition occurred in approximately 20% of patients with AIDS-associated systemic Kaposi sarcoma.

Histopathologic investigation shows spindle cells mixed with vascular structures (Fig 12-8). Recent evidence suggests that AIDS-related Kaposi sarcoma may have an infectious origin. Human herpesvirus 8 has been isolated from patients with Kaposi sarcoma. That HIV may play a role in the pathogenesis of Kaposi sarcoma is evident from studies of transgenic mice bearing the HIV-1 transactivator *(tat)* gene under the control of the virus regulatory region (HIV-LTR). The HIV-*tat* protein has been shown to be a potent mitogen for human Kaposi sarcoma–derived cell lines. As in humans, these lesions in mice occur predominantly in males, which suggests that their development may be hormonally controlled.

Three clinical stages of ocular adnexal Kaposi sarcoma have been described:

- Stage I and stage II tumors are patchy, flat (<3 mm in height), and of less than 4 months' duration.
- Stage III tumors are nodular, elevated (>3 mm in height), and of greater than 4 months' duration (Fig 12-9).

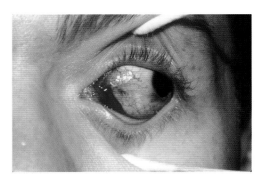

Figure 12-9 Conjunctival involvement in Kaposi sarcoma; hemorrhagic conjunctival tumor. *(Courtesy of Elaine Chuang, MD.)*

Treatment of Kaposi sarcoma is based on the clinical stage of the tumor as well as its location and the presence or absence of disseminated lesions. If the lesion is confined to the ocular adnexa, local treatment is appropriate. If the tumor is confined to the bulbar conjunctiva, is at stage I or II, and is symptomatic, an excisional biopsy with 1–2 mm tumor-free margins should be considered. Stage III Kaposi sarcoma of the bulbar conjunctiva should be surgically excised, preferably after delineation by fluorescein angiography. Stage I and II Kaposi sarcoma involving the eyelid may be treated with cryotherapy. Stage III Kaposi sarcoma of the eyelid may be treated with either radiation or cryotherapy, although radiation is preferred because of a lower recurrence rate. However, there are radiation-related complications. To avoid these, cryotherapy may be used, but the patient must be made aware that recurrence is more likely and may necessitate retreatment.

When evaluating a patient with AIDS who has ocular adnexal Kaposi sarcoma, the physician should perform a full systemic examination for tumor dissemination. If chemotherapy is administered for systemic Kaposi sarcoma, the ophthalmologist should wait at least 4–6 weeks to observe response to treatment before deciding whether further therapy is warranted.

Molluscum contagiosum

Molluscum contagiosum is caused by a DNA virus of the poxvirus family. The characteristic skin lesions show a small elevation with central umbilication. Molluscum lesions in healthy individuals are few, are unilateral, and involve the eyelids. In patients with AIDS, however, these lesions may be numerous and bilateral. If molluscum lesions in patients with AIDS are symptomatic or cause conjunctivitis, surgical excision may be necessary. However, surgery and cryotherapy sometimes fail to treat these viral lesions.

Herpes zoster

People younger than 50 years presenting with herpes zoster lesions of the face or eyelids should be tested for HIV. Corneal involvement can cause a persistent, chronic epithelial keratitis; treatment consists of intravenous and topical acyclovir. See the discussion of PORN earlier in this chapter. Although PORN is rare, these patients should be followed periodically with retinal examination.

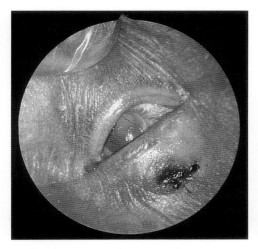

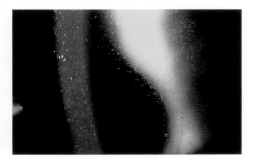

Figure 12-10 Lesions of the eyelid and cornea in a patient with AIDS and disseminated herpes simplex.

Figure 12-11 Superficial punctate keratitis caused by Microsporida.

Other infections

HIV infection does not appear to predispose patients to bacterial keratitis. However, infections appear to be more severe and are more likely to cause perforation in patients with AIDS than in immunocompetent patients. Bacterial and fungal keratitis can occur in patients with AIDS with no obvious predisposing factors such as trauma or topical corticosteroid use. Although herpes simplex keratitis does not appear to have a higher incidence in patients with AIDS, it may have a prolonged course or multiple recurrences and involve the limbus in these patients (Fig 12-10). Microsporida organisms have been shown to cause a coarse, superficial punctate keratitis with a minimal conjunctival reaction in patients with AIDS (Fig 12-11). Electron microscopy of the epithelial scrapings has revealed the organism, which is an obligate, intracellular, protozoal parasite.

Solitary granulomatous conjunctivitis from cryptococcal infection, tuberculosis, or other mycotic infections can occur in HIV-infected persons. As with all other infections in AIDS, the possibility of dissemination must be considered, aggressively investigated, and, if present, treated. Orbital lymphomas and intraocular lymphomas have been described in patients with AIDS. These neoplasms are mostly large B-cell lymphomas. Conjunctival squamous cell carcinomas have been reported, and in some patients these neoplasms show spindle cells with frequent abnormal mitotic figures.

The Ophthalmologist's Role

The role of the ophthalmologist is to diagnose and treat opportunistic infections and malignancies affecting the ocular system. Occasionally, the ophthalmologist is the first health care provider to suspect HIV infection on the basis of an ocular opportunistic infection such as cytomegalovirus retinitis or microangiopathy in a nondiabetic patient. It is the responsibility of the ophthalmologist to provide not only an ophthalmic examination but also a pertinent systemic evaluation, timely referrals, and periodic follow-up care.

Precautions in the Health Care Setting

Specific precautionary measures against HIV infection have been advocated in the United States by the CDC and other governmental agencies, including the Occupational Safety and Health Administration (OSHA). These agencies insist on adoption of bloodborne pathogen standards, commonly referred to as *universal precautions*. These precautions should be followed whether or not a patient is known to be HIV-positive and include the following:

- Take measures to prevent accidental needle-stick injury.
- Wear gloves routinely when collecting and handling specimens.
- Dispose of contaminated sharp objects in puncture-resistant (sharps) containers.
- Ensure that the eyes and mouths of clinical and laboratory workers are properly shielded.
- Thoroughly disinfect examination equipment that touches mucosal surfaces after each use.
- Ensure that a gloved person using 10% chlorine bleach solution promptly cleans all blood spills in the examining rooms and waiting area.
- Make hepatitis B vaccine available to all personnel who come in contact with patient blood.

Precautions in Ophthalmic Practice

Although it appears that ophthalmology is at less risk than some other, more hazardous specialties, the American Academy of Ophthalmology has advocated that ophthalmic practices follow precautionary measures against HIV infection. These measures are meant to provide protection to patients, ancillary health care personnel, and ophthalmologists. To be effective, precautions must be identical for all patients, not just those who are known to be HIV-infected.

Even though there are no published reports of HIV transmission in ophthalmic health care settings, hand washing or use of a hand sterilizer solution is recommended between various tests on an individual and between patients. If an open wound or weeping lesion is present, disposable gloves should be worn and discarded appropriately.

Tonometers and diagnostic contact lenses should be wiped with an alcohol sponge. Similarly, the Schiøtz tonometer can be disassembled and cleaned with an alcohol sponge. The CDC recommends household chlorine bleach (1:10 dilution) for 10 minutes to clean such instruments. The contact surface of diagnostic contact lenses should be soaked in dilute bleach for 10 minutes. These items must be carefully rinsed after the use of either alcohol or chlorine. BCSC Section 10, *Glaucoma,* gives more specific instructions for infection control in tonometry.

Contact lens trial sets need to be disinfected between patients. For hard contact lenses and rigid gas-permeable contact lenses, hydrogen peroxide disinfection or a chlorhexidine-containing disinfectant system should be used. For soft contact lenses, hydrogen peroxide or a heat disinfection system should be used.

Barrier precautions, such as disposable gloves, should be used during diagnostic procedures such as injection of dye for fluorescein angiographic studies. During surgical procedures, particularly when contact with blood or blood-contaminated fluids is likely, all health care personnel in attendance should wear disposable gloves, masks, and protective eyewear.

Corneal and scleral tissue used for transplantations should be screened for HIV and hepatitis B virus, in accordance with the guidelines provided by the Eye Bank Association of America. See BCSC Section 8, *External Disease and Cornea.*

Minimizing transmission of bloodborne pathogens and surface infectious agents in ophthalmic offices and operating rooms. Information Statement. San Francisco: American Academy of Ophthalmology; 2002.

Basic Texts

Intraocular Inflammation and Uveitis

Albert DM, Jakobiec FA, eds. *Principles and Practice of Ophthalmology*. 6 vols. 2nd ed. Philadelphia: Saunders; 2000.

Delves PJ, Martin S, Burton D, Roitt IM. *Roitt's Essential Immunology*. 11th ed. Malden, MA: Blackwell; 2006.

Foster CS, Vitale AT. *Diagnosis and Treatment of Uveitis*. Philadelphia: Saunders; 2002.

Giles CL. Uveitis in childhood. In: Tasman W, Jaeger EA, eds. *Duane's Clinical Ophthalmology*. Philadelphia: Lippincott; 2001.

Michelson JB. *Color Atlas of Uveitis Diagnosis*. 2nd ed. St Louis: Mosby; 1992.

Nussenblatt RB, Whitcup SM. *Uveitis: Fundamentals and Clinical Practice*. 3rd ed. St Louis: Mosby; 2004.

Pepose JS, Holland GN, Wilhelmus KR, eds. *Ocular Infection and Immunity*. St Louis: Mosby; 1996.

Rao NA, ed. Uveitis and other intraocular inflammations. In: Yanoff M, Duker JS. *Ophthalmology*. 2nd ed. St Louis: Mosby; 2004:chap 159–184.

Rao NA, Forster DJ, Augsburger JJ. *The Uvea: Uveitis and Intraocular Neoplasms*. New York: William C Brown Communications; 1992.

Smith RE, Nozik RA. *Uveitis: A Clinical Approach to Diagnosis and Management*. 2nd ed. Baltimore: Williams & Wilkins; 1989.

Related Academy Materials

Focal Points: Clinical Modules for Ophthalmologists

Ahmed M, Foster CS. Steroid therapy for ocular inflammatory disease (Module 7, 2006).

Arellanes-Garcia L. Infectious posterior uveitis (Module 3, 2005).

Buggage RR. White dot syndrome (Module 4, 2007).

Cunningham ET. Diagnosis and management of anterior uveitis (Module 1, 2002).

Dodds EM. Ocular toxoplasmosis: clinical presentations, diagnosis, and therapy (Module 10, 1999).

Doft BH. Managing infectious endophthalmitis: results of the Endophthalmitis Vitrectomy Study (Module 3, 1997).

Dunn JP. Uveitis in children (Module 4, 1995).

Jampol LM. Nonsteroidal anti-inflammatory drugs (Module 6, 1997).

Lightman S, McCluskey P. Cystoid macular edema in uveitis (Module 8, 2003).

Margo CE. Nonpigmented lesions of the ocular surface (Module 9, 1996).

Moshfeghi DM, Muccioli C, Belfort R Jr. Laboratory evaluation of patients with uveitis (Module 12, 2001).

Read RW. Sympathetic ophthalmia (Module 5, 2005).

Rosenbaum JT, Smith JR. Immune-mediated systemic diseases associated with uveitis (Module 10, 2003).

Samples JR. Management of glaucoma secondary to uveitis (Module 5, 1995).

Smith JR, Rosenbaum JT. Immune-mediated systemic diseases associated with uveitis (Module 11, 2003).

Tessler HH, Goldstein DA. Update on systemic immunosuppressive agents (Module 11, 2000).

Publications

Cunningham ET Jr, Belfort R Jr. *HIV/AIDS and the Eye: A Global Perspective* (Ophthalmology Monograph 15, 2002).

Lane SS, Skuta GL, eds. *ProVision: Preferred Responses in Ophthalmology*. Series 3 (Self-Assessment Program, 1999; includes 2005 update).

Schwab L. *Eye Care in Developing Nations*. 3rd ed. (1999).

Wilson FM II, ed. *Practical Ophthalmology: A Manual for Beginning Residents*. 5th ed. (2005).

Academy MOC Essentials

MOC Exam Self-Assessment: Core Ophthalmic Knowledge and Practice Emphasis Areas (2005).

MOC Exam Study Guide: Comprehensive Ophthalmology and Practice Emphasis Areas (2005).

Multimedia

Johns KJ, ed. *Eye Care Skills: Presentations for Physicians and Other Health Care Professionals.* Contains all 7 titles from the Eye Care Skills for the Primary Care Physician Series (CD-ROM; 2005).

Smith JR, Buggage RR, Goldstein DA, Van Gelder RN. *LEO Clinical Update Course on Uveitis* (CD-ROM; 2004).

Continuing Ophthalmic Video Education

Kelly MP. *Basic Techniques of Fluorescein Angiography* (1994; reviewed for currency 2004).

Osher RH. *More Challenging Cases in Cataract Surgery* (2001).

To order any of these materials, please call the Academy's Customer Service number at (415) 561-8540, or order online at www.aao.org.

Study Questions

Although a concerted effort has been made to avoid ambiguity and redundancy in these questions, the authors recognize that differences of opinion may occur regarding the "best" answer. The discussions are provided to demonstrate the rationale used to derive the answer. They may also be helpful in confirming that your approach to the problem was correct or, if necessary, in fixing the principle in your memory.

1. Which of the following statements about innate immunity is correct?
   a. It comprises recognition, processing, and effector phases.
   b. It is triggered by bacterial toxins and cell debris.
   c. It demonstrates specificity for each unique offending antigen.
   d. It demonstrates memory, with an accelerated and more vigorous response to a second antigenic exposure.

2. Characteristics of the adaptive immune response include which of the following?
   a. identifies various offensive stimuli in an antigen-independent manner
   b. responds in a preprogrammed fashion determined by preexisting receptors for the stimulus
   c. generates generic cytokines that recruit nonspecific effector cells
   d. generates unique antigen-specific effector cells and specific antibodies to remove a specific offending antigen

3. Which of the following ocular inflammatory diseases is correctly matched to the corresponding predominant reactivities of the adaptive immune response in the eye?
   a. sympathetic ophthalmia—Th1-mediated delayed hypersensitivity
   b. necrotizing scleritis in Wegener granulomatosis—acute IgE-mediated mast-cell degranulation
   c. allergic conjunctivitis—stimulatory antibodies
   d. acute anterior uveitis—circulating immune complexes

4. The epidemiologic studies of uveitic entities from around the world suggest that uveitis occurs
   a. most commonly in the first and second decades of life
   b. most commonly in the posterior or intermediate segment of the eye
   c. most commonly in patients over the age of 65
   d. most commonly in men

5. Which of the following immunomodulatory agents belongs to the T-cell inhibitors?

    a. azathioprine

    b. cyclophosphamide

    c. tacrolimus

    d. infliximab

6. Trans pars plana intravitreal injection of triamcinolone in a phakic patient with chronic, noninfectious uveitis and cystoid macular edema can result in

    a. curing the uveitis

    b. cataract

    c. hypotony from ocular fistula at the injection site

    d. exudative retinal detachment

7. Which of the following statements regarding HLA disease associations is true?

    a. HLA haplotypes are good diagnostic markers.

    b. The strongest HLA disease association in humans is the HLA-B51 haplotype in Adamantiades-Behçet disease.

    c. HLA molecules may act as peptide-binding molecules to etiologic antigens or infectious agents.

    d. HLA genes on chromosome 6 are unique in that they can never be coinherited with other disease-related genes.

8. The most common cause of hypopyon anterior uveitis in the United States is

    a. Adamantiades-Behçet disease

    b. idiopathic

    c. HLA-B27–associated disease

    d. endogenous endophthalmitis

9. Which of the following is *true* regarding early-onset, pauciarticular JRA/JIA-associated iridocyclitis?

    a. Patients present with redness, pain, and photophobia.

    b. Iridocyclitis is more common in the subset of patients who are ANA negative.

    c. Girls are much more commonly affected than boys.

    d. Intraocular lens implantation can never be performed during cataract surgery.

10. Which of the following is *true* regarding late-onset, pauciarticular JRA/JIA-associated iridocyclitis?

    a. Patients present with redness, pain, and photophobia.

    b. Most patients are HLA-B27 negative.

    c. Girls are much more commonly affected than boys.

    d. The iridocyclitis is chronic and has a very poor prognosis.

11. Fuchs heterochromic iridocyclitis is characterized by

    a. anterior uveitis that resolves without recurrence when treated with topical corticosteroids

    b. sectoral iris transillumination defects

    c. zonular dehiscence and capsular rupture during cataract surgery

    d. glaucoma in more than 50% of patients

12. Patients with which of the following are most likely to present with granulomatous uveitis?

    a. sarcoidosis

    b. Adamantiades-Behçet syndrome

    c. juvenile rheumatoid arthritis/juvenile idiopathic arthritis

    d. Reiter syndrome

13. Which of the following topical agents is most effective in controlling intraocular inflammation in anterior uveitis?

    a. loteprednol (Lotemax)

    b. fluorometholone 0.25% (FML Forte)

    c. dexamethasone 0.1% (Decadron)

    d. prednisolone 1% (Pred Forte, Inflammase Forte)

14. Periocular depot corticosteroid injections should *not* be used in which of the following uveitic syndromes?

    a. pars planitis with cystoid macular edema

    b. sarcoidosis

    c. toxoplasmosis

    d. Reiter syndrome

15. Reiter syndrome is associated with all *except* which of the following?

    a. nonspecific urethritis

    b. polyarthritis

    c. conjunctivitis

    d. ankylosing spondylitis

16. Major diagnostic criteria for Adamantiades-Behçet syndrome include all *except* which of the following?

    a. aphthous stomatitis

    b. arthritis

    c. genital ulceration

    d. retinal vasculitis

17. In which of the following uveitic syndromes is the indication for early institution of immunomodulatory therapy considered absolute?

    a. Adamantiades-Behçet retinal vasculitis

    b. HLA-B27–associated iridocyclitis

    c. pars planitis

    d. sarcoid panuveitis

18. Which of the following types of intraocular lenses are most associated with recurrent uveitis?

    a. rigid, closed-loop anterior chamber intraocular lenses

    b. iris plane intraocular lenses

    c. sulcus-placed posterior chamber intraocular lenses

    d. silicone intraocular lenses

19. Which of the following is the most common cause of intermediate uveitis?

    a. multiple sclerosis

    b. idiopathic disease

    c. Lyme disease

    d. syphilis

20. Which of the following is the major cause of visual loss in pars planitis?

    a. band keratopathy

    b. posterior subcapsular cataract

    c. epiretinal membrane

    d. cystoid macular edema

21. Acute retinal necrosis syndrome is characterized by

    a. severe peripheral periphlebitis

    b. little or no vitreous inflammation

    c. severe occlusive retinal arteriolitis

    d. extensive retinal hemorrhages, giving a "pizza-pie" appearance to the retina

22. Characteristic clinical features of the ocular histoplasmosis syndrome include

    a. vitritis

    b. multiple, large, confluent areas of retinal and choroidal whitening

    c. choroidal neovascularization

    d. optic papillitis

23. Which of the following is the most common ophthalmic manifestation of systemic lupus erythematosus (SLE)?

    a. anterior uveitis

    b. intermediate uveitis

    c. sclerokeratitis

    d. retinal and choroidal vasculopathy

24. The presence of c-ANCA directed against proteinase 3 is highly specific for the diagnosis of which condition?
    a. polyarteritis nodosa (PAN)
    b. Wegener granulomatosis
    c. relapsing polychondritis
    d. microscopic polyangiitis

25. Multiple evanescent white dot syndrome (MEWDS) is characterized by
    a. bilateral involvement at presentation
    b. greatest prevalence among males
    c. recurrence in more than half of patients
    d. spontaneous resolution in 2–10 weeks

26. Characteristics of acute posterior multifocal placoid pigment epitheliopathy (APMPPE) include which of the following?
    a. The disease may be associated with cerebral vasculitis, which may be fatal if untreated.
    b. It is usually not associated with a viral prodrome.
    c. Choroidal neovascularization is a common complication of APMPPE.
    d. It is almost always unilateral at presentation.

27. Which of the following commonly occurs in an immunocompromised host?
    a. cytomegalovirus retinitis
    b. herpes simplex keratouveitis
    c. acute retinal necrosis syndrome
    d. ocular histoplasmosis syndrome

28. Which of the following medications should be avoided as initial treatment for vision-threatening ocular toxoplasmosis?
    a. pyrimethamine and sulfadiazine
    b. trimethoprim/sulfamethoxazole
    c. azithromycin and pyrimethamine
    d. systemic or periocular corticosteroids

29. Which of the following is the best laboratory test for a newly acquired ocular toxoplasmosis infection?
    a. IgM antibody titer
    b. IgG antibody titer
    c. *Toxoplasma* dye test of Sabin and Feldman
    d. hemagglutination test

30. Which of the following statements about syphilis and uveitis is *not* correct?

    a. A salt-and-pepper fundus may be seen in congenital syphilis.

    b. Uveitis may be seen in secondary-stage syphilis.

    c. Syphilitic uveitis cannot be cured in patients with AIDS.

    d. A lumbar puncture should be performed in patients with uveitis and syphilis.

31. The treatment of syphilitic uveitis requires which of the following regimens?

    a. 18–24 million units (MU) of aqueous crystalline penicillin G per day, administered as 3–4 MU intravenously every 4 hours or as a continuous infusion for 10–14 days

    b. benzathine penicillin G 2.4 MU IM as a single dose

    c. benzathine penicillin G 2.4 MU IM, weekly × 3 doses

    d. doxycycline 100 mg PO bid × 4 weeks

32. Ocular manifestations of various stages of Lyme disease include

    a. retinal vasculitis in stage 1

    b. follicular conjunctivitis in stage 3

    c. intermediate uveitis in stage 2

    d. multifocal choroiditis in stage 1

33. Which of the following is the most common cause of neuroretinitis?

    a. *Treponema pallidum*

    b. *Borrelia burgdorferi*

    c. *Bartonella henselae*

    d. malignant hypertension

34. A patient with bilateral granulomatous panuveitis whose workup revealed a positive PPD skin test would require treatment with which of the following medications?

    a. isoniazid alone because multidrug-resistant tuberculosis is rare in the United States

    b. isoniazid, rifampin, and pyrazinamide

    c. isoniazid, rifampin, pyrazinamide, and corticosteroids

    d. corticosteroids alone if the induration from the PPD skin test is less than 15 mm

35. A definitive diagnosis of sarcoid uveitis is confirmed by which of the following?

    a. hilar adenopathy on chest radiography or computed tomography

    b. elevated serum angiotensin-converting enzyme (ACE) and lysozyme levels

    c. abnormal gallium scan of minor salivary glands

    d. demonstration of noncaseating granuloma on histopathology

36. A 41-year-old Japanese man with a remote history of blunt ocular trauma in 1 eye but good vision and no history of ocular surgery presents with decreased vision and severe pain in both eyes. He has bilateral uveitis, alopecia, vitiligo, and recent cerebrovascular accident. There is an exudative retinal detachment in 1 eye. Which of the following diagnoses is most likely?

    a. sarcoidosis

    b. sympathetic ophthalmia

    c. Vogt-Koyanagi-Harada syndrome

    d. Adamantiades-Behçet syndrome

37. A 67-year-old white female presents with mild uveitis with a mild vitritis and subretinal infiltrates. The condition has been minimally responsive to topical corticosteroid treatment. She has recently experienced weakness and confusion. Which of the following tests would be the most important to obtain at this time?

    a. gallium scan

    b. Westergren sedimentation rate and C-reactive protein

    c. PPD and chest x-ray

    d. CT scan or MRI of the head

38. What is the most likely diagnosis in a 50-year-old male with a recent history of fever, fatigue, headache, myalgias, and a rash involving the trunk of the body who presents with ocular pain, photophobia, and blurred vision, together with mild, bilateral, nongranulomatous anterior uveitis, vitritis, and a multifocal choroiditis characterized by targetoid lesions (hyperpigmentation surrounded by hypopigmentation) and linear hypopigmented streaks randomly distributed throughout the retinal periphery?

    a. sarcoidosis

    b. West Nile virus

    c. syphilis

    d. multifocal choroiditis and panuveitis

39. Retinal vasculitis involving primarily retinal venules occurs in which of the following conditions?

    a. systemic lupus erythematosus

    b. sarcoidosis

    c. polyarteritis nodosa

    d. necrotizing herpetic retinitis (acute retinal necrosis)

40. A 60-year-old patient presents with a 1-year history of decreased peripheral vision in the left eye, with anterior chamber cell and flare, an elevated IOP of 28, and evidence of retinal detachment *without* shifting subretinal fluid. The most appropriate management of this patient would include

    a. laboratory workup, including HLA-DR4 testing

    b. a lumbar puncture to look for cerebrospinal fluid pleocytosis

    c. careful evaluation of the peripheral retina for retinal breaks

    d. B-scan ultrasonography looking for presence of a T sign

41. Which of the following organisms is a frequent cause of endophthalmitis after ocular trauma but is an uncommon cause of endophthalmitis after cataract surgery or in bleb-related endophthalmitis?

    a. *Staphylococcus epidermidis*

    b. *Staphylococcus aureus*

    c. *Haemophilus influenzae*

    d. *Bacillus cereus*

42. Which of the following is the most common cause of endogenous fungal endophthalmitis?

    a. *Candida*

    b. *Aspergillus*

    c. *Rhizopus*

    d. *Cryptococcus*

43. Mild, acute postoperative endophthalmitis is characteristic of infections due to

    a. *Propionibacterium acnes*

    b. streptococcal spp

    c. coagulase-negative *Staphylococcus*

    d. *Staphylococcus aureus*

44. In contrast to the management of acute postoperative endophthalmitis after cataract surgery, the management of *Propionibacterium acnes* chronic endophthalmitis usually requires which of the following?

    a. intravitreal antibiotics

    b. removal of white plaque and capsulectomy

    c. systemic antibiotics

    d. periocular corticosteroids

45. Which of the following glaucoma medications should probably be avoided in a healthy patient with uveitis, cystoid macular edema, and uncontrolled glaucoma?

    a. dorzolamide (Trusopt)

    b. timolol (Timoptic)

    c. brimonidine (Alphagan)

    d. latanoprost (Xalatan)

46. Which procedure is *not* indicated in patients with medically uncontrolled glaucoma associated with uveitis?

    a. laser trabeculoplasty

    b. trabeculectomy

    c. glaucoma implant (aqueous drainage device)

    d. trabeculodialysis

47. The initial management of a patient with uveitis and iris bombé should include which of the following?

    a. laser iridotomy

    b. surgical iridectomy

    c. trabeculectomy

    d. glaucoma implant

48. Appropriate management for a patient with rapid progression of cataract with active, chronic anterior uveitis would include

    a. urgent removal of the cataract because of the risk of phacoantigenic uveitis

    b. complete control of the uveitis for 1 month with aggressive anti-inflammatory therapy prior to elective cataract surgery

    c. elective cataract surgery at any time because clear corneal phacoemulsification does not worsen or cause intraocular inflammation

    d. complete control of uveitis for 3 months with aggressive anti-inflammatory therapy prior to elective cataract surgery

49. Florid bilateral cystoid macular edema (CME) in a patient with bilateral, chronic, granulomatous anterior uveitis with 2+ cells in the anterior chamber, posterior synechiae, and 2+ vitreous cells is most effectively managed by which of the following?

    a. oral acetazolamide

    b. topical ketorolac

    c. systemic corticosteroids and immunomodulators

    d. pars plana vitrectomy

50. Which of the following is the most frequent mode of transmission of HIV infection?

    a. intravenous drug abuse

    b. sexual intercourse

    c. perinatal transmission

    d. blood transfusion

51. The granular pattern of cytomegalovirus retinitis with few retinal hemorrhages is associated with

    a. very low $CD4^+$ T-lymphocyte counts

    b. anemia

    c. peripheral location

    d. increased risk of retinal detachment

52. Which of the following is the most common ocular finding in patients with AIDS?

    a. herpes zoster
    b. HIV retinopathy
    c. *Candida*
    d. toxoplasmosis

53. The most common ocular opportunistic infection in AIDS in the era of highly active anti-retroviral therapy (HAART) is which of the following?

    a. *Toxoplasma* retinochoroiditis
    b. *Pneumocystis* choroiditis
    c. cytomegalovirus (CMV) retinitis
    d. cryptococcal choroiditis

54. Which of the following tests is imperative to perform *prior* to initiating therapy with infliximab in order to avoid potential treatment-related complications?

    a. serum alanine aminotransferase level
    b. PPD skin test
    c. serum blood urea nitrogen and creatinine levels
    d. cardiac catheterization

Answers

1. **b.** Innate immunity is genetically preprogrammed and triggered by bacterial toxins and cell debris. Adaptive, not innate, immunity requires recognition, processing, and effector phases and demonstrates specificity and memory.

2. **d.** Choices *a, b,* and *c* are characteristics of innate immunity. Adaptive immunity is an antigen-specific, tailored response to an offending antigen. See Chapter 1.

3. **a.** Necrotizing scleritis in Wegener granulomatosis occurs due to cell- and tissue-bound immune complexes that stimulate translocated cytoplasmic proteinase 3 molecules on the neutrophil cell membrane. Acute allergic conjunctivitis is due to IgE-mediated (Coombs and Gell Type I) mast-cell degranulation. Acute anterior uveitis is probably not due to circulating immune complexes. The exact effector mechanisms for anterior uveitis are not well understood. Sympathetic ophthalmia is a helper T cell (subset 1)–mediated delayed hypersensitivity reaction probably due to melanocyte-associated tyrosinase and melanin-associated protein complexes.

4. **c.** Anterior uveitis is the most common morphologic form of uveitis worldwide. Men and women appear to be equally affected. The pediatric age group has the lowest incidence and prevalence and the group over 65 years of age has the highest prevalence and incidence.

5. **c.** Tacrolimus, cyclosporine, and serolimus are all T-cell inhibitors although the mechanism of action of sirolimus is different from that of the other 2. Azathioprine, mycophenolate mofetil, and methotrexate are antimetabolites that interfere with DNA synthesis. Cyclophosphamide and chlorambucil are alkylating agents that cross-link DNA, inhibiting replication and cell division. Infliximab, adalimumab, and etanercept are biologic response modifiers that inhibit TNF-α by different mechanisms.

6. **b.** Cataract may occur in phakic patients, especially if multiple injections are given. Ocular hypertension may occur in 25% of patients requiring topical therapy, but up to 10% may need surgical treatment of their glaucoma. Endophthalmitis and rhegmatogenous retinal detachment are rare complications. Patients with uveitic cystoid macular edema seem to benefit most from intravitreal corticosteroid injection, but the effect rarely lasts more than 6 months. Intravitreal injection of corticosteroids is not curative of chronic uveitic conditions and should never be used as the sole agent in the treatment of infectious uveitic conditions.

7. **c.** The HLA association identifies persons at risk and is not a diagnostic marker. The strongest HLA disease association in humans is HLA-A29 and birdshot retinochoroidopathy. The associated haplotype is not necessarily present in all persons affected with the specific disease, and its presence in a person does not ensure the correct diagnosis. The concept of linkage disequilibrium proposes that if 2 genes are physically near on the chromosome, they may be inherited together rather than undergo genetic randomization in a population. Thus, HLA may be coinherited with an unrelated disease gene, and sometimes

2 HLA haplotypes can occur together more frequently than is predicted by their independent frequencies in the population. Many theoretical explanations have been offered for HLA disease associations. The most direct theory postulates that HLA molecules act as peptide-binding molecules for etiologic antigens or infectious agents.

8. **c.** Hypopyon anterior uveitis is most often associated with HLA-B27 positivity in the United States. Idiopathic anterior uveitis will not typically result in hypopyon. Adamantiades-Behçet anterior uveitis and hypopyon is less common in the United States than in other parts of the world. The hypopyon in Adamantiades-Behçet is often transient and may not be associated with fibrin in the anterior chamber or much conjunctival injection. Endogenous endophthalmitis is, in comparison, exceedingly rare.

9. **d.** The early-onset, pauciarticular, ANA-positive subgroup is most likely to develop chronic iridocyclitis, which is insidious in onset. Girls are much more commonly affected than boys. It is asymptomatic, can be very difficult to detect early, and can be recalcitrant to treatment. Long-term complications can include cataract (>80%), glaucoma (25%), calcific band keratopathy (70%), and cystoid macular edema (46%). Intraocular lens implantation is possible in these patients as long as meticulous and aggressive long-term and perioperative control of iridocyclitis is achieved.

10. **a.** Late-onset, pauciarticular, JRA/JIA-associated iridocyclitis is usually acute, recurrent, and symptomatic. It has a somewhat better long-term visual prognosis than the ANA-positive, early-onset pauciarticular group. Seventy-five percent of patients are HLA-B27 positive. Many go on to develop seronegative spondyloarthropathy later in life. Older boys are most often affected.

11. **d.** Fuchs heterochromic iridocyclitis is characterized by asymptomatic, mild to moderate anterior uveitis that is only mildly responsive to steroids. It is chronic and is associated with cataract in 50% and glaucoma in 60% of patients. In classic cases, patients have diffuse dendritic keratic precipitates and loss of iris crypts and stroma. Sectoral iris transillumination defects are characteristic of herpes simplex– and varicella-zoster–associated iridocyclitis and not of Fuchs heterochromic iridocyclitis. Unlike with pseudoexfoliation, cataract surgery is not associated with any greater incidence of zonular or capsular disruption and vitreous loss in patients with Fuchs heterochromic iridocyclitis compared to normal controls.

12. **a.** Patients with rheumatoid arthritis, Adamantiades-Behçet syndrome, and Reiter syndrome are more likely to have a nongranulomatous uveitis, and patients with sarcoidosis, a granulomatous uveitis.

13. **d.** Prednisolone acetate 1% (Pred Forte) and prednisolone phosphate 1% (Inflammase Forte) are more effective than loteprednol (Lotemax), fluorometholone 0.25% (FML Forte), and dexamethasone 0.1% (Decadron) in treating intraocular inflammation in uveitis.

14. **c.** Periocular corticosteroid injections may benefit patients with uveitis and vitritis or cystoid macular edema. However, periocular corticosteroid injections should not be used in patients with infectious uveitis (eg, toxoplasmosis) and should also be avoided in patients with scleritis.

15. **d.** Reiter syndrome is associated with nonspecific urethritis, polyarthritis, and conjunctivitis, often accompanied by iritis. Ankylosing spondylitis is not a part of Reiter syndrome.

16. **b.** Adamantiades-Behçet syndrome is associated with aphthous stomatitis, genital ulceration, erythema nodosum, hypopyon uveitis, and retinal vasculitis. Arthritis is usually not associated with Adamantiades-Behçet syndrome.

17. **a.** Although any of these diseases could require immunomodulatory therapy, Adamantiades-Behçet disease, necrotizing scleritis (especially if associated with systemic vasculitis syndromes such as Wegener granulomatosis), sympathetic ophthalmia, and chronic recurrent Vogt-Koyanagi-Harada disease are considered absolute indications for early institution of immunomodulatory therapy.

18. **a.** Rigid, closed-loop anterior chamber intraocular lenses are most associated with recurrent uveitis. Iris plane intraocular lenses occasionally cause inflammation, and, less commonly, a sulcus-placed posterior chamber intraocular lens causes inflammation from iris chafing or uveitis-glaucoma-hyphema (UGH) syndrome. Silicone intraocular lenses have been associated with iritis in the past.

19. **b.** Intermediate uveitis of unknown etiology, pars planitis, accounts for 85%–90% of cases. Other, less common causes include multiple sclerosis, Lyme disease, syphilis, and tuberculosis.

20. **d.** Cystoid macular edema is the major cause of visual loss in pars planitis. Other reasons for visual loss include band keratopathy, cataract, vitreous hemorrhage, epiretinal membrane, and retinal detachment.

21. **c.** The classic triad of acute retinal necrosis (ARN) syndrome includes occlusive arteriolitis, vitritis (often severe), and a multifocal yellow-white peripheral retinitis. Extensive retinal hemorrhages are usually not present. The "pizza-pie" appearance of the retina is seen more commonly in cytomegalovirus retinitis.

22. **c.** Peripapillary pigment changes, peripheral atrophic chorioretinal ("histo") spots, and choroidal neovascularization associated with histo spots in the posterior pole are all seen in ocular histoplasmosis syndrome; optic papillitis, vitritis, anterior uveitis, and large areas of retinitis are not.

23. **d.** Ocular manifestations occur in 50% of SLE cases and include cutaneous manifestations on the eyelids (discoid lupus erythematosus), secondary Sjögren syndrome occurring in approximately 20% of patients, all subtypes of scleral inflammatory disease, neuro-ophthalmic lesions (cranial nerve palsies, optic neuropathy, retrochiasmal and cerebral visual disorders), retinal vasculopathy, and, rarely, uveitis. Lupus retinopathy, the most well-recognized posterior segment manifestation, is considered an important marker of systemic disease activity, with a prevalence ranging from 3% among outpatients with mild disease to 29% among those with more active disease. Its clinical spectrum is characterized by cotton-wool spots, sometimes with retinal hemorrhages; retinal vascular occlusions, with and without retinal vasculitis; and lupus choroidopathy.

24. **b.** The cytoplasmic pattern, or c-ANCA, is both sensitive and specific for Wegener granulomatosis, whereas the perinuclear pattern, or p-ANCA, is associated with PAN, microscopic polyarteritis nodosa, relapsing polychondritis, and renal vasculitis. Between 85% and 95% of all ANCA found in Wegener granulomatosis is c-ANCA with antigen specificity for proteinase 3 (PR-3), which is highly specific for the disease; the remainder is p-ANCA directed against myeloperoxidase (MPO). In contrast, the diagnostic sensitivity of c-ANCA and p-ANCA for PAN is only 5% and 15%, respectively; in patients with microscopic polyarteritis nodosa, p-ANCA (MPO) positivity is more common (50%–80%), with a smaller percentage (40%) having the c-ANCA (anti-PR-3) marker.

25. **d.** MEWDS is an idiopathic inflammatory condition of the retina that typically presents with acute, unilateral (80%) blurred or decreased vision with central or peripheral scotomata in otherwise healthy, young (14–47 years), moderately myopic females (90%), frequently surrounding a flulike prodrome. Recurrences are uncommon, occurring in 10%–15% of patients, and bilateral disease is rare. The prognosis is excellent, with vision recovering completely in 2–10 weeks without treatment.

26. **a.** Characteristics of APMPPE include vitreous cells; optic disc edema; and bilateral, multiple, cream-colored, plaquelike homogenous lesions, which are seen beneath the retina. APMPPE often follows a prodromal influenza-like illness. It is commonly seen in adolescents and young adults and not those in the fifth or sixth decade of life. It presents most often as a bilateral disease. Cerebral vasculitis is a rare association that can be fatal if not treated with systemic corticosteroids. Choroidal neovascularization is a very rare complication of APMPPE; it is a much more common complication of serpiginous choroidopathy.

27. **a.** Cytomegalovirus retinitis is seen in immunocompromised patients with AIDS, as well as in those who have received organ transplants or are receiving chemotherapy. Herpes simplex, ocular histoplasmosis, and acute retinal necrosis syndrome each may be seen in otherwise healthy individuals.

28. **d.** The use of systemic corticosteroids without appropriate antimicrobial cover and the use of long-acting periocular or intraocular corticosteroid preparations such as triamcinolone acetonide are contraindicated, as they have been associated with severe, uncontrollable intraocular inflammation and loss of the eye. Systemic corticosteroids are generally begun either at the time of antimicrobial therapy or within 48 hours in immunocompetent patients.

29. **a.** The IgM antibody titer is the best laboratory test for a newly acquired toxoplasmosis infection. The IgM antibody titer will be elevated early after the infection but will not be detectable 2–6 months after the initial infection.

30. **c.** A salt-and-pepper fundus may be seen in congenital syphilis, and uveitis may be seen in secondary syphilis and in other stages. A lumbar puncture should be performed in patients with uveitis and syphilis. Syphilic uveitis can be cured with proper treatment, even in patients with AIDS.

31. **a.** Parenteral penicillin G is the preferred treatment for all stages of syphilis. Although the formulation, dose, route of administration, and duration of therapy vary with the stage of the disease, patients with syphilitic uveitis should be considered as having CNS dis-

ease and so require neurologic dosing regimens irrespective of immune status. There are no proven alternatives to penicillin for the treatment of neurosyphilis, so patients with penicillin allergy require desensitization before treatment with penicillin. Alternative treatments in penicillin-allergic patients without evidence of neurosyphilis and who are HIV negative include doxycycline 200 mg orally once daily or tetracycline 500 mg orally 4 times daily for 30 days.

32. **c.** The spectrum of ocular findings in Lyme disease is expanding and varies with the stage of the disease. The most common ocular manifestation of early *stage 1* disease is a follicular conjunctivitis that occurs in approximately 11% of patients. Intraocular inflammatory disease is reported most often in *stage 2* and, less frequently, in *stage 3* and may manifest as anterior uveitis, intermediate uveitis (very common), posterior uveitis, or panuveitis. A distinct clinical entity of peripheral multifocal choroiditis has been described in association with Lyme disease and is characterized by multiple small, round, punched-out lesions associated with vitritis, similar to those seen with sarcoidosis. Keratitis and, much less commonly, episcleritis, presenting months to years after the onset of infection, are the most common ocular manifestations of stage 3 disease.

33. **c.** *Bartonella henselae* is the etiologic agent of cat-scratch disease and the most common cause of neuroretinitis, a constellation of findings that include abrupt visual loss, unilateral optic disc swelling, and macular star formation. Other causes of neuroretinitis vary widely and include infectious entities, such as syphilis, Lyme disease, tuberculosis, DUSN, toxoplasmosis, toxocariasis, leptospirosis, salmonella, and varicella-zoster and herpes simplex viruses. Among noninfectious inflammatory conditions, sarcoidosis may present as unilateral optic nerve head swelling, macular edema, and multifocal retinochoroiditis. Other conditions that may present with unilateral or bilateral optic nerve edema and macular star formation include acute systemic hypertension, diabetes mellitus, increased intracranial pressure (pseudotumor cerebri), anterior ischemic optic neuropathy, and leukemia infiltration of the optic nerve.

34. **c.** Systemic antibiotic therapy is clearly indicated for patients with uveitis, a recently converted TB skin test, an abnormal chest radiograph, positive bacterial cultures, or positive PCR results. Multiple-agent therapy is recommended because of the increasing incidence of resistance to isoniazid (INH), as well as adherence problems associated with long-term therapy. This, together with the extremely slow growth rate of TB, contributes to the acquisition of drug resistance, known as *multidrug-resistant tuberculosis* (MDRTB). Patients at risk for MDRTB include noncompliant patients on single-agent therapy; migrant or indigent populations; immunocompromised patients, including those with HIV; and recent immigrants from countries where INH and rifampin are available over the counter. More difficult is the management approach to patients with uveitis consistent with TB, a normal chest radiograph, and a positive PPD. In this situation, a diagnosis of extrapulmonary TB may be entertained and treatment initiated, particularly in the setting of medically unresponsive uveitis or other findings supportive of the diagnosis, such as recent exposure or inadequately treated disease, a large area of induration, or new conversion on skin testing. Topical and systemic corticosteroids are frequently used in conjunction with antimicrobial therapy to treat the inflammatory component of the disease. Because intensive

corticosteroid treatment administered without appropriate antituberculous cover may lead to progressive worsening of ocular disease, any patient suspected of harboring tuberculous disease should undergo appropriate testing prior to beginning such therapy.

35. **d.** A chest radiograph is the single best screening test for the diagnosis of sarcoidosis because it is abnormal in approximately 90% of patients with this disease. Thin-cut, spiral computed tomographic (CT) imaging is a more sensitive imaging modality and may be particularly valuable in the setting of a normal chest radiograph in which there remains a high clinical index of suspicion for disease. Although serum ACE and lysozyme levels may be abnormally elevated, neither are diagnostic or specific. Gallium scanning in combination with an elevated ACE level appears to be highly specific for sarcoidosis in patients with active disease in whom the clinical suspicion of sarcoidosis is high; however, routine screening of patients with uveitis with both ACE levels and gallium scanning may be inappropriate given the low positive predictive value in this clinical setting. Ultimately, the diagnosis of sarcoidosis is made histopathologically from tissue obtained from the lungs, mediastinal lymph nodes, skin, peripheral lymph nodes, liver, conjunctiva, or minor salivary glands (lacrimal gland).

36. **c.** In the patient described, Vogt-Koyanagi-Harada syndrome is the most likely diagnosis. Sarcoidosis and Adamantiades-Behçet syndrome are less likely. Blunt trauma is not likely to incite sympathetic ophthalmia.

37. **d.** In an older patient with a nonresponsive uveitis, vitritis, subretinal infiltrates, and neurologic signs, a large cell, non-Hodgkin lymphoma should be suspected. A CT scan or MRI of the head would be the first important step in this patient's management. Cerebrospinal fluid analysis or vitreous biopsy can confirm the diagnosis. Sarcoidosis, tuberculosis, and giant cell arteritis are possible; however, it is important to rule out the possibility of a large cell lymphoma.

38. **b.** Systemic West Nile virus infection is marked by the acute onset of a febrile illness, often accompanied by myalgias, arthralgias, headache, conjunctivitis, lymphadenopathy, and a maculopapular or roseolar rash arising in approximately 20% of infections. Severe infection may cause meningitis or encephalitis. Presenting ocular symptoms include ocular pain, photophobia, conjunctival hyperemia, and blurred vision. A characteristic multifocal chorioretinitis is observed in the majority of patients, together with nongranulomatous anterior uveitis and vitreous cellular infiltration. Chorioretinal lesions are distributed most often in the retinal periphery in a random distribution or in linear arrays, following the course of the choroidal blood vessels or, less frequently, in the posterior pole. Many lesions exhibit a "target-like" appearance angiographically, with central hypofluorescence due to blockage from pigment. The presence of the unique pattern of multifocal chorioretinal lesions in patients with systemic symptoms suggestive of West Nile virus can help establish the diagnosis while serologic testing is pending. Conversely, a systemic ocular evaluation,

including dilated funduscopy and fluorescein angiography may be very helpful in suggesting the diagnosis of West Nile virus infection in patients presenting with meningoencephalitis. Differential diagnosis includes syphilis, multifocal choroiditis and panuveitis, histoplasmosis, sarcoidosis, and tuberculosis, all of which may be distinguished on the basis of history, systemic signs and symptoms, serology, and the pattern of chorioretinitis.

39. **b.** Sarcoidosis, multiple sclerosis, birdshot retinochoroidopathy, and Eales disease are associated with retinal vasculitis affecting venules. Systemic lupus erythematosus, polyarteritis nodosa, and necrotizing herpetic retinitis are associated with retinal vasculitis primarily affecting arterioles.

40. **c.** Chronic peripheral rhegmatogenous retinal detachment can be associated with anterior segment cell and flare and vitreous inflammatory and pigment cells. Patients often have good vision but can sometimes develop decreased vision due to cystoid macular edema. The key to the diagnosis of peripheral retinal detachment is the dilated fundus examination with scleral depression. Peripheral pigment demarcation lines, subretinal fluid, retinal breaks, subretinal fibrosis, and peripheral retinal cysts may be present. In some cases, the anterior segment cells may represent not true inflammation but rather the presence of photoreceptor outer segments that have been liberated from the subretinal space. In these situations, IOP can be elevated. Photoreceptor outer segments are phagocytosed by the endothelial cells in the trabecular meshwork and result in secondary open-angle glaucoma. This condition is called *Schwartz syndrome*. The other choices are incorrect because this case does not represent VKH syndrome or posterior scleritis, entities that are associated with exudative retinal detachments and shifting subretinal fluid.

41. **d.** The *Bacillus cereus* organism is frequently (26%–46% of the time) found in traumatic endophthalmitis and may cause a fulminant endophthalmitis. *Staphylococcus epidermidis* and *Staphylococcus aureus* are the most common agents in post–cataract surgery endophthalmitis. *Haemophilus influenzae* and *Streptococcus* species are important causes of late bleb-related endophthalmitis.

42. **a.** *Candida albicans* is the most common cause of endogenous fungal endophthalmitis.

43. **c.** *Propionibacterium acnes* is an uncommon cause of acute endophthalmitis. Streptococcal species and *Staphylococcus aureus* cause more virulent infections than coagulase-negative *Staphylococcus*.

44. **b.** In contrast to the management of acute postoperative endophthalmitis after cataract surgery, the management of *P acnes* chronic endophthalmitis usually requires removal of white plaque and capsulectomy. Both forms of endophthalmitis require intravitreal antibiotics, and neither requires systemic antibiotics. Periocular corticosteroids are sometimes used in severe acute postoperative endophthalmitis but not in *P acnes* endophthalmitis.

45. **d.** Latanoprost (Xalatan) should probably be avoided in a patient with uveitis and cystoid macular edema. It may worsen both the intraocular inflammation and the cystoid macular edema. The other 3 agents listed should each pose no problem with respect to uveitis and cystoid macular edema.

46. **a.** Laser trabeculoplasty in any form (argon, diode, selective) is not indicated in patients with uveitis and glaucoma. It is ineffective, may exacerbate intraocular inflammation, and may cause severe IOP elevation in these patients. Trabeculectomy, glaucoma implant (aqueous drainage device), and trabeculodialysis have all been successfully used in the surgical management of these patients.

47. **a.** The initial management of patients with uveitis and iris bombé should include laser iridotomy, glaucoma medications as needed, and intensive topical corticosteroids. Surgical iridectomy occasionally becomes necessary if a patent laser iridotomy cannot be successfully maintained. A trabeculectomy or glaucoma implant could later become necessary if there is a patent laser iridotomy and medically uncontrolled IOP.

48. **d.** Cataract surgery in uveitic eyes is generally complex and, thus, more likely to lead to postoperative complications when improperly managed. The key to a successful visual outcome in these cases is careful long-term control of pre- and postoperative inflammation. The absence of inflammation preoperatively for 3 or more months is a prerequisite for any elective intraocular surgery in uveitic eyes. The control of perioperative inflammation is as important as the technical feat of performing successful complex cataract extraction in uveitic eyes.

49. **c.** Uveitic CME is best managed by first aggressively controlling intraocular inflammation with corticosteroids and immunomodulatory agents. Topical nonsteroidal anti-inflammatory drugs (NSAIDs) and acetazolamide (Diamox) have marginal benefits in controlling CME in an eye that is actively inflamed. Intravitreal triamcinolone shows promise in eliminating CME, at least temporarily, and is under active investigation. The value of pars plana vitrectomy in the management of uveitic CME is controversial, although it may have some role in refractory cases.

50. **b.** In one study, heterosexual and homosexual intercourse was the most common mode of transmission (70% of cases), followed by intravenous drug abuse (27%) and blood transfusions (2%–3%). Perinatal transmission was the least frequent (1%) mode of HIV transmission.

51. **c.** Granular vs fulminant appearance is a function of retinal thickness, which is less in the periphery. Peripheral CMV retinitis appears granular.

52. **b.** HIV retinopathy is the most common ocular finding in patients with AIDS, although many other infections can also affect the eye in AIDS.

53. **c.** In the era of HAART, despite a reduction in the incidence of new CMV retinitis cases by 80%, CMV retinitis is still the most common opportunistic infection in patients with AIDS.

54. **b.** A PPD skin test is imperative prior to therapy with infliximab because miliary or disseminated tuberculosis may occur in patients treated with infliximab who have latent undetected tuberculosis. Congestive heart failure, lupuslike syndrome, and multiple sclerosis–like demyelinating disease may also occur as complications of treatment. It is, however, unnecessary to perform cardiac catheterization in these patients unless cardiac symptoms warrant. Hepatotoxicity and nephrotoxicity are uncommon with infliximab therapy.

Index

(*f* = figure; *t* = table)